Value-Based Health Care in Orthopaedics

EDITORS

Eric C. Makhni, MD, MBA, FAAOS
Clinical Associate Professor of Orthopedic Surgery
Michigan State University
Senior Staff Surgeon, Orthopedic Service Line
Division of Sports Medicine
Senior Clinical Advisor
Center for Patient-Reported Outcome Measures
Henry Ford Health
Detroit, Michigan

Benedict U. Nwachukwu, MD, MBA
Attending Orthopedic Surgeon
Hospital for Special Surgery
Associate Professor, Orthopedic Surgery
Weill Cornell Medical College
New York, New York

Kevin J. Bozic, MD, MBA, FAAOS
Department Chair
Department of Surgery and Perioperative Ca[...]
Dell Medical School
The University of Texas at Austin
Austin, Texas

T0395064

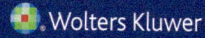

Wolters Kluwer

Philadelphia · Baltimore · New York · London
Buenos Aires · Hong Kong · Sydney · Tokyo

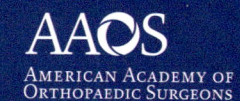

AAOS
AMERICAN ACADEMY OF
ORTHOPAEDIC SURGEONS

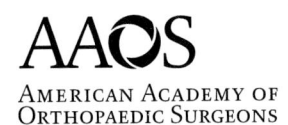

AAOS
AMERICAN ACADEMY OF ORTHOPAEDIC SURGEONS

ISBN 978-1-9752-2308-3

Library of Congress Control Number: Cataloging in Publication data available on request from publisher.

Printed in the United States of America

Published 2025 by the American Academy of Orthopaedic Surgeons
9400 West Higgins Road
Rosemont, Illinois 60018

Copyright 2025 by the American Academy of Orthopaedic Surgeons

Contributors

John P. Andrawis, MD, MBA
Director of Value-Based Care
Department of Orthopaedics
Harbor-UCLA Medical Center
Torrance, California

Kenoma Anighoro, MD, MBA
Connecticut Orthopaedics
Hamden, Connecticut

Wael K. Barsoum, MD, FAAOS
Professor of Surgery, Cleveland Clinic
    Lerner College of Medicine
Department of Orthopaedic Surgery
    Cleveland Clinic Florida
Weston, Florida

David N. Bernstein, MD, MBA, MEI
Orthopaedic Surgery Resident
    Physician
Harvard Combined Orthopaedic
    Residency Program
Massachusetts General Hospital
Boston, Massachusetts

Kevin J. Bozic, MD, MBA, FAAOS
Department Chair
Department of Surgery and
    Perioperative Care
Dell Medical School
The University of Texas at Austin
Austin, Texas

James A. Browne, MD
Alfred R. Shands Professor of
    Orthopaedic Surgery
Department of Orthopaedic Surgery
University of Virginia
Charlottesville, Virginia

Kassandra S. Carter, MD
Medical Resident
Department of Internal Medicine
TriStar Centennial Medical Center
Nashville, Tennessee

Ashley E. Chacko, MHA
Vice President
Market Intelligence and Strategic
    Planning
Healthcare Outcomes Performance
    Company (HOPCO)
Fort Lauderdale, Florida

**Toby Colegate-Stone, MA (Oxon), MBBS,
    MRCS, MSc, FRCS (Tr and Orth)**
Clinical Lead
Department of Ortopaedic and Trauma
    Surgery King's Health Partners
Consultant, Orthopaedic and Trauma
    Surgeon
King's College Hospital
London, England

Ryan Desgrange, DMSc, MPAS, PA-C
Advanced Practice Provider
    Orthopaedic Service Line
Department of Orthopaedic Surgery
Henry Ford Health
Detroit, Michigan

Elizabeth Duckworth, MD, MBA
Orthopaedic Surgery Resident
Department of Surgery and
    Perioperative Care
Dell Medical School
The University of Texas at Austin
Austin, Texas

Heather S. Haeberle, MD
Resident Physician
Orthopaedic Trauma Service
Hospital for Special Surgery
New York, New York

Jeremy T. Hines, MD
Orthopaedic Surgeon
Department of Orthopaedic Surgery
EmergeOrtho
Wilmington, North Carolina

Jessica M. Hooper, MD
Clinical Assistant Professor
Department of Orthopaedic Surgery
Stanford University
Stanford Health and Clinics
Redwood City, California

James I. Huddleston III, MD, FAAOS
Professor of Orthopaedic Surgery
Division Director, Adult Reconstruction
Department of Orthopaedic Surgery
Stanford Healthcare
Stanford, California

Prakash Jayakumar, MD, PhD
Assistant Professor
Department of Surgery and
   Perioperative Care
Dell Medical School
The University of Texas at Austin
Austin, Texas

Brandy Keys, MPH
Director, Health Policy
American Academy of Ophthalmology
Washington, DC

Karl Koenig, MD, MS, FAAOS
Division Chief, Orthopaedic Surgery
Department of Surgery and
   Perioperative Care
Dell Medical School
The University of Texas at Austin
Austin, Texas

Dylan S. Koolmees, MD
Orthopaedic Surgery Resident
Department of Orthopeadic Surgery
Campbell Clinic
Memphis, Tennessee

Kevin A. Lawson, MD
Orthopaedic Surgeon
Department of Orthopeadics
MultiCare Health System
Tacoma, Washington

Harry M. Lightsey IV, MD
Orthopaedic Surgery Resident
Department of Orthopardic Surgery
Harvard Combined Orthopaedic
   Residency Program
Massachusetts General Brigham
Boston, Massachusetts

Eugenia Lin, MD
Resident Physician
Department of Orthopaedic Surgery
Mayo Clinic Arizona
Phoenix, Arizona

Bryan C. Luu, MD
Resident
Department of Internal Medicine
Baylor College of Medicine
Houston, Texas

Catherine H. MacLean, MD, PhD
Professor, Department of Medicine
Weill Cornell Medical College
Chief Value Medical Officer
Value Management Office
Hospital for Special Surgery
New York, New York

Eric C. Makhni, MD, MBA, FAAOS
Clinical Associate Professor of
    Orthopedic Surgery
Michigan State University
Senior Staff Surgeon, Orthopedic Service
    Line
Division of Sports Medicine
Senior Clinical Advisor
Center for Patient-Reported Outcome
    Measures
Henry Ford Health
Detroit, Michigan

Melvin C. Makhni, MD, MBA
Assistant Professor
Director of Complex Spine Surgery
Department of Orthopaedic Surgery
Brigham and Women's Hospital
Boston, Massachusetts

Olivia Manickas-Hill, BA
University of Minnesota Medical School
Minneapolis, Minnesota

Richard C. Mather III, MD, MBA
Clinical Assistant Professor
Department of Orthopaedic Surgery
Duke University and Hospital
Durham, North Carolina

Raquel Mayne, MPH, MS, RN, CPHQ
Assistant Vice President, Quality
    Management
Department of Quality and
    Accreditation
Hospital for Special Surgery
New York, New York

Samuel Gray McClatchy, MD
Surgeon
Department of Orthopaedics
Ozark Orthopaedics
Fayetteville, Arkansas

Stephanie Muh, MD, FAAOS
Deputy Chief, Orthopaedic Surgery
    Service, Henry Ford West Bloomfield
    Hospital
Residency Associate Program Director
Clinical Associate Professor
Wayne State University School of
    Medicine
Service Chief, Shoulder and Elbow
    Surgery Department of Orthopaedics
Henry Ford Health
Detroit, Michigan

Daniel B. Murrey, MD, MPP
Chief Physician Executive, SCA Health
Senior Vice President, Optum Specialty
    Care
Asheville, North Carolina

Christopher Naso, MPH
Alexandria, Virginia

Wendy M. Novicoff, PhD
Professor
Department of Orthopaedic Surgery and
    Public Health Sciences
University of Virginia School of
    Medicine
Charlottesville, Virginia

Benedict U. Nwachukwu, MD, MBA
Attending Orthopedic Surgeon
Hospital for Special Surgery
Associate Professor, Orthopedic Surgery
Weill Cornell Medical College
New York, New York

Nicholas S. Piuzzi, MD
Associate Professor of Orthopaedic
  Surgery
Cleveland Clinic Lerner College of
  Medicine
Musculoskeletal Research Center
  (MSRC) Co-Director
Cleveland Clinic Adult Reconstruction
  Research (CCARR) Director
Department of Orthopaedic Surgery
Cleveland Clinic
Cleveland, Ohio

Prem N. Ramkumar, MD, MBA
Attending Physician
Department of Orthopaedic Surgery
Long Beach Orthopaedic Institute
Orthopaedic Surgeon
Joint Preservation and Reconstruction
Long Beach Memorial Hospital
Long Beach, California

Paul Rizk, MD
Resident
Department of Orthopaedic Surgery
University of Florida
Gainesville, Florida

Ran Schwarzkopf, MD, MSc, FAAOS
Professor, Department of Orthopaedic
  Surgery
NYU Langone Health
New York, New York

Ahmed Siddiqi, DO, MBA
Orthopaedic Surgeon
Orthopaedic Institute Brielle
  Orthopaedics, A Division of OrthoNJ
Assistant Professor
Department of Orthopeadic Surgery
Hackensack Meridian Health
Manasquan, New Jersey

**Christopher Doria Skeehan, MD,
  FAAOS**
Medical Director, Adult Reconstruction
Department of Orthopedic Surgery
Southcoast Health
Fall River, Massachusetts

James D. Slover, MD, MS, FAAOS
Chief of Adult Reconstruction
Lenox Hill Hospital
New York, New York

Spencer W. Sullivan, BS
Medical Student
School of Medicine
University of North Carolina
Chapel Hill, North Carolina

**Thomas (Quin) Throckmorton, MD,
  FAAOS**
Professor, Department of Orthopaedic
  Surgery
University of Tennessee - Campbell
  Clinic
Memphis, Tennessee

Erik Y. Tye, MD
Resident Physician
Department of Orthopaedic Surgery
Harbor-UCLA Medical Center
Torrance, California

Kevin Wang, MHA
Doctoral Candidate
Department of Health Policy and
  Management
Johns Hopkins University
Baltimore, Maryland
Senior Director, Performance Programs
Value Management Officer
Hospital for Special Surgery
New York, New York

Mary Lynch Witkowski, MD, MBA
Fellow, Institute for Strategy and
  Competitiveness
Harvard Business School
Boston, Massachusetts

Rory R. Wright, MD, FAAOS
President of Medical Staff
Department of Surgery
Orthopaedic Hospital of Wisconsin
Glendale, Wisconsin

Caleb M. Yeung, MD
Resident Physician
Harvard Combined Orthopaedic
  Residency Program
Harvard Medical School
Boston, Massachusetts

Preface

The challenges facing the US healthcare system are considerable. Costs continue to climb at unsustainable rates, access remains challenging for many, and quality metrics continue to lag relative to our global counterparts. At the core of these challenges is a transactional infrastructure that rewards volume of care delivered without emphasis on health outcomes nor on improving access to high-value care. The result is a system that is simultaneously overutilized, underutilized, and inappropriately utilized.

Unsurprisingly, due to these and other issues, health care has been thrust into the public and political spotlight. The need for transformation of the US healthcare system has never been more pressing. Such improvements require complete alignment across all stakeholders – clinician, patient, payer – which is in stark contrast to the status quo. Currently, the transactional nature of the fee-for-service system places excessive emphasis on specialty care utilization, which directly results in increased costs without commensurate improvements in health outcomes. In contrast, a value-based health care delivery and payment system aligns the incentives of all stakeholders, including payers, clinicians, and most importantly patients, by prioritizing health over care, and facilitating competition across health care providers based on health outcomes and cost.

It is with this context in mind that we decided to create a resource for orthopaedic surgeons who are navigating the transition to value-based health care. Even though the focus of this text is on musculoskeletal care, we believe that the underlying principles can be applied to all aspects of modern health care. We are especially grateful to our team of contributing authors, whose deep expertise in value-based health care we have leaned on heavily. We hope you will enjoy reading and synthesizing the lessons contained herein as much as we did as we assembled the textbook, and we wish you great success on your journey to value.

Eric C. Makhni, MD, MBA, FAAOS
Benedict U. Nwachukwu, MD, MBA
Kevin J. Bozic, MD, MBA, FAAOS

Table of Contents

What Does Value-Based Health Care Mean? An Overview of Key Concepts

Eric C. Makhni, MD, MBA, FAAOS • Kassandra S. Carter, MD
Kevin J. Bozic, MD, MBA, FAAOS

INTRODUCTION

The United States healthcare system has been focused on transactional care, both in its delivery and its payment. Medical providers are paid for the services rendered rather than outcomes delivered. A clinician will get paid the same amount for a given service, regardless of the effect of that service on the patient's outcome. This is especially clear in volume-driven fields such as orthopaedics, in which the priority is to maximize the number of procedures performed safely, not to optimize health outcomes after surgery.

It is no surprise, therefore, that behavior follows incentive. Healthcare systems have been designed to provide care at maximal efficiency from a volume perspective under the fee-for-service (FFS) payment model. This has resulted in continuously increasing costs of health care as demand for health care services continues to grow. Under the FFS model, providers bill separately for individual services such as appointments, treatments, and tests ordered. This health care model defines success as achieving high profit margins.[1] Because financial incentives are based on volume and the price of each service provided, providers often prioritize the quantity of services over the quality of those services.[2]

Dr. Makhni or an immediate family member has stock or stock options held in Protera Health and serves as a board member, owner, officer, or committee member of American Academy of Orthopaedic Surgeons and American Orthopaedic Society for Sports Medicine. Dr. Bozic or an immediate family member serves as a paid consultant to or is an employee of CMS/CMMI; serves as an unpaid consultant to Harvard Business School; has stock or stock options held in Carrum Health; has received nonincome support (such as equipment or services), commercially derived honoraria, or other non–research-related funding (such as paid travel) from OM1; and serves as a board member, owner, officer, or committee member of American Academy of Orthopaedic Surgeons. Neither Dr. Carter nor any immediate family member has received anything of value from or has stock or stock options held in a commercial company or institution related directly or indirectly to the subject of this chapter.

There are clear ramifications to the FFS model; some are apparent and some are less obvious. In an FFS model, the incentive is to increase volume of high-margin services. This results in an enormous investment into processes, technologies, and personnel that aid in this type of "productivity." Conversely, this limits the investments in necessary services such as preventive care or measurement of health outcomes. As demand for these procedures and interventions increases over time, such a model invariably causes ballooning costs. There are many hidden dangers of such a system, such as burnout. Physicians, providers, and health care staff are pressed to take on more patients and burdened by copious amounts of paperwork, resulting in higher rates of burnout and lower rates of job satisfaction.

The framework of value-based health care discards the fragmented, flawed model of FFS and creates a team-based, integrated approach to health care that focuses on delivering value to the patient. Value-based health care defines success as improving health outcomes for patients.[3] Providers are incentivized to treat patient needs effectively rather than providing services, whether appropriate or not. Delivery of care is organized around patient needs and conditions rather than individual providers, and team-based approaches are encouraged. Improving health outcomes requires investment into processes and technology that accurately measure patient outcomes and costs. Unlike FFS, where providers are paid for individual services, value-based health care reimburses providers based on the value of care delivered over an entire care cycle. Providers are then incentivized to focus on services that produce the best outcomes for patients rather than prioritizing treatments based on reimbursement and/or providing unnecessary services that ultimately may not improve patient health.

Because FFS incentivizes the volume and intensity of services, FFS has led to an increase in overall health care utilization and cost over time. Compared to other countries with similar gross domestic product and gross domestic product per capita, data from the Organisation of Economic Co-operation and Development show that the United States spends nearly twice as much on health care per person as compared to other developed countries ($10,637 to $5,527 per person, on average). Despite spending more, the United States ranks last in many measures of health care access and quality, indicating higher rates of preventable mortality. Additionally, the United States also has higher rates of medical, medication, and laboratory errors than other Organisation of Economic Co-operation and Development member countries.[4] Therefore, the state of the US healthcare system requires change. Current models project that health care expenditures are projected to increase at an average annual rate of 5.6% until 2025 and will encompass 19.9% of gross domestic product by 2025.[5] Rising health care costs without commensurate gains in health have led to transformation of the healthcare system to one that promotes and rewards value delivered to patients.

DEFINING VALUE FOR PATIENTS

Value is defined by outcomes that matter to patients over total costs of care. Attention must be placed on outcomes that matter to patients so that clinicians can successfully deliver necessary and effective care. Outcomes are the result of the care rendered to patients, families, and populations. Outcomes range from survival to improved function to reduced pain. For example, outcome measures for patients who have undergone total hip arthroplasty include the number of days it will take them to walk after surgery, or if surgery will lead to less pain after surgery than before surgery.[6] Providers are encouraged to organize interactions around patient conditions such as musculoskeletal pain rather than a clinician's individual expertise such as orthopaedic surgery. Teams created around a set of patients with shared problems share a core set of critical concerns.[7] Health care teams that are aligned around common conditions have shared goals, which facilitates measuring outcomes, continuous learning, and increased improvements to delivered care.

Outcome measures can help elucidate areas of success and opportunities for improvement. This insight allows providers to focus on improving ineffective aspects of care and thus enhance the value of care delivered to patients. Value permanently exists within the context of costs spent to deliver certain outcomes. Value can be improved in a variety of ways; for example, by improving outcomes for patients without raising costs, and by maintaining good outcomes while decreasing costs or improving outcomes dramatically for a smaller increase in costs.[2] Overall, a value-based healthcare system focuses on improved patient-centric outcomes and decreased episode costs.

INTEGRATED PRACTICE UNITS

Currently, most health care organizations and their corresponding budgets are grouped by clinical departments (surgery, medicine), care locations (operating rooms, emergency department), and ancillary departments (pharmacy, radiology, pathology). Using this framework, a patient undergoing total hip arthroplasty, for example, shows up on each department budget. If a particular department wants to lower the cost of care and improve outcomes by using a new process or technology, they must do so either by spending their own resources or with buy-in from the other departments.[7] This decentralized model of organization slows innovation, inhibits quick adaptation, and makes it difficult to track improvement across cycles of care. Value-based health care moves away from fragmented, decentralized care organized by individual units or departments to integrated care across facilities centered around patient medical needs.

Integrated practice units (IPUs) manage the care of a patient over the entire cycle of care for a particular condition, such as arthritis or low back pain. IPUs are composed of dedicated, multidisciplinary teams within dedicated facilities, if possible, for each service line. Each service line should have a clinical leader, common scheduling and intake processes, and a unified financial structure. Because service lines integrate care for common conditions, it is easier to routinely measure outcomes, costs, care processes, and patient and clinician experience. Health systems that organize care by service lines have demonstrated that they were able to increase margins while improving clinical outcomes such as complication rates and readmission rates.[8]

Accountable for complete care cycles and their related costs, IPUs can be more easily compensated through bundle payments, which is a single reimbursement for all services provided by all members of the clinical team across the entire cycle of care. IPUs, combined with bundle payments, have greater incentive to invest in innovative techniques and technologies if they result in improved outcomes and/or reduced episode costs of care. Thus, IPUs can use the unique factors in their specific patient populations to develop standardized processes that allow each patient to receive consistent and high-quality care. Ultimately, innovative technology plus standardized processes will allow IPUs to assess and reduce episode costs per patient. Adopting this organizational structure allows for a true value-based system of health care.

FOCUS ON PATIENT-REPORTED OUTCOMES

Traditionally, orthopaedics relied on process metrics and claims data to measure outcomes associated with specific interventions. Examples of process metrics include adherence to evidence-based practice guidelines for administration of perioperative antibiotic prophylaxis or anticoagulation prophylaxis. Claims-based data include data from billing sources that can be used to capture readmission, re-operation, and mortality rates. Although these outcomes are valuable, they do not necessarily indicate whether a patient has benefited from the given intervention or care process. Having outcomes that indicate patient improvement and patient benefit is an essential step to understanding the value of care delivered, as experienced by the patient.

Within orthopaedics, care is largely directed toward improving symptoms such as pain or lack of function. Therefore, outcomes should focus on improvement in these symptoms before and after care. Such measures include patient-reported outcome measures (PROMs), which are questionnaires completed by patients that encapsulate their perception of their symptoms. PROMs generally determine a patient's general health or health-related quality of life by assessment of the patient's physical, mental, and social aspects of health. They can also focus specifically on a particular disease, symptom, treatment, or body function.[9] Despite their importance and relevance, PROMs are challenging to implement in daily practice because of numerous logistical, operational, financial, and technical challenges. As health care continues to emphasize value over volume, these measures are essential to understanding value and thus are increasingly used in daily health care operations and analyses.

COST ACCOUNTING

In addition to measuring outcomes, accurate cost measurement is essential to a value-based healthcare system. However, cost analysis in modern health care can be extremely challenging due to the lack of clarity surrounding true costs and challenges of measuring costs in the presence of complex workflows.

Traditionally, cost accounting has been performed using activity-based costing (ABC) techniques. In this method, overhead and indirect costs are applied to products or processes based on the percentage of time spent on each process. This time is typically determined through surveys or interviews. Although effective in other fields, the workflows in modern health care are often too complex and complicated for ABC to assess costs accurately. For any given surgical episode, there are numerous members of the health care team caring for the patient, sometimes simultaneously, thus making it difficult to assess cost drivers.

Recently, a new method for cost accounting, time-driven activity-based costing (TDABC), was introduced to health care by Harvard Business School professor Robert Kaplan.[10] This method develops an accurate assessment of the true costs associated with treating a patient over an entire cycle of care. The amount of time spent by each health care team member is evaluated, thus a cost per minute of their time, termed time cost rates, can be determined. TDABC also creates capacity rates by estimating costs of other resources used, such as radiologic imaging or time in the operating room. By using time and capacity cost rates to determine resource costs, the true costs of healthcare delivery can be separated and analyzed from the costs of overhead.[10] The TDABC method allows for a more accurate understanding of the cost of care per patient and disease condition. Through the implementation of more accurate cost accounting systems, clinicians and hospitals can better understand and account for their costs of care.

In addition to reevaluating the way that costs are tracked and itemized, the information technology systems used to process and bill these costs require a major overhaul. Current billing systems do not measure the costs per patient over a cycle of care. Most accounting systems rely on separate charges and thus require that payments to a group of providers involved in an episode of care be manually separated and submitted. Additionally, most cost accounting systems allocate costs arbitrarily rather than with the use of time-driven data. Because of the need to track costs and outcomes over individual patient care cycles, a value-based costing system should be able to identify which provider is providing each service, the time taken to provide the service, and other key inputs involved in the care. By creating systems that can track patient care cycles, healthcare systems dramatically reduce administrative costs of billing and adapt to value-based reimbursement models such as bundled payments.

A QUALITY IMPROVEMENT METHOD

The quality improvement landscape in health care has been shaped by the work of Avedis Donabedian, a public health professor at the University of Michigan who wrote more than 100 manuscripts and 11 books that provided the foundation for quality processes and systems management. The Donabedian Method of Quality[11] offers a framework to launch effective quality improvement efforts that positively affect outcomes.

This method outlines how to classify and understand three sequential factors of quality: structure, process, and outcomes. First, the structure or the resources available must be accounted for, such as the equipment, facilities, the staff, and the complexity of health care services. Second, the process or technical quality of care is examined. This means assessing the use of diagnostic testing and procedures, delays in treatment, the quality of interpersonal care, and anything else related to how care is delivered by providers and received by patients. New process measures must be able to demonstrate that they can produce better outcomes. Third, desired outcomes can be created by establishing benchmarks and setting goals for the department or organization.[11] Use of the Donabedian Method of Quality allows for the creation and implementation of effective processes that will meet established outcomes that ultimately improve the quality of the care delivered.

Using the structure-process-outcomes framework,[12] providers and quality teams can better examine complex clinical processes and determine effective improvements in the context of their own system. Additionally, successful quality teams regularly evaluate quality improvement changes through audits and feedback. Successful quality initiatives must concentrate on aligning the goals and outcomes of the quality improvements at the patient, surgeon, hospital, and payer levels, so that each stakeholder perceives that the new systems are providing better quality health care.

PAYMENT MODELS THAT REWARD INCREASING VALUE DELIVERED TO PATIENTS

By definition, value-based health care payment models reward improved patient outcomes and incentivize lowering costs. There are four types of value-based payment models that are in current use: shared savings, shared risk, global capitation, and bundles. In 2018, the Centers for Medicare & Medicaid Services (CMS) estimated that 50% of Medicare payments were tied to alternative payment models based on quality and value.[13] The first payment model is shared savings, which holds providers accountable by offering financial incentives if providers can lower costs. Under this payment model, the healthcare system or provider only shares in the savings and does not have any downside risk. If the actual cost of care is less than the predicted costs, and quality thresholds are met, the provider receives a percentage of the difference between the actual costs and predicted costs as a reward for lowering costs.[1] However, if the actual total costs are greater than the predicted costs, the provider is not responsible for the difference in costs. An example of this model can be seen in the Medicare Shared Savings Program.[14]

The second payment model, shared risk, is very similar to shared savings except that if actual costs are greater than predicted costs, the provider is responsible for the difference. This payment model requires that the provider or healthcare system keep health care costs at or below a prespecified target.[1] Medicare uses this payment model through the Hospital Readmission Reduction Program. CMS penalizes hospitals for readmissions over a set level of expected readmissions. Since 2010, Medicare data show that hospitals have prevented more than 565,000 readmissions and experienced approximately $2.5 billion in penalties, including an estimated $564 million in fiscal year 2018.[15] Additionally, CMS also piloted the Pioneer Accountable Care Organization (ACO) model, which targeted organizations experienced in coordination of care. This pioneer program was structured similarly to the shared savings model with higher levels of shared savings and consequently a higher level of risk. The organizations that performed well were then allowed to move their payments to a population-based model.[16]

The third payment model, global capitation, resembles a subscription model where providers received a fixed, per member per month fee for the care of a defined population of patients. An ACO is a group of health care providers (doctors and/or hospitals) that share financial and medical responsibility for providing coordinated care to patients in hopes of reducing unnecessary spending. An ACO brings together the different components of care—including primary care, specialists, hospitals, and home health care—to facilitate effective coordinated care.[17] ACOs employ global capitation to incentivize providers to reduce costs of care. ACOs also offer bonuses when providers reduce costs. Additionally, doctors and hospitals must meet specific quality benchmarks that focus on prevention and treatment of patients with chronic diseases. Moreover, data show that patients treated through global capitation models rather than traditional FFS models are screened for breast and colon cancer at higher rates and have superior health outcomes such as better controlled blood sugar levels, more eye examinations, and higher rates of functional status assessments.[18]

The most common type of value-based payment model currently in use in the United States is bundled payments, in which a group of providers or health system is paid one price for a full episode of care. This payment model financially rewards providers based on their ability to reduce total cost of care for an episode below a predetermined target price.[1] Bundled payments began as early as 1983 when CMS introduced the Inpatient Prospective Payment System, in which hospitals received a single payment per discharge while orthopaedic surgeons received separate fees. This program expanded into the Acute Care Episode program, which bundled both inpatient and outpatient costs of orthopaedic and cardiovascular care episodes.

Medicare introduced a bundled payment program in 2013 called Bundled Payments for Care Improvement Initiative, which was composed of four broadly defined models of care that linked payments for all care associated with a specific clinical episode, such as total joint arthroplasty. The four models varied in whether they included acute care, postacute care, or both. They also varied in terms of payments being prospective or retrospective and whether they included upside risk only or downside risk. In general, CMS assessed both quality metrics and costs per clinical episode and compared the costs to predetermined target prices. If the hospital was liable for downside risk, then it would have to pay a portion of all payments that exceeded the target pricing set for the clinical episodes. If there was only upside risk and the costs for the care episode were less than the target pricing, then the risk-bearing entity would earn a surplus on the bundled episode. This initiative capped risk for both providers and CMS at greater than or less than 20%.[19]

Private insurers and employers are also offering bundled payments as alternatives to more traditional payment methods. The ProvenCare program at Geisinger Health System in Pennsylvania accepts a single payment for several procedures, including total joint arthroplasty. Geisinger Health System has defined critical patient care steps that must be in each bundle and has demonstrated improved outcomes. The Prometheus Payment model takes into account three components: evidence-based base payment, patient-specific severity adjustment, and allowance for complications.[20] In a value-based system organized by IPUs, bundled payments incentivize health care organizations to invest in new technology or innovate at some part of the care cycle. These four payment models allow health care entities to be financially rewarded by providing more value to their patients.

VALUE-FOCUSED HEALTH INFORMATION TECHNOLOGY

In the FFS system, health information technology is dedicated to complex billing processes and reporting metrics. In a value-based healthcare system, health information technology is optimized to streamline care and accurately measure both clinical and financial results. Clinical registries are organized data systems that can evaluate specified outcomes for specific patient populations defined by a particular disease, condition, or health care resource.[21] They can be used for collecting data on patients who use particular health services for a short time, such as patients undergoing total hip arthroplasty, or for chronic conditions over time or across multiple providers, such as a patient with scoliosis. The intent of clinical registries is to pinpoint differences across treatments and outcomes, provide feedback on performance, and then use this feedback to create more standardized care. Predictive modeling offers a proactive way to assess and manage costs by assessing the risk in certain patient populations to determine appropriate clinical action. By identifying trends from existing clinical data, predictive modeling can consider the health of a specific patient population and identify proper preventive care measures.[22]

SUMMARY

Value-based health care is a model that prioritizes patient health over an abundance of tests and procedures. Because of the rising costs and overutilization of health care services in the United States, implementation of a value-based health care model helps organizations reduce costs and provide value. Value is defined as patient-centric outcomes over costs of delivered care. A value-based healthcare system requires healthcare organizations to think about care not as a breakdown of services and procedures, but as coordination of clinicians focused on the health of patients with specific conditions. Value-based health care introduces concepts such as service lines, bundled payments, and patient-reported outcomes to create frameworks and incentives that prioritize patient health over care. Outcome measures help healthcare organizations improve outcomes whereas TDABC and value-based payment models help align the goal of delivering better outcomes per health care dollar spent. Together, this framework provides hope that the problems currently plaguing the healthcare system can be overcome, allowing both patients and clinicians to thrive.

REFERENCES

1. American Academy of Pediatrics: Alternative payment models. Available at: https://www.aap.org/en-us/professional-resources/practice-transformation/getting-paid/Pages/Payment-Models.aspx. Accessed June 10, 2021.

2. Porter ME: What is value in health care? *N Engl J Med* 2010;363(26):2477-2481.

3. Peterson-KFF Health System Tracker: How does the quality of the U.S. healthcare system compare to other countries? 2020. Available at: https://www.healthsystem-tracker.org/chart-collection/quality-u-s-healthcare-system-compare-countries/#item-start. Accessed October 20, 2020.

4. Keehan SP, Stone DA, Poisal JA, et al: National health expenditure projections, 2016-25: Price increases, aging push sector to 20 percent of economy. *Health Aff (Millwood)* 2017;36(3):553-563.

5. Le Manach Y, Collins G, Bhandari M, et al: Outcomes after hip fracture surgery compared with elective total hip replacement. *J Am Med Assoc* 2015;314(11):1159-1166.

6. Porter ME, Teisberg EO: *Redefining Health Care: Creating Value-Based Competition on Results.* Harvard Business School Press, 2006.

7. Haas D, Jellinek M, Kaplan R: *Hospital Budget Systems are Holding Back Innovation. Harvard Business Review.* April 2018.

8. Lee TH, Kaplan R, Porter ME: *The Strategy That Will Fix Health Care. Harvard Business Review.* September 2015.

9. Wilson I, Bohm E, Lübbeke A, et al: Orthopaedic registries with patient-reported outcome measures. *EFORT Open Rev* 2019;4(6):357-367.

10. Kaplan R, Anderson S: *Time-Driven Activity-Based Costing. Harvard Business Review.* November 2004.

11. Auerbach A: Healthcare quality measurement in orthopaedic surgery: Current state of the art. *Clin Orthop Relat Res* 2009;467(10):2542-2547.

12. Donabedian A: *The Criteria and Standards of Quality.* Health Administration Press, 1982.

13. Centers for Medicare & Medicaid Services: Medicare, 2020. Available at: https://www.cms.gov. Accessed October 21, 2020.

14. Centers for Medicare & Medicaid Services: Shared Savings Program, 2020. Available at: https://www.cms.gov/Medicare/Medicare-Fee-for-Service-Payment/sharedsavingsprogram. Accessed October 30, 2020.

15. Centers for Medicare & Medicaid Services: Hospital Readmissions Reduction Program (HRRP), 2020. Available at: https://www.cms.gov/Medicare/Medicare-Fee-for-Service-Payment/AcuteInpatientPPS/Readmissions-Reduction-Program. Accessed October 30, 2020.

16. Centers for Medicare & Medicaid Services: Pioneer ACO model, 2021. Available at: https://innovation.cms.gov/innovation-models/pioneer-aco-model. Accessed June 10, 2021.

17. Gold J: *Accountable Care Organizations, Explained. Kaiser Health News.* July 13, 2016. Available at: https://khn.org/news/aco-accountable-care-organization-faq/. Accessed June 10, 2021.

18. United Health Group: Global capitation payments result in the highest quality primary care for seniors, 2020. Available at: https://www.unitedhealthgroup.com/content/dam/UHG/PDF/2020/UHG-Global-Capitation-Research.pdf. Accessed June 10, 2021.

19. Centers for Medicare & Medicaid Services: Bundled Payments for Care Improvement (BPCI) Initiative, 2020. Available at: https://innovation.cms.gov/innovation-models/bundled-payments. Accessed October 30, 2020.

20. Evans J: The current state of bundled payments. *Am Health Drug Benefits* 2010;3(4):292.

21. American Medical Association: 5 things to know about clinical data registries. October 15, 2014. Available at: https://www.ama-assn.org/practice-management/digital/5-things-know-about-clinical-data-registries. Accessed June 10, 2021.

22. Vogenberg FR: Predictive and prognostic models: Implications for healthcare decision-making in a modern recession. *Am Health Drug Benefits* 2009;2(6):218-222.

CHAPTER 2

Cost Accounting in Orthopaedic Surgery: A Review of Current Methods

Prem N. Ramkumar, MD, MBA • Spencer W. Sullivan, BS
Dylan S. Koolmees, MD • Benedict U. Nwachukwu, MD, MBA

INTRODUCTION

In the setting of fixed payments for certain conditions and procedures with alternative payment models, hospital organizations have shifted from analyzing revenue metrics to scrutinizing cost of care for organizational decision-making. However, substantial variability exists in the cost of care for even the most basic orthopaedic diagnoses such as osteoarthritis. A deeper dive into the methods by which costs of care, or cost accounting, are determined is therefore critical in understanding the drivers of cost with the goal of lowering the denominator in the value equation. It is important to explore both legacy and novel cost accounting methods and discuss their merits in the shift toward clarifying cost in value-based orthopaedic surgery.

TRADITIONAL LEGACY COST ACCOUNTING

The cost of health care in the United States is expected to reach 20% of the gross domestic product by 2025.[1] Therefore, it is important to understand the best methods for cost accounting. There are two commonly used traditional methods of cost accounting in health care: the ratio of costs to charges (RCC) and the relative value unit (RVU).[2] Both of these approaches are considered top-down accounting methods because they attempt to derive the cost of care from revenue, which maintains

Dr. Ramkumar or an immediate family member has received royalties from Globus Medical; serves as a paid consultant to or is an employee of Globus Medical and Stryker; has stock or stock options held in ConforMIS, Johnson & Johnson, and Overture; has received nonincome support (such as equipment or services), commercially derived honoraria, or other non–research-related funding (such as paid travel) from Stryker; and serves as a board member, owner, officer, or committee member of American Association of Hip and Knee Surgeons. Dr. Nwachukwu or an immediate family member serves as a paid consultant to or is an employee of Figur8 and has stock or stock options held in BICMD. Neither of the following authors nor any immediate family member has received anything of value from or has stock or stock options held in a commercial company or institution related directly or indirectly to the subject of this chapter: Dylan Koolmees and Spencer W. Sullivan.

a somewhat predictable but inexact relationship with cost.[3] These methods have been widely adopted because of their relative simplicity and ease of use.

The RCC is the ratio of the cost for a single service to the charge of that service, as determined by the payer. Conversely, if the RCC is known using historical data, the cost of a given procedure can be estimated using the product of the RCC and the charge of a given procedure. Using an RCC multiplier derived from the cost of all procedures in a given period divided by the charges in the same period and applying it to a future procedure can be interpreted as a rough estimate at best.[4] Certainly, this approach is limited by numerous case-specific variables. Moreover, the cost of different support staff throughout the continuum of care is absent from the equation. This results in a highly inaccurate true cost of care.

The RVU method estimates the physician's cost of service based on the value of the RVU and number of RVUs for that service.[5] The RVU has become a national standard of measurement for clinical productivity commonly used for physician evaluation and reimbursement for these services.[2,6,7] The Centers for Medicare & Medicaid Services (CMS) is responsible for updating and revising the RVUs assigned within the medical field at least every 5 years.[7] The current method for cost accounting utilizes determination of payment under the CMS resource-based relative value scale, and the Current Procedural Terminology (CPT®) and International Classification of Diseases (ICD) codes.[6] A simple equation is calculated to generate the compensation using the total RVU multiplied by the conversion factor listed by the CMS. With corresponding assignments to respective ICD and CPT® codes, RVUs allow for a quantitative comparison of productivity between different physicians among the services they provide. Universal understanding and straightforward compensation analytics are one of the largest benefits of RVU accounting.

However, arriving at cost from revenue remains nebulous, making it difficult for surgeons and hospital administrator to optimize spending and reduce overhead costs.[5] Within orthopaedic surgery, high variability in reimbursement has been noted based on insurance providers. Lalezari et al[8] reported in 2018 that variability of Medicaid reimbursement among the states was substantial for the 10 most commonly performed inpatient orthopaedic procedures. Casper et al[9] found the most interstate variation was noted for anterior cruciate ligament (ACL) reconstruction, ranging from 20.6% to 229% of local Medicare reimbursement. On average, Medicaid insurance reimburses at a rate of 81.9% of Medicare reimbursement.[9] Lack of consistency not only affects physician reimbursement, but also decreases access to optimal care when comparing Medicaid to Medicare alone.[9] In the case of total hip arthroplasty and total knee arthroplasty (TKA), primary cases are valued over complex revision cases. Using the RVU system, surgeons are reimbursed at a substantially higher rate per minute for primary TKA compared to revision TKA, resulting in a reimbursement difference approaching $140,000 per year.[10] Using this methodology of RVU accounting, surgeons are incentivized to select the easier primary cases and avoid the complex revision cases.[11] Moreover, the RVU cost accounting methodology may imply primary cases therefore carry more procedural cost, highlighting the misalignment between this form of legacy cost accounting and arriving at the true cost of care. Moreover, this form of cost accounting wholly fails to take into account the cost of support staff and surgical materials, from instrumentation to implants.

ACTIVITY-BASED COSTING

Activity-based costing (ABC) represents an alternative form of cost accounting more commonly used outside medicine. Using this cost accounting system, there are three cost drivers: total expenses, the quantity of a particular activity or proce-dure, and the percentage of time spent on the activity.[12] Total expenses and quan-tities of a procedure or activity are totaled from administrative bookkeeping, and time spent on each activity is derived from employee surveys. Thus, in theory, ABC allows a department to break down costs to a per-procedure basis. This small scope allows for close inspection of each procedure or service rendered and pro-vides areas for improving cost reduction and decreasing waste of resources.[13]

However, many other issues can arise when relying on an ABC system. When examining larger scale organizations, this system fails to accurately capture the percentage of time spent when surveying a large number of employees and the difficulty performing subsequent analyses of data processing. Using employee estimates for the time required to complete a certain task or activity can result in an inaccurate depiction of the actual time required for a procedure due to recall bias. This can lead to a cost-driver rate that is often overestimated. ABC systems require consistent upkeep to continually update the cost allocation for services provided, which results in a substantial amount of time and resources to update the cost-of-care model.

TIME-DRIVEN ACTIVITY-BASED COSTING

Time-driven activity-based costing (TDABC) is a variation of ABC but imple-ments the direct use of time as the driving factor. However, unlike ABC, manag-ers estimate the time required for a specific procedure through direct observation and prior knowledge.[12] With this method of cost accounting, only two factors are needed to calculate the cost expenditure: cost per unit of time and the time required to complete a specific task or procedure.[14] Unlike ABC, which determines employee time by survey, TDABC estimates time based on direct observation by a supervisor. Additionally, the supervisor can factor in idle time by assuming an employee works at 80% of capacity. This improves on the previous ABC model to better capture the complexities of a given procedure and more easily implement changes or variations to the model through use of a time map, which details how long it takes each person to complete discrete steps of a procedure. Thus, the cost per unit time is calculated based on an employee's salary over the amount of time spent performing the discrete steps of each activity.[4] Likewise, the TDABC model is easier to validate, allows for quicker calculation of the cost of procedures, and involves significantly less work to manage than the ABC model.[15] Unlike legacy cost accounting, such as RVU and RCC-based methods, TDABC builds cost at the individual level and adopts a more patient-centered view. This cost accounting methodology sheds light on variation, offers granularity in cost differentiation, mitigates risk, sparks opportunities for operational efficiency and waste reduction, and challenges the status quo by upholding the value-based tenets that provide accurate reference.[16] Jayakumar et al[16] herald TDABC as a form of agile innovation that focuses on individual and complex interactions, rather than processes and tools, to build in modularity with iterative development of constituent components, responsiveness to change, and the need for multidisciplinary collaboration.

Unlike the RVU-based cost accounting methodology that favors primary arthroplasty, TDABC studies of arthroplasty of the lower extremity aptly highlight implants as the primary cost driver and take the complexity of the procedure into account using time as a surrogate.[4] More than yielding procedural-level insights, TDABC is versatile enough to render clinical insights that evaluate pathways along the phase of care. For example, TDABC is capable of identifying cost drivers, whether it be cost of labor or cost of implant. Moreover, it offers easy cost comparison when adopting novel technologies and adapting to change, such as the rapid adoption of telemedicine during the COVID-19 pandemic. The data provided by broad adoption of TDABC may provide the blueprint for alternative payment models, such as risk stratification and navigation around gainsharing.[17,18] Pathak et al[17] applied TDABC to highlight a wide variation of cost estimates for total hip arthroplasty and TKA, from $7,081 to 29,557, derived from the timeframe of the procedure and the implant cost. For ankle fracture fixation, the TDABC model generated substantially lower costs for every cost category, except for implant cost, when compared with traditional hospital cost accounting.[19] Similar cost reductions with TDABC were also seen in both open and endoscopic carpal tunnel surgery[20] as well as with many pediatric distal radius fracture treatment methods.[21] Not only has TDABC been shown to help reduce overhead costs in orthopaedic surgery, but it was also used during the implementation of a new electronic medical record system at an outpatient orthopaedic clinic.[22] Although labor costs and overall clinical efficiency increased dramatically after implementation of the electronic medical record, productivity and costs returned to preintroduction levels at the 6-month time point under a TDABC model.[22]

Although the TDABC may be a viable model for more complex companies or employees in health care, there are some drawbacks to this model. TDABC requires some initial knowledge for model implementation. This also includes research into the cost of each employee's time to complete a specific task, as well as other time-driven variables. Additionally, there is more initial start-up work to be done in implementing a time map to track each aspect of a specific procedure. Thus, additional cost is necessary to properly implement a TDABC model in a company or institution. Pathak et al[17] called for standardized principles to guide TDABC implementation, especially for indirect costs that may be undervalued. Certain indirect costs, specifically structural and administrative costs, are not easily captured in a bottom-up approach but are, conversely, captured in the top-down ABC approach.[14,19]

SUMMARY

Four key cost accounting approaches are used to quantify cost in orthopaedics. RVU and RCC-based accounting approaches are traditional legacy methods that are broadly adopted for simplicity but only further obfuscate the true drivers of cost. ABC assigns value to activities performed by an organization based on the sum of total expenses, the quantity of a particular activity or procedure, and the percentage of time spent on the activity. However, there still is room for over-estimation and inaccuracy without providing a process map that identifies critical cost drivers. TDABC holds the most promise by accounting for salaries and resources along a meticulously established episode of care, while still offering the flexibility to readily identify true cost drivers and examine modular changes that may optimize value. However, this bottom-up approach fails to capture the indirect costs associated with structural maintenance and administration. Although no cost accounting approach is perfect, understanding the strengths and weaknesses of each approach will lead to more appropriate measures that result in the delivery of value-based orthopaedic care.

REFERENCES

1. Keehan SP, Stone DA, Poisal JA, et al: National health expenditure projections, 2016-25: Price increases, aging push sector to 20 percent of economy. *Health Aff (Millwood)* 2017;36(3):553-563.

2. Yun BJ, Prabhakar AM, Warsh J, et al: Time-driven activity-based costing in emergency medicine. *Ann Emerg Med* 2016;67(6):765-772.

3. Kaplan RS, Haas D: Defining, measuring, and improving value in spine care. *Semin Spine Surg* 2018;30(2):80-83.

4. Koolmees D, Bernstein DN, Makhni EC: Time-driven activity-based costing provides a lower and more accurate assessment of costs in the field of orthopaedic surgery compared with traditional accounting methods. *Arthroscopy* 2021;37(5):1620-1627.

5. Najjar PA, Strickland M, Kaplan RS: Time-driven activity-based costing for surgical episodes. *JAMA Surg* 2017;152(1):96-97.

6. Baadh A, Peterkin Y, Wegener M, Flug J, Katz D, Hoffmann JC: The relative value unit: History, current use, and controversies. *Curr Probl Diagn Radiol* 2016;45(2):128-132.

7. Rosner MH, Falk RJ: Understanding work: Moving beyond the RVU. *Clin J Am Soc Nephrol* 2020;15(7):1053-1055.

8. Lalezari RM, Pozen A, Dy CJ: State variation in Medicaid reimbursements for orthopaedic surgery. *J Bone Joint Surg Am* 2018;100(3):236-242.

9. Casper DS, Schroeder GD, Zmistowski B, et al: Medicaid reimbursement for common orthopedic procedures is not consistent. *Orthopedics* 2019;42(2):e193-e196.

10. Peterson J, Sodhi N, Khlopas A, et al: A comparison of relative value units in primary versus revision total knee arthroplasty. *J Arthroplasty* 2018;33(7 suppl):S39-S42.

11. Samuel LT, Grits D, Acuña AJ, Piuzzi NS, Higuera-Rueda CA, Kamath AF: Work relative value units do not adequately support the burden of infection management in revision knee arthroplasty. *J Bone Joint Surg Am* 2020;102(3):230-236.

12. Kaplan RS, Anderson SR: *Time-Driven Activity-Based Costing. Harvard Business Review.* November 2004. Available at: https://hbr.org/2004/11/time-driven-activity-based-costing. Accessed January 10, 2023.

13. Jalalabadi F, Milewicz AL, Shah SR, Hollier LH, Reece EM: Activity-based costing. *Semin Plast Surg* 2018;32(4):182-186.

14. Akhavan S, Ward L, Bozic KJ: Time-driven activity-based costing more accurately reflects costs in arthroplasty surgery. *Clin Orthop Relat Res* 2016;474(1):8-15.

15. Keel G, Savage C, Rafiq M, Mazzocato P: Time-driven activity-based costing in health care: A systematic review of the literature. *Health Policy* 2017;121(7):755-763.

16. Jayakumar P, Triana B, Bozic KJ: Editorial commentary: The value of time-driven, activity-based costing in health care delivery. *Arthroscopy* 2021;37(5):1628-1631.

17. Pathak S, Snyder D, Kroshus T, et al: What are the uses and limitations of time-driven activity-based costing in total joint replacement? *Clin Orthop Relat Res* 2019;477(9):2071-2081.

18. Keswani AH, Snyder DJ, Ahn A, et al: Metric selection, metric targets, and risk adjustment should be considered in the design of gainsharing models for bundled payment programs in total joint arthroplasty. *J Arthroplasty* 2021;36(3):801-809.

19. McCreary DL, White M, Vang S, Plowman B, Cunningham BP: Time-driven activity-based costing in fracture care: Is this a more accurate way to prepare for alternative payment models? *J Orthop Trauma* 2018;32(7):344-348.

20. Koehler DM, Balakrishnan R, Lawler EA, Shah AS: Endoscopic versus open carpal tunnel release: A detailed analysis using time-driven activity-based costing at an academic medical center. *J Hand Surg Am* 2019;44(1):62.e1-62.e9.

21. Waters PM: Value in pediatric orthopaedic surgery health care: The role of Time-Driven Activity-Based Cost accounting (TDABC) and Standardized Clinical Assessment and Management Plans (SCAMPs). *J Pediatr Orthop* 2015;35(5 suppl 1):S45-S47.

22. Scott DJ, Labro E, Penrose CT, Bolognesi MP, Wellman SS, Mather RC: The impact of electronic medical record implementation on labor cost and productivity at an outpatient orthopaedic clinic. *J Bone Joint Surg Am* 2018;100(18):1549-1556.

Clinical Outcomes Measurement

Eric C. Makhni, MD, MBA, FAAOS • Kassandra S. Carter, MD

INTRODUCTION

Because outcomes are core to understanding value in healthcare, organizations must have sophisticated processes for measuring, analyzing, and modifying care delivery based on clinical outcomes. Numerous types of clinical outcomes are available for measurement, and each type has its own unique application and method for collection. Organizations must understand how each type of clinical outcome contributes to a successful value-based operation.

ADMINISTRATIVE CLAIMS-BASED OUTCOMES

Administrative claims-based outcomes are clinical outcomes derived from bills, also known as claims, submitted by physicians and hospitals to private and public payers. Administrative claims databases hold millions of transactions between provider and patient. Consequently, claims-based data can be analyzed for large patient populations at relatively low costs.[1] For some clinical measures, claims data can be more accurate than chart reviews because it shows whether tests were ordered or prescriptions were filled. However, claims data can have limitations due to coding errors or inconsistencies; in addition, these data can only examine conditions for which the patient was treated and submitted a claim.[2] For example, a noncompliant patient with diabetes may have no claim history of the disease. Because of their representation of large populations and relatively low costs, the use of administrative claims data as a surrogate for clinical outcomes has increased in recent years.

Public and private payers interpret the quality of healthcare organizations by examining claims-based outcomes such as incidence of death, nonfatal complications, and hospital-acquired conditions (HACs). Measured by patient safety indicators (PSIs), HACs are viewed as costly expenditures representative of hospital quality. In an effort to reduce health care spending, the Centers for Medicare & Medicaid Services (CMS) through the Inpatient Prospective Payment System in

Dr. Makhni or an immediate family member has stock or stock options held in Protera Health and serves as a board member, owner, officer, or committee member of American Academy of Orthopaedic Surgeons and American Orthopaedic Society for Sports Medicine. Neither Dr. Carter nor any immediate family member has received anything of value from or has stock or stock options held in a commercial company or institution related directly or indirectly to the subject of this chapter.

2008 refused to pay for several HACs.[3] Encouraged by the reduction in the rates of HACs as a result of this program, CMS announced it would penalize the lowest-quartile health systems 1% of total reimbursements based on a composite rate known as PSI 90 and five high-cost HACs. The PSI 90 went into effect in 2015 and consists of 10 PSIs (including iatrogenic pneumothorax, in-hospital fall with hip fracture, and postoperative respiratory failure). The five high-cost HACs are *Clostridium difficile* infection, surgical site infection, catheter-associated urinary tract infection, central line-associated bloodstream infection, and methicillin-resistant *Staphylococcus aureus* bacteremia.[4] Following this lead, private insurance companies also implemented ways to reduce costs by driving consumers away from high-cost, low-quality hospitals to low-cost, high-quality hospitals. For example, some employer-based insurance plans encourage employees to receive treatment at centers of excellence or high-value health care facilities, rather than visit in-network hospitals. A 2019 survey showed 16% of firms with 50 or more workers were designated centers of excellence as part of employee health plans.[5] Overall, entities such as Medicare, employers, and private insurers use claims-based data to favor higher performing organizations and penalize lower performing organizations.

Because of their ability to assess the cost and quality of health care provided, claims-based outcomes are playing increasingly significant roles in financial compensation and consumer decision-making. CMS uses claims-based quality data to assess reimbursements, whereas private insurers implement claims-based data to design plans with financial incentives such as lower copays to drive customers to high-value providers. It is to the benefit of providers to understand metrics such as PSI 90 and the five high-cost HACs. These claims-based metrics not only represent the quality of a healthcare organization to CMS and private insurers, but they also determine the compensation that a healthcare organization may or may not receive. To create a successful value-based organization, providers need to be aware of the metrics used to evaluate them and the influence that they have on their organization.

NATIONAL RANKING METRICS

Each year, factors such as patient satisfaction, clinical outcomes, and quality of health care providers are analyzed and converted into scores used to compare and rank hospitals in order of best to worst performance. These scores and rankings are then disseminated to the public to guide decisions on where patients choose to receive care. The four main national ranking bodies are Quality Rating System, US News & World Report, Leapfrog, and Healthgrades.[6] Although each rating system operates a little differently, these rankings systems possess the power to influence both consumer and payer behavior.

Arguably the most influential of the national ranking systems, the Quality Ratings are a five-star rating system to track the experience of Medicare beneficiaries with their health plans. These ratings are based on measures in three categories with Medical Care given the greatest weight: (1) Medical Care, (2) Member Experience, and (3) Plan Administration.[7] Medicare patients use the Quality

Ratings as a way to compare and select health care plans and providers. CMS and private insurers also use these ratings to assign bonus payments, structure reimbursement rates, dole out penalties, and decide which health care provider organizations should receive contracts. Because of the wide influence of these ratings from consumer choice to reimbursement, organizations must be aware of their rating and aim for ways to improve quality and value.

According to a 2018 Deloitte survey, 39% of respondents considered reputation when choosing a physician, whereas almost 25% reported that they had used a quality rating when choosing a physician or hospital, an increase of 5% from a 2013 survey.[8] US News & World Report aims to help consumer decision making by listing the top 50 hospitals in the United States and within 16 specialties. It also regionally ranks hospitals and provides scores (out of 100) for each hospital. It breaks down the scoring of hospitals into three categories: outcomes and experience; key programs, services, and staff; and professional recognition. Using Medicare data, it incorporates clinical outcomes such as 30-day survival, discharging patients to home, and patient experience via survey into the total hospital score.[9]

Led by the mission of increasing transparency in health care, Healthgrades, a popular consumer site for hospital and physician ratings, ranks America's best 250, 100, and 50 hospitals. To determine these rankings, Healthgrades establishes an overall performance score based on in-hospital mortality, 30-day mortality, and influence of mortality and complication outcomes on overall performance.[10] Leapfrog provides safety grades for more than 2,600 hospitals using both process/structural and outcome measures.[11] As the influence of national rankings expands and the demand for increased health care transparency grows, healthcare organizations must be aware of the evaluation criteria used for the rankings and of their rankings and scores on the various consumer-facing national ranking systems.

CLINICAL OUTCOMES

In a value-based healthcare system, there is an advantage to using comprehensive, user-friendly platforms that can synthesize and interpret data for real-time clinical decision making and improvement. These platforms extract data from electronic medical records and health information technology systems. These data, specifically termed electronic clinical quality measures (eCQMs), measure the value of care provided through indicators such as length of stay, readmissions, complications, cost per case, or cost per supplies.

These platforms and by extension, eCQMs, can be leveraged to improve value of care through comparison by service line, surgeon, or hospital. For example, these platforms allow a total joint arthroplasty service line to compare the cost of case by surgeon and examine cost drivers. This analysis might show that one surgeon is using more costly implants or supplies, thus driving up the total cost of that surgeon's cases. Moreover, eCQMs can shed light on specific patient factors such as comorbidities or age that can increase readmissions or length of stay, so that hospitals and physicians can be more attuned when managing specific patient populations. These platforms, if implemented correctly, have the potential to ease the burden of quality reporting and bolster quality improvement through increasing access to real-time information.

eCQMs are essential to the improvement of care and quality. For these measures to be justifiable in regard to use of resources needed to collect and analyze, eCQMs must be feasible to collect in an automated fashion, generate valid and reliable results, and demonstrate a benefit that outweighs costs.[12] Electronic health record-based automated quality measure reporting has the potential, if implemented correctly, to ease the burden of quality reporting while simultaneously increasing access to real-time information to bolster quality improvement.

The American College of Surgeons has indicated that surgical quality could not be improved if it could not be measured, which led to the creation of the National Surgical Quality Improvement Program (NSQIP) to help hospitals detect potentially preventable adverse events. As a national, outcomes-based registry, the American College of Surgeons NSQIP helps surgeons determine the quality of their surgical programs and measurable improvement in surgical outcomes. NSQIP is a 20% sample that tracks outcomes for randomly selected patients until 30 days after hospital admission. The program uses eCQMs rather than administrative or claims data. One study compared NSQIP data to administrative and claims data and found that NSQIP data identified 61% more adverse events, including 97% more surgical site infections.[13] The tools, analyses, and reports provided by the American College of Surgeons NSQIP allow surgeons and hospitals to make informed decisions about improving care quality.

PATIENT-CENTRIC OUTCOMES

Although administrative and claims-based data are relatively easy to measure, they do not necessarily represent the most meaningful outcomes to patients.[14] As providers place increasing focus on value, they must similarly focus on outcomes that matter most to patients. For instance, a healthy patient undergoing a total hip replacement will likely care more about postoperative pain and function outcomes and less so about 90-day mortality rates. Therefore, organizations must install processes and systems whereby patient-centered outcomes data can not only be collected but analyzed and acted on as well.

In general, there are three types of patient-centric outcomes that orthopaedic health care leaders must be aware of: patient-reported outcomes, patient-reported outcome measures (PROMs), and patient-reported outcomes-based performance measures (PRO-PMs).

Patient-Reported Outcomes

Patient-reported outcomes (PROs) are representative of the patient's perspective. They are directly answered by the patient and relate to his or her perception of care. Commonly measured parameters for PROs include pain, satisfaction, or adverse reactions. For example, a routinely assessed PRO is pain (often on a visual analog scale). These responses can then be compared before and after treatment rendered. These measures can be administered by any member of the health care team. Often, they are collected upon patient check-in or rooming (particularly pain scores for orthopaedic patients). Because they measure the patient perspective, they can be particularly helpful in a value-based health care environment focused on improving outcomes that matter most to patients.

Although PROs are valuable in understanding patient experience and symptoms, they have certain limitations.[15,16] Despite a quantitative numeric rating system, PROs are prone to subjectivity that can limit their utility. In one recent study of numeric rating scale pain scores measured in a cohort of musculoskeletal patients, these scores were only moderately correlated with more robust measures of pain, and inclusion of these robust scores was recommended as part of routine pain assessment in patients.[17] These findings were corroborated by other similar studies that compared pain assessments to pain measurements from PROMs. For example, in a study of spine patients by Bernstein et al,[18] they found that the Patient-Reported Outcomes Measurement Information System (PROMIS) Pain Interference scale, which is a PROM that measures the impact of pain on a patient's quality of life, had improved correlation with physical function PROMs when compared to Likert pain scales.

Regardless of these limitations, PROs still serve valuable purposes. Because they are easy to measure, they provide an opportunity for clinicians to longitudinally track metrics such as pain and satisfaction easily (and affordably) in the busy ambulatory setting.

Patient-Reported Outcome Measures

There are two major types of PROMs: general health and diagnosis-specific measures. General health PROMs focus on broad measures, or domains, of patient health, such as pain, function, satisfaction, quality of life, and general health. In contrast, diagnosis-specific measures focus on individual patient cohorts or pathologies, such as knee osteoarthritis or rotator cuff tear. Advantages of general health measures include the ability to use a single measure across different patient groups (ie, using a pain PROM for all orthopaedic patients), thereby promoting automation of PROM assignments (to be discussed in detail later in this chapter).[19,20] However, general forms may misrepresent outcomes following a given surgery or intervention if there was a concomitant injury. For example, a patient who has recovered successfully from a knee ligament reconstruction but later injures the hip will report poor scores on a physical function assessment. Conversely, if that patient was administered a knee ligament PROM and a hip function PROM, their score would likely reflect improved knee function and decreased function in the hip. One main disadvantage of diagnosis-specific PROMs is that a clinician must first make a diagnosis, thereby requiring some manual effort in properly assigning questionnaires to patients. This limits the ability to automate PROM assignment on a population perspective.

National Institutes of Health PROMIS Assessment Tools

Recently, in collaboration with Northwestern University, the National Institutes of Health created the PROMIS assessment tools,[21] general health and domain-specific tools designed by incorporating questions from various existing legacy PROMs of numerous disease states. One goal of PROMIS was to create a PROM assessment tool that could be standardized across groups, as numerous studies have demonstrated significant variability in PROM selection across clinical trials within a given diagnosis.[22-24] This variability in PROM selection makes it difficult to compare clinical outcomes and findings from studies that utilize disparate measures. Therefore, PROMIS was created as a method by which all clinical centers could use a single, standardized measure.

The PROMIS assessments are scored using T-scores, whereby a score of 50 represents the score of a reference population of control patients, with 10 points representing a standard deviation. Moreover, the scores reflect how much of that functional capacity or symptom level the patient reports. For example, a patient who scores 60 on a physical function assessment has one standard deviation more of function than the reference population, whereas a patient who scores a 60 on a depression assessment has one standard deviation more of depressive symptoms than the reference population. In this manner, high scores are not necessarily good or bad, but simply a reflection of the domain being measured. Further explanation of score interpretations can be found online.[22]

Best Practices of Successful PROM Administration and Collection

Practical measurement of PROMs in the busy ambulatory and surgical settings can be challenging. Numerous factors, such as financial constraints, workflow considerations, logistics with personnel, and patient/provider education make such collection challenging. However, there are defined best practices that can aid in collection, regardless of practice size.

Information from PROMs is most valuable at the time of the initial clinical evaluation with the patient. These data, when combined with patient history, physical examination, and imaging findings, can guide decision making and facilitate shared decision making. Traditionally, many provider groups only measure PROMs on surgical patients; however, these data are collected after surgery has been indicated and scheduled and are thereby unavailable for shared decision making. In order to incorporate PROM data into shared decision-making efforts, they must be collected prior to the clinical evaluation.

Pre-evaluation PROM capture relies on several key attributes and assumptions.[23,24] PROM collection must be seamlessly integrated into the clinical workflow. As mentioned previously, automatic collection relies on utilization of general health or domain-specific measures, and for this reason the use of NIH PROMIS tools is emphasized. The PROMs are available for completion in the patient's electronic health record portal up to 1 week prior to the scheduled visit. While checking in for the appointment, all patients who still have pending questionnaires then complete them on a tablet computer prior to being called into the examination room.

Successful capture of universal PROMs also relies on standardization and collaboration across orthopaedic divisions and health system teams. PROM selection should be standardized within a division, department, or practice in order to successfully aggregate and compare outcomes by provider. Ideally, patients should need no more than 5 minutes to complete questionnaires. Any attempts to improve workflow (eg, utilize the PROM platform for forms that were previously collected on paper) will help make the process manageable for office staff. Significant effort must be made to educate providers, office staff, and clinical support staff on the importance of PROMs and how they should be collected within the clinical space.

Finally, data from PROMs should be readily available to all providers in real time in order to review with patients. **Figure 1** demonstrates a sample screenshot from an electronic medical record that displays the PROM scores for a patient who underwent injection treatment and physical therapy for the diagnosis of adhesive capsulitis (frozen shoulder). This score improvement can then be discussed between patient and provider when determining when or if any further treatment is needed.

Using PROMs to Improve Value

As mentioned previously, value-based care consists of improving health outcomes that matter most to the patient. Therefore, PROMs play a central role in measuring value of care, as these outcomes reflect the patient's perceptions of their functional capacity and symptom severity. When considering how to incorporate these measures into value-based care, there are numerous options to consider.

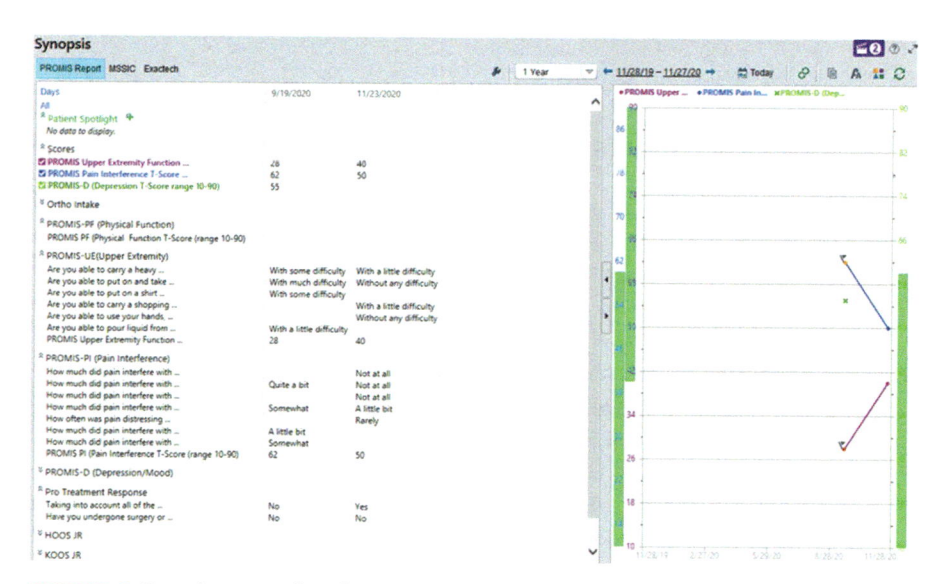

FIGURE 1 Sample screenshot from an electronic medical record that shows PROM scores for a patient who underwent injection treatment and physical therapy for the diagnosis of adhesive capsulitis (frozen shoulder).

Measuring Quality Through PROMs

PROMs can be used to measure quality of care across a division, department, practice, or service line. The goal of most orthopaedic interventions is to improve function, decrease pain, improve quality of life, or any combination of these metrics. Therefore, PROMs can be incorporated into quality improvement initiatives within an orthopaedic practice. For example, a director can identify select procedures that are high value or high volume within a given specialty (ie, total hip and knee replacement, anterior cruciate ligament reconstruction, spinal fusion, ankle reconstruction, etc.) and focus PROM collection preoperatively and postoperatively on those key metrics. PROM scores can then be compared across provider, site, and hospital to ensure PROM improvement across key specialties.

Care should be taken to consider factors that could affect PROM scores outside of the surgeon's control. One such factor could include patient characteristics (which can be mitigated through risk stratification). Directors should also ensure that efforts are made to comprehensively collect preoperative and follow-up data with robust completion rates.

Patient-Reported Outcomes-Based Performance Measures

PRO-PMs may serve additional value when these metrics are incorporated into value-based accountability and payment programs. One method for doing so is through incorporation of PRO-PMs. Although these measures are infrequently utilized in current orthopaedic practice, they do have the potential to transform payment and delivery models.

The use of PRO-PMs was detailed in a 2013 report from the National Quality Forum (NQF)[25] entitled Patient-Reported Outcomes (PROs) in Performance Measurement. In this report, the National Quality Forum outlines how these measures can improve the value of care. In the example provided, the assessment for clinical depression is the Patient Health Questionnaire (PHQ)-9, with a score greater than 9 indicating an intervention is warranted. The PRO-PM is subsequently the proportion of affected patients whose PHQ-9 scores improve by a minimal clinically important difference (MCID) at 6 months following the initial test.

PROMs and Predictive Analytics

As increasing amounts of data become available, PROM scores may be used for shared decision making using predictive analytics. An improvement in PROM scores may not necessarily denote clinical improvement. Therefore, the score change may denote statistical significance but not clinical significance, meaning that the patient has not improved sufficiently enough to warrant a state of meaningful change. In order to better understand this distinction, researchers have identified score changes for various PROMs and treatments that denote MCID. For example, if a PHQ-9 score change of 5 points denotes MCID for a given PROM following a particular surgery, any patient improving at least 5 points postoperatively would have been considered to have meaningfully improved from a clinical perspective. Patients whose PHQ-9 score improves by 4 points—even if this represents a statistically meaningful change—would not be considered as improved clinically.

With this in mind, research has recently been directed at identifying predictive factors that correspond to likelihood of achieving MCID following surgery. There have been numerous examples within orthopaedic literature that have successfully performed these analyses.[26,27] There are also commercial vendors and applications that assimilate patient data preoperatively into predictive models for postoperative score changes.[28] Successful incorporation of predictive analytics into preoperative decision making will not only identify possible modifiable factors that can be improved on, but also provide invaluable guidance to patients who are considering various treatment options.[29-31]

SUMMARY

Value-based health care is dependent on measurement of clinical outcomes that are meaningful to patients and clinicians. Administrative claims-based outcomes provide relatively low-cost data for large patient populations. Because these outcomes can be used to assess the cost and quality of provided care, claims-based data play consequential roles in reimbursement and hospital-reported metrics. Factors such as patient satisfaction, clinical outcomes, and quality of health care providers influence national ranking metrics that guide patient decisions and shape perception of healthcare organizations. Electronic clinical measures use data from electronic health records or health information technology to measure the quality of health care. PROMs are outcomes that are representative of the patient's perspective because they are derived from questionnaires directly answered by the patient. Because they relay patient perceptions, PROMs can be utilized effectively in a value-based health care environment focused on improving outcomes that matter most to patients.

Although effort and investment are required to implement a sustainable and effective outcomes measurement platform, there are numerous benefits with regard to improving value delivered to patients. Ultimately, clinical outcomes measurement is paramount to making a successful transition to a value-based healthcare system.

REFERENCES

1. Wennberg JE, Roos N, Sola L, Schori A, Jaffe R: Use of claims data systems to evaluate health care outcomes: Mortality and reoperation following prostatectomy. *J Am Med Assoc* 1987;257(7):933-936.

2. Crews H, Pronovost PJ, Helft PR, Austin JM: Improving the quality of data for inpatient claims-based measures used in public reporting and pay-for-performance programs. *Jt Comm J Qual Patient Saf* 2017;43(12):671-675.

3. Centers for Medicare and Medicaid Services (CMS), HHS: Medicare program: Changes to the hospital inpatient prospective payment systems and fiscal year 2009 rates; payments for graduate medical education in certain emergency situations; changes to disclosure of physician ownership in hospitals and physician self-referral

rules; updates to the long-term care prospective payment system; updates to certain IPPS-excluded hospitals; and collection of information regarding financial relationships between hospitals. Final rules. *Fed Regist* 2008;73(161):48433-49084.

4. Centers for Medicare & Medicaid: Hospital-Acquired Condition Reduction Program (HACRP), 2020. Available at: https://www.cms.gov/Medicare/Medicare-Fee-for-Service-Payment/AcuteInpatientPPS/HAC-Reduction-Program#:~:text=The%20Hospital%2DAcquired%20Condition%20(HAC,in%20the%20inpatient%20hospital%20setting. Accessed April 24, 2023.

5. Claxton G, McDermott D, Cox C, Hudman J, Kamal R, Rae M: Employer strategies to reduce health costs and improve quality through network configuration. Peterson-KFF Health System Tracker, 2019. Available at: https://www.healthsystemtracker.org/brief/employer-strategies-to-reduce-health-costs-and-improve-quality-through-network-configuration/. Accessed January 18, 2023.

6. Bae JA, Curtis LH, Hernandez AF: National hospital quality rankings: Improving the value of information in hospital rating systems. *J Am Med Assoc* 2020;324(9):839-840.

7. Centers for Medicare & Medicaid Services: Provider enrollment and certification, 2020. Available at: https://www.cms.gov/files/document/quality-rating-system-101-20221014.pdf. Accessed April 24, 2023.

8. Betts D, Korenda L: Inside the patient journey: Three key touch points for consumer engagement strategies. Deloitte Insights, 2018. Available at: https://www2.deloitte.com/us/en/insights/industry/health-care/patient-engagement-health-care-consumer-survey.html. Accessed January 18, 2023.

9. FAQ: How and why we rank and rate hospitals. U.S. News & World Report, 2020. Available at: https://health.usnews.com/health-care/best-hospitals/articles/faq-how-and-why-we-rank-and-rate-hospitals. Accessed January 18, 2023.

10. Healthgrades: America's best hospitals for clinical excellence awards 2020 methodology. Available at: https://www.healthgrades.com/quality/americas-best-hospitals-for-clinical-excellence-2020-methodology. Accessed January 18, 2023.

11. The Leapfrog Group: Hospital ratings and reports. Available at: https://www.leapfroggroup.org/ratings-reports. Accessed January 18, 2023.

12. eCQI Resource Center: Getting started with eCQMs, 2021. Available at: https://ecqi.healthit.gov/ecqms. Accessed January 18, 2023.

13. American College of Surgeons: About ACS NSQIP, 2021. Available at: https://www.facs.org/quality-programs/acs-nsqip/about. Accessed January 18, 2023.

14. Bentler SE, Morgan RO, Virnig BA, Wolinsky FD: Do claims-based continuity of care measures reflect the patient perspective? *Med Care Res Rev* 2014;71(2):156-173.

15. Morasco B, Lovejoy T, Hyde S, Shull S, Dobscha S: Limitations of pain numeric rating scale scores collected during usual care: Need for enhanced assessment. *J Pain* 2018;19(3):S57-S58.

16. Tishelman JC, Vasquez-Montes D, Jevotovsky DS, et al: Patient-reported outcomes measurement information system instruments: Outperforming traditional quality of life measures in patients with back and neck pain. *J Neurosurg Spine* 2019;30(4):1-6.

17. Morasco BJ, Yarborough BJ, Smith NX, et al: Higher prescription opioid dose is associated with worse patient-reported pain outcomes and more health care utilization. *J Pain* 2017;18(4):437-445.

18. Bernstein DN, St John M, Rubery PT, Mesfin A: PROMIS pain interference is superior to the Likert pain scale for pain assessment in spine patients. *Spine (Phila Pa 1976)* 2019;44(14):E852-E856.

19. Gulledge CM, Smith DG, Ziedas A, Muh SJ, Moutzouros V, Makhni EC: Floor and ceiling effects, time to completion, and question burden of PROMIS CAT domains among shoulder and knee patients undergoing nonoperative and operative treatment. *JB JS Open Access* 2019;4(4):e0015.1-7.

20. Franovic S, Gulledge CM, Kuhlmann NA, Williford TH, Chen C, Makhni EC: Establishing "normal" patient-reported outcomes measurement information system physical function and pain interference scores: A true reference score according to adults free of joint pain and disability. *JB JS Open Access* 2019;4(4):e0019.

21. Makhni EC, Meadows M, Hamamoto JT, Higgins JD, Romeo AA, Verma NN: Patient Reported Outcomes Measurement Information System (PROMIS) in the upper extremity: The future of outcomes reporting? *J Shoulder Elbow Surg* 2017;26(2):352-357.

22. Makhni EC, Padaki AS, Petridis PD, et al: High variability in outcome reporting patterns in high-impact ACL literature. *J Bone Joint Surg Am* 2015;97(18):1529-1542.

23. Guo EW, Elhage K, Cross AG, et al: Establishing and comparing reference preoperative Patient-Reported Outcomes Measurement Information System (PROMIS) scores in patients undergoing shoulder surgery. *J Shoulder Elbow Surg* 2021;30(6):1223-1229.

24. Makhni EC, Meyer MA, Saltzman BM, Cole BJ: Comprehensiveness of outcome reporting in studies of articular cartilage defects of the knee. *Arthroscopy* 2016;32(10):2133-2139.

25. HealthMeasures: PROMIS 2020. Available at: https://www.healthmeasures.net/score-and-interpret/interpret-scores/promis. Accessed January 19, 2023.

26. Nwachukwu BU, Rasio J, Beck EC, et al: Patient-reported outcomes measurement information system physical function has a lower effect size and is less responsive than legacy hip specific patient reported outcome measures following arthroscopic hip surgery. *Arthroscopy* 2020;36(12):2992-2997.

27. Makhni EC: Meaningful clinical applications of patient-reported outcome measures in orthopaedics. *J Bone Joint Surg Am* 2021;103(1):84-91.

28. Cella D, Hahn E, Jensen S, et al: *Patient-Reported Outcomes in Performance Measurement.* RTI Press, 2015.

29. Anderson MR, Houck JR, Saltzman CL, et al: Validation and generalizability of preoperative PROMIS scores to predict postoperative success in foot and ankle patients. *Foot Ankle Int* 2018;39(7):763-770.

30. Franovic S, Kuhlmann N, Pietroski A, et al: Preoperative patient-centric predictors of postoperative outcomes in patients undergoing arthroscopic meniscectomy. *Arthroscopy* 2021;37(3):964-971.

31. Jayakumar P, Bozic KJ: Advanced decision-making using patient-reported outcome measures in total joint replacement. *J Orthop Res* 2020;38(7):1414-1422.

Clinical Registries in Orthopaedics

Jeremy T. Hines, MD • Wendy M. Novicoff, PhD
James A. Browne, MD

INTRODUCTION

The development of clinical registries in medicine has resulted in numerous advancements in a wide variety of health care domains. Such domains include, but are not limited to, understanding the course of particular diseases and various treatments affecting outcomes; identifying specific factors that influence quality of life or prognosis; monitoring safety; evaluating socioeconomic effect; and studying quality of care, quality improvement, and more recently, patient-reported outcome measures (PROMs). Modern clinical registries play an increasingly important role in orthopaedic surgery and have the potential to further advance the field.

Clinical registries, also referred to as patient registries, are organized bodies of information collected in a uniform manner to evaluate specific outcomes in a patient population. Registries allow collection, storage, retrieval, and analysis of information on individuals based on a disease, condition, or exposure of interest. Data may be collected from a specific geographic region or nationwide, and only a limited amount of information that reflects the purpose of the registry is captured. Clinical registries have evolved from the pooled data of single surgeon's series or small clinical trials to large databases of patients, which provide valuable epidemiologic data that can be analyzed, disseminated, and compared throughout global orthopaedic communities.

The components of a clinical registry follow a specific design and rationale to collect data on particular outcomes of interest. The data collected are scrutinized regarding internal and external validity, compliance, and generalizability during collection, analysis, and reporting. Implementing and maintaining a registry can be complex and requires substantial effort and resources. This chapter focuses on the history, purposes, composition, application, and implications of clinical registries in orthopaedics. Specific examples will show how clinical registries can affect the delivery of value-based health care. A thorough discussion of all significant registries in orthopaedics is beyond the scope of this chapter; however, a few select registries are highlighted to provide an overview of this topic.

COMPONENTS OF A REGISTRY

Multiple facets are required to create a successful registry. At initiation, there must be a clearly articulated purpose or objective of the registry, an identified target population to study, and specifically identified data that can be collected accurately and efficiently. An established governance is imperative to ensure proper guidance and decision making on behalf of the registry, clear communication with the stakeholders involved, transparent funding proposals and acquisition, and data collection, reporting, and dissemination of results. This requires a variety of participating teams, with representative individuals who have expertise in multiple domains.[1,2]

A committee involved in project management is necessary for registry coordination, time management, expense budgets, funding, and communication with both stakeholders and participating data collection sites. Clinical experts must delineate the appropriate target population to study and data collected aligning with registry goals. An infrastructure for data collection and management serves as the core of the clinical registry; information collected from multiple target sources at participating units must be accurately documented, stored appropriately, and accessible for extraction. This database management requires trained personnel to ensure data validity and completeness: as technology has enabled much of this work to be done electronically, management of specific registry-driven programs and algorithms require regular assessment for quality assurance and validation. Additionally, specialists in the field of epidemiology, statistics, and health outcomes are vital in data analysis. Legal counsel is necessary to provide guidance on patient eligibility within the registry and protection of identifiable information. Finally, the clinical registry team must be able to effectively communicate and corroborate results with other organizations, the orthopaedic community, and patients to increase knowledge and quality of care.[1-3]

The components of a clinical registry are a reflection of the defined focus of the registry; therefore, the rationale, design, and goals of the registry must align to assess a variety of related issues regarding epidemiology, safety, efficacy, and practice policy, among others. Registries at various levels, from institutional to national, may be different regarding the type and amount of data collected. For example, total joint arthroplasty registries record specific patient identification and corresponding demographic, surgical, implant, and clinical outcome information. There are four recognized levels of data that can be collected by registries that, in turn, determine potential application[4] (**Table 1**).

In total joint arthroplasty registries that record data on primary and revision arthroplasty, level I data include identifiers on patients, surgeons, and hospitals as well as procedural data to monitor rates of revisions. Level II data include patient

TABLE 1 Levels of Data Collection in Orthopaedic Clinical Registries

Data Level	Data Collected	Significance
I	Patient, surgeon, and hospital identifiers; procedural data	Monitor revision rates
II	Patient factors and comorbidities, surgical information, perioperative care, complications	Assessment of type and rate of complications, changes in patterns over time
III	Patient-reported outcome measures focusing on patient health, function, pain, and satisfaction	Identification of factors affecting patient outcomes; value in assessment of association socioeconomic implications, cost analysis, and policy making
IV	Radiographic/imaging assessment	Assessment of component alignment/positioning, implant wear, osteolysis over time

Data from Hansen VJ, Greene ME, Bragdon MA, et al: Registries collecting level-I through IV data: Institutional and multicenter use: AAOS exhibit selection. *J Bone Joint Surg Am* 2014;96(18):e160. and Malchau H, Garellick G, Berry D, et al: Arthroplasty implant registries over the past five decades: Development, current, and future impact. *J Orthop Res* 2018;36(9):2319-2330.

factors and comorbidities, surgical information, perioperative care, and complications; this allows for assessment in the types and rates of complications associated with a particular standard of care, and respective changes in these patterns with time. Level III data include PROMs by using questionnaires focusing on the patient's perceived health, function, pain, and satisfaction. These data have implications in the identification of factors driving poor or successful patient outcomes, as well as socioeconomic implications of the procedures performed that inherently affect cost analysis and policy making. The addition of radiographs for further assessment of implants denotes level IV data; such information, collected and stored for a large number of patients, can be influential in analyzing technically driven alignment and component positioning, as well as implant wear and osteolysis over time.[4,5]

Two examples of dataset recommendations to meet the specific aims of the organization include those proposed by the International Society of Arthroplasty Registries (ISAR) and American Joint Replacement Registry (AJRR). The ISAR has developed a minimum dataset recommended for collection by national arthroplasty registries. This dataset represents the core minimum required to effectively compare specific prosthesis and patient outcomes, limited in an attempt to increase coverage, accuracy, and efficiency of recorded information. The ISAR minimum dataset includes prosthesis, patient, surgery, and hospital details[6] (**Table 2**). In comparison, elements currently collected by the AJRR focus on three categories:

TABLE 2 The International Society of Arthroplasty Registries Minimum Dataset

Data Type	Data Collected
Prosthesis data	Catalogue number
	Lot number
Patient data	National identity number
	Full name
	Age
	Sex
	Address
	Operative hospital patient identifier
Surgical data	Date of surgery
	Site/side of procedure
	Diagnosis
	Primary or revision procedure type
Hospital data	Identity number OR name/address

Data from International Society of Arthroplasty Registries: Available at: https://www.isarhome.org/bylaws. Accessed March 15, 2021.

procedural, postoperative, and PROMs. Within the procedure category, data are collected on the patient, site of service, surgeon, specific procedure performed, patient comorbidities, and surgical complications. The postoperative category includes data on postoperative complications and 90-day readmissions. A variety of patient-reported outcomes are collected, with recommendations on using a measure of health-related quality of life and specific hip- or knee-related surveys.[7] Registries may elect to add data elements that become clinically relevant (such as robotics or computer navigation) or sunset the collection of those that are no longer of interest.

DATA QUALITY AND VALIDITY

The foundation of clinical registries relies on the input of quality data. Five dimensions, as reported by Malchau et al,[5] that are fundamental to clinical registry reporting are coverage, completeness, response rate, missing values, and validation. In an attempt to maximize internal and external validity of the studies conducted, clinical registries must control for potential bias influencing results.[8]

Clinical registries are subject to accurate and comprehensive reporting. Coverage, as defined by the ratio of the number of participating units to the total number of units producing data for a procedure of interest, is particularly relevant to achieve more representative data collections. Participating institutions are also subject to the completeness of data reporting, as underreporting at the singular level may deleteriously affect analysis into misleading conclusions.[4,5] As previously mentioned, the ISAR attempts to achieve such quality by requiring accurate data collection, more than 80% contribution of national hospitals, with at least 90% procedural reporting from each site.[6] Similarly, the use of PROMs risk incomplete or unanswered variables prior to analysis—this poses a requirement to be included in statistical analysis, as well as response rates recorded at individual follow-up times. At each step of the process, from defining the purpose of the registry to data acquisition, completeness of data reporting, and finally, analysis, efforts are required to adequately structure, staff, and fund the registry to enhance overall compliance.[4,5]

The concept of validity is essential to understand. Internal validity, in essence, is a measure of bias influencing results of a study. Reducing potential bias, or systematic errors influencing results, increases the internal validity of a study in that there are fewer implications due to unmeasured variables not controlled for in reported associations between exposure and outcomes. Registry data are subject to random and systematic error, notably during data collection and storage. Validation of registry data to clinical records or an external dataset representative of criterion validity and regular assessment of new data are methods to resolve such error. Registry data should be cross-compared to clinical data and even a similar database that has been recognized as criterion validity (cross comparing to a gold standard database) can help to reduce errors; consistent assessment of incoming or new data decreases unrecognized error.[4] Randomized controlled trials, for example, attain a high degree of internal validity given the process of treatment randomization among groups of similar measured or unmeasured characteristics. Resultant outcome differences are therefore attributed to differences in the efficacy and safety of the different treatments and less subject to bias. Clinical registries, however, tend to focus on external validity instead of a more homogenous patient population of randomized controlled trials that inherently limits generalizability.[8]

External validity refers to the generalizability of the inferences made of a study, translating to a wider population beyond the population under study. Clinical registries often achieve high external validity given the population heterogeneity under study. As such, registry data may be more applicable and realistic of disease epidemiology, treatment, and outcomes. An argument can therefore be made that the inferences made from observational studies in clinical registries are more representative of the diverse patient population in current medical practices, and more relevant in driving decision making and policymaking to improve outcomes.[8] Clinical registries are inherently different from one another regarding processes for estimating internal and external validity, but such processes should be publicly and clearly available for review.[5]

The current progression of clinical registries to utilize PROMs requires special consideration. As discussed later in the chapter, PROMs are derived from questionnaires filled out by patients regarding aspects of generalized health, pain, function, and quality of life, among others. These tools are subject to thorough assessment to ensure standards of validity, reliability, and responsiveness are met. Validity, the ability to measure an intended outcome, requires specific content to address the concept of interest; the tool should provide comparable measurements to known standards and among different groups of interest. Reliability is the consistency and reproducibility of the tool's ability to produce similar measurements in different scenarios in which an element is unchanged. Finally, the responsiveness of the outcome measure is the actual ability to detect change in a particular area of interest in the patient. Intrinsic to standards of responsiveness are principles of minimal clinically important difference and minimal detectable change. The minimal clinically important difference is the minimal change in outcome scoring that is clinically important or significant to the patient; the minimal detectable change is the minimal change necessary to ensure the resultant score is outside the scope of standard error within the outcome measure, and that the change in score is true and not due to internal error.[9-11]

VALUE AND USEFULNESS OF REGISTRIES

Clinical registries have been central to the understanding of disease epidemiology and treatment patterns. As one of the earliest registries, the Swedish Hip Arthroplasty Registry (SHAR) has documented an increase in incidence and corresponding change in prevalence of total hip arthroplasties (THAs) over time; by the end of 2019, 3.6% of the population older than 40 years underwent THA, of whom 27% underwent bilateral THA with a higher prevalence in women (4.1%) than men (3.0%). In men and women, primary osteoarthritis was the primary diagnosis for THA, but a greater proportion of women underwent THA secondary to acute trauma (hip fracture) during this same timeframe. In addition, there was a higher rate of cemented femoral stems in women compared with men.[12] This registry has been able to trend multiple epidemiologic and demographic data points with corresponding treatment patterns, which is representative of how clinical registries serve as a valuable tool for analysis and future projections.

Similarly, registries have expanded understanding regarding etiologies of primary arthroplasty failure. The recent Australian Orthopaedic Association National Joint Replacement Registry (AOANJRR) 2020 report identified the revision burden (defined as the ratio of implant revisions to the total number of arthroplasties in a specific period) of primary total knee arthroplasty (TKA) and THA at 8.0% and 8.4%, respectively[13]; the recent AJRR 2020 report identified revision rates of 4% in TKA and 3.1% in THA from years 2012 through 2019.[14] The registries have identified major etiologies for failure as well as risk factors for revision surgery including patient factors, implant factors, and surgeon factors such as surgical approach. Registries are uniquely situated to follow failure rates of primary procedures and help identify areas where improvement is needed for survivorship.

Registries have also been instrumental in the surveillance of specific implants used in orthopaedic surgery, providing critical information on implant performance, survivorship, and adverse events. Currently, orthopaedic devices comprised more than 16% of all class I and II medical device recalls in the United States from the years 2015 through 2019.[15] There has been a focus on revision as an endpoint as it can serve as an indicator for the quality of an implant, poses considerable burden to the patient and healthcare system (time and expense), and is a reproducible and comparable data point. The United Kingdom National

Joint Registry (NJR) provided early insight on the poor implant survivorship of metal-on-metal (MoM) hip resurfacing with more than 13% requiring revision after 10 years, recognized by other registries such as the AOANJRR, notably in women, irrespective of femoral head size.[16] These two registries also identified similar findings regarding MoM bearing surfaces in THA, for which 1 in 5 of these articulations needed revision 10 years after the index procedure because of MoM wear-related issues. In a similar mechanism of failure, femoral stems with a modular neck in the 2012 AOANJRR report showed a 7.4% revision rate at 5 years across all similar featured stem designs, 10.6% at 10 years, which was twice the failure rate of other contemporary stems.[17] These results are just a few examples of the value of clinical registries in implant surveillance, which has led to corroboration of results within the orthopaedic community, resulting in improvement of quality, safety, and efficacy of care.

Fundamental to value-based health care is the idea that an intervention should be measured by the outcome achieved for the patient and whether or not it successfully meets their needs. Substantial progress has been made in the past decade to measure and understand clinical parameters in orthopaedics more relevant to patients through use of PROMs, and PROMs are increasingly being collected in clinical registries: to date, approximately 18 current orthopaedic arthroplasty registries are collecting PROMs.[18] Measurements that include the patient's perspective, often in the form of surveys/questionnaires, have become more relevant as the focus of health care systems transitions to improving quality, value, and outcome-based patient care. Generalized PROMs focus on assessing physical, mental, and social qualities of health to gauge overall health and quality of life. More specific PROMs aim to measure additional features related to a specific disease or intervention, such as osteoarthritis in a patient who underwent TKA[18] (**Table 3**). To the patient, PROMs increase communication to clinicians regarding treatment outcomes and effects on quality of life, facilitating open decision making between both patient and clinician on future decision making together. Clinicians utilize PROMs to compare performance with established standards of care and regulate changes in the health of patients, again facilitating improved communication with the patient. Healthcare organizations also use PROMs collectively to monitor and compare performance with other organizations; this allows recognition in areas of deficit and subsequent vital feedback to quality improvement initiatives. At the highest level, PROMs allow health system policymakers to understand outcomes at local to international levels over time. By using this information, the advantages and disadvantages of the different models of care can be compared, prompting necessary changes to increase value-based health care.[10,11,18]

In value-based health care, PROMs can help achieve understanding of what is of value from a patient's perspective. Quality-adjusted life years is one method of understanding the generic measure of disease burden, incorporating general PROMs of quality of life such as the EQ-5D and quantity of time lived, providing insight into more rational allocation of health care resources.[11] Therefore, PROMs can be used to confirm the cost effectiveness of arthroplasties as number and cost of quality-adjusted life years, integral in healthcare systems as resources are

TABLE 3 Common Patient Reported Outcome Measure Surveys

Survey	Abbreviation	Year Established	Validation in Arthroplasty	No. of Items	Analysis
EuroQol 5 Dimension Health Outcome Survey 3-Level Version	EQ-5D-3L	1990	Hip and knee	6	Mobility, self-care, usual activities, pain/discomfort, anxiety/depression
Short Form 12 Health Survey	SF-12	1996	Unknown	12	Vitality, physical functioning, bodily pain, general health perceptions, physical role functioning, emotional role functioning, social role functioning, mental health
Western Ontario and McMaster Universities Arthritis Index	WOMAC	1982	Hip and knee	24	Pain, disability, and joint stiffness in hip and knee osteoarthritis
Knee Injury and Osteoarthritis Outcome Score	KOOS	1998	Knee	42	Pain, other symptoms, function in activities of daily living, function in sport and recreation, knee-related quality of life, quality of life
KOOS Physical Function Short Form	KOOS-PS	2007	Unknown	7	Function, daily living, sport, recreation
Hip Disability and Osteoarthritis Outcome Score	HOOS	2003	Hip	40	Pain, other symptoms, function in activities of daily living, function in sport and recreation, hip-related quality of life, quality of life
HOOS Physical Function Short Form	HOOS-PS	2008	Unknown	5	Function, daily living, sport, recreation
Oxford Knee Score	OKS	1998	Knee	12	Joint pain and function
Oxford Hip Score	OHS	1996	Hip	12	Joint pain and function
University of California at Los Angeles Activity Score	UCLA	1984	Hip and knee	10 levels	Level of activity

Data from Rolfson O, Bohm E, Franklin P, et al: Patient-reported outcome measures in arthroplasty registries Report of the Patient-Reported Outcome Measures Working Group of the International Society of Arthroplasty Registries Part II. Recommendations for selection, administration, and analysis. *Acta* directed to higher value care. In a recent study analyzing PROMs data from the AJRR, it was identified that patients with higher mental health and lower physical function preoperative scores preoperatively were more likely to clinically benefit from THA or TKA. However, patients with poor preoperative mental health scores undergoing TKA were more likely to undergo early revision TKA.[19] Insight into value and quality improvement strategies in health care continue to emerge as orthopaedic registries increase collection of patient-reported outcomes.

HISTORY OF ORTHOPAEDIC REGISTRIES

Many existing orthopaedic registries have been modeled from the successes garnered by initial clinical registries focusing on total joint arthroplasty. These registries aimed to collect specific data on hip and knee arthroplasty to analyze patient- and implant-associated risk factors as well as variations in surgical technique affecting outcomes. The mission and structure of these early registries has led to the development of other registries from an institutional to national level worldwide.

The Mayo Clinic Total Joint Registry

The Mayo Clinic total joint registry was established by Dr. Mark Coventry in 1969 to collect clinical, surgical, and radiographic data on THA and TKA in a uniform and methodical manner; this information would then be used to communicate, not only to the individual, but to the orthopaedic community, outcomes of the procedures performed. This is the largest institutional registry in the United States, with detailed data on more than 100,000 primary and revision arthroplasties entailing patient-specific demographics, detailed surgical and implant-related information, and any revision or reoperation procedures performed. Additionally, patients can be cross-referenced for further analysis within other institutional databases including oncologic, medical, anesthesia, and billing databases.[3,5]

In 1985, reports from the registry regarding revision THA identified that first-generation cemented acetabular and femoral component techniques were associated with high failure rates.[20] Collaboration with results from other registries led the transition away from cemented acetabular components in the 1980s to newly available noncemented porous coated implants. Similarly, initial proximally porous coated monoblock femoral implants used in revision THA were noted to have high implant failure secondary to aseptic loosening and osteolysis.[21] The Mayo Clinic registry has been instrumental in the evolution of surgical technique to improve survivorship and patient outcomes in THA and TKA; current techniques include use of noncemented modular fluted tapered stems and highly porous noncemented acetabular components with highly cross-linked polyethylene liners.[22-24]

Nationwide Orthopaedic Registries

Several countries have established orthopaedic registries over the past 50 years. The first nationwide orthopaedic registry, established in Sweden in 1975, focused on TKA. Many other countries subsequently followed suit, with the first

English-language nationwide orthopaedic registry formed in New Zealand in 1998. A chronological summary of several of the major nationwide registries is depicted in **Figure 1**.

The Swedish Knee and Hip Arthroplasty Registries

The Swedish Knee Arthroplasty Registry (SKAR) and the SHAR, founded in 1975 and 1979, respectively, represent two of the earliest influential national orthopaedic registries. Over time, the SKAR has been able to estimate implant survivorship and delineate implant failures, epidemiology of periprosthetic joint infection (and, in turn, efficacious and cost-effective preventative and treatment strategies), and outcomes of specific surgical techniques.[5,25] Reports from the SKAR in the 1970s on infection as a revision etiology in TKA still influence current practice: the identification of systemic prophylactic antibiotics and antibiotic-laden bone cement were found to be safe and efficacious in infection prevention.[26]

The SHAR initially sought to identify complications associated with revision hip arthroplasty, in turn identifying data on implant survivorship, etiology for revision, and associated complications that helped in understanding and mitigating

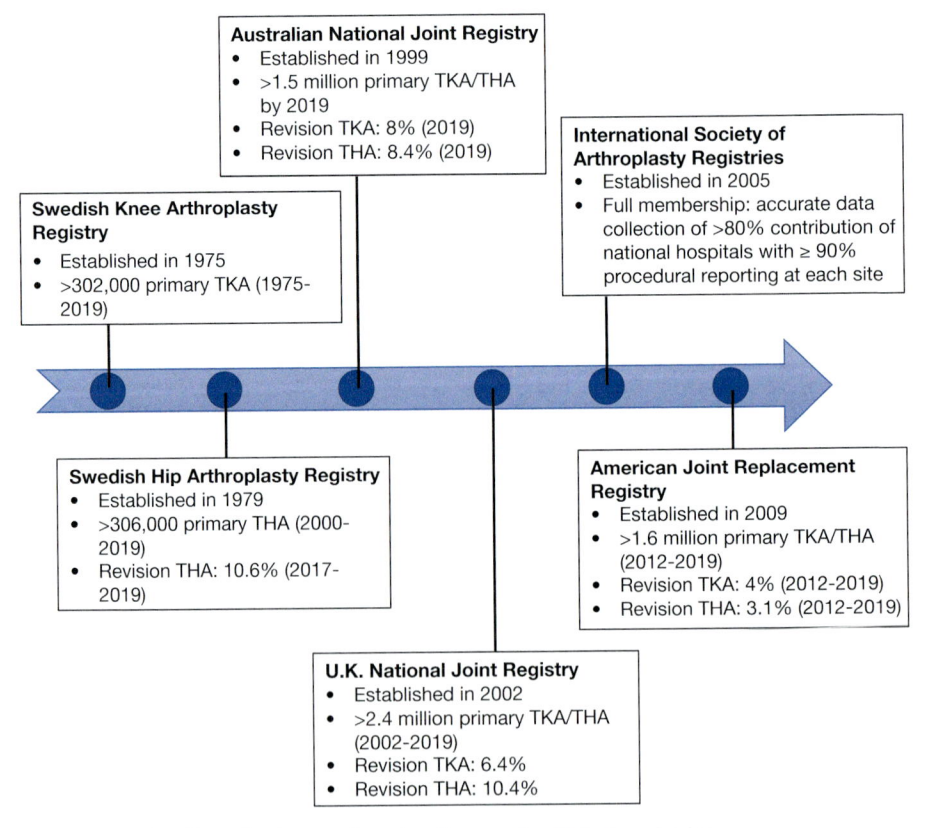

FIGURE 1 Timeline of select national orthopaedic clinical registries.

such adversities, improving overall quality of care. In time, the SHAR adopted measures to assess patient-reported outcomes dealing with quality of life, pain, and satisfaction, which led to the creation of publicly accessible annual reports at the local and national levels, a common practice that has been adopted by other registries.[25,27] The SHAR's focus on implant survivorship and outcomes led to the cautious adoption of new techniques as evidenced by the limited femoral stems (6 designs) and acetabular components (10 designs) accounting for more than 92% and more than 82% component use, respectively, as of 2017.[28,29] The evidence-based guidance of this clinical registry allowed the nation to avoid calamities faced by other nations, namely those associated with MoM THA articulations.

Australian Orthopaedic Association National Joint Replacement Registry

The AOANJRR, founded in 1999, uses a defined minimum dataset to enable efficient analysis, including patient characteristics, prosthesis type and features, method of prosthesis fixation, and surgical technique; principal outcome of the registry is revision surgery, and mortality rates are monitored. Implementation of data collection has expanded to include other orthopaedic procedures of the wrist, ankle, elbow, shoulder, and spine.[25,29,30]

The AOANJRR has been pivotal in the identification of outlier prosthesis and techniques, setting precedence to improve standard of care. This registry reported on the use of the DePuy Articular Surface Replacement hip prosthesis, utilizing MoM bearing surfaces, highlighting that the rate of revision secondary to aseptic loosening, osteolysis, and metal sensitivities has more than doubled compared with a conventional prosthesis at 5 years in both the Articular Surface Replacement acetabular and hip-resurfacing systems.[31] This information affirmed results of other registries, which led to the consensus within the orthopaedic community worldwide to abandon use of these specific components, given the heightened complications and poor survivorship, increasing awareness of the impediments of MoM articulations.

United Kingdom NJR

The NJR of England and Wales was established in 2002 by the United Kingdom Department of Health, expanding in 2013 to include Northern Ireland and in 2015 to include the Isle of Man.[32] The registry was initially founded with the intent to collect appropriate information of implanted prosthesis performance, spurred by the early failure of a cemented THA femoral component (3M Capital Hip) that drew substantial public scrutiny and concern.[33] The NJR now includes registry data on more than 2.4 million hip and knee arthroplasties, as well as 50,000 shoulder, elbow, and ankle arthroplasties.

The NJR values transparency and accountability. Restricted access clinician feedback online portals, provided by the NJR, allow clinicians and surgeons to review multiple domains of procedure-level data and outcomes on a personal and hospital level; similar annual clinical reports are given to affiliated hospitals to assess and compare outcomes in attempt to improve care. In 2013, the NJR developed a public website, as part of the National Health Service England Consultant

Outcomes Publication initiative, allowing the public to review the number and types of cases performed by surgeon/hospital, outcomes achieved, revision rates, and certain collected PROMs. All implants are monitored on a 6-month basis in terms of revision rate; appropriate action is taken by the Medicines and Healthcare products Regulatory Agency for any prosthesis with elevated revision rates in comparison to the group average. Data from the registry and a variety of other sources are provided to an independent organization, the Orthopaedic Data Evaluation Panel, which provides a benchmark at 3, 5, 7, and 10 years and grade of evidence at each timepoint for specific prostheses, a practice that has been shown to influence subsequent implant use.[32]

American Joint Replacement Registry

The AJRR, founded in 2009, was established as a multistakeholder, independent, not-for-profit organization. The AJRR was fully integrated into the American Academy of Orthopaedic Surgeons (AAOS) in 2017 and became the cornerstone of the AAOS Registry Program. Data collected on hip and knee arthroplasties include procedural data, postoperative data, and patient-reported outcomes. A variety of surveys are captured regarding patient self-assessment related to physical function, mental health, mobility, social function, and pain; specific hip and/or knee measures are also included. In 2018, AJRR received claims data from the Centers for Medicare & Medicaid Services that were linked to the existing AJRR database, further expanding the amount of data available for analysis. The registry allows for continual patient follow-up and outcome measure assessment vital to the evolving changes in orthopaedic standards of care as well as implications in policymaking. The AJRR has been recognized and validated as a Qualified Clinical Data Registry that satisfies reporting requirements by the Centers for Medicare & Medicaid Services.[7,34,35]

Despite the concerns with data submission being voluntary, the AJRR has grown rapidly. The AJRR's recent report included more than 1,300 enrolled sites with data on more that 2.2 million knee and hip arthroplasty procedures. The report highlighted important epidemiologic data on revision arthroplasty procedures, patient-related risk factors, evolving techniques, and implant survivorship. Recent analysis of the registry data suggests that it is representative of the broader practice of total joint arthroplasty in the United States despite only capturing approximately 40% of all procedures performed across the country. The AJRR recently introduced a surgeon dashboard feature that allows surgeons and site administrators at participating AJRR sites to access their individual data and compare against national deidentified information and benchmarks. These dashboards can help clinicians better understand their outcomes and add value to quality improvement efforts.[14,36]

In addition to the AJRR, the AAOS Registry Program now includes a Musculoskeletal Tumor Registry (MsTR), Shoulder and Elbow Registry (SER), Fracture and Trauma Registry (FTR), and American Spine Registry in collaboration with the American Association of Neurological Surgeons (AANS). The AAOS Registry Program has partnered with the Centers for Medicare & Medicaid Services on its Bundled Payments for Care Improvement (BPCI) Advanced Program, which will utilize the AAOS reported registry data as part of an Alternate Quality Measure Set. As BPCI Advanced qualifies as an Advanced Alternative Payment Model under the Quality Payment Program, registry data will be instrumental in the ongoing emphasis of value-based care and payment models that can better guide decision-making. Participation in the AAOS Registry supports a multitude of quality certification programs, federal quality initiatives, insurer's distinction programs, and state collaboratives. For example, registry program participation supports reuse of date for payer incentive programs such as the Centers for Medicare & Medicaid Services Merit-based Incentive Payment System (MIPS), which counts toward the Quality Payment Program focusing on high-value, high-quality care.[37,38]

The International Society of Arthroplasty Registries

The ISAR was established in 2005 to improve outcomes for patients undergoing total joint arthroplasty globally. The society emphasizes the need to establish conformity in terminology and standardization of statistical analysis to allow for more applicable and accurate data assessment among registries. Full membership in the ISAR on the national level adheres to a nomination process that requires clinical registries to have accurate data collection of more than 80% contribution of national hospitals, with at least 90% procedural reporting from each site. Examples of such registries include the SKAR and SHAR, the AOANJRR, and the Kaiser Permanente Total Joint Replacement Registry (TJRR), among others.[5,6]

Regional Orthopaedic Registries

Orthopaedic registries have been highly effective at the regional level and do not require nationwide coverage to be influential in the practice of value-based care.

The Michigan Arthroplasty Registry Collaborative Quality Initiative

At the state registry level, the Michigan Arthroplasty Registry Collaborative Quality Initiative (MARCQI) was founded in 2011 and comprises data from more than 50 participating hospitals in Michigan. The registry aims to improve patient safety and quality of arthroplasties by promoting continuous quality improvement activities, reporting results and identifying devices and techniques with superior outcomes, and demonstrating that participating sites are improving the value of arthroplasty services. Specific initiative focus includes infection and venous thromboembolic event prevention, complication reduction, device analysis, postoperative readmission analysis and reduction, and PROMs.[34,35,39]

The use of tranexamic acid is an example of a recent collaborative quality improvement initiative analyzed by MARCQI. The clinical registry aimed to assess the safety and efficacy of tranexamic acid in total joint arthroplasty and identified reductions in transfusion rates without increased risk of venous thromboembolic events, cardiovascular events, length of hospitalization, or readmission rates. The analysis of these results was shared to collaboratively adopt the use of tranexamic acid in standardized surgical protocols, and similar initiatives have been established regarding appropriate discharge planning, evidence-based pain management protocols in collaboration with tracking of opiate prescribing and use, and anticoagulation prophylaxis guidelines, among others.[39-42] These examples show how a regional registry can influence local clinical practice.

The Kaiser Permanente TJRR

The Kaiser Permanente TJRR was developed in 2001 to identify and evaluate short- and long-term complications of total joint arthroplasties utilizing data from the electronic health care system of Kaiser Permanente, one of the largest managed care organizations in the United States that services a multitude of health care plans. Goals of the registry include identification of patient risk factors, best care practice, and implant efficacy and safety, which extend to other specific orthopaedic registries focusing on sports-related procedures, spine surgery, and fracture care. Advancements in this registry have allowed particular focus on short- and long-term complications, radiographic assessment, and patient-reported outcomes serving as a tool for quality improvement.[35,43,44]

A recent analysis using the TJRR focusing on the direct anterior approach and the posterior approach for THA was conducted in a cohort of more than 38,000 primary THAs. The registry identified that the direct anterior approach, when compared with the posterior approach, was significantly associated with lower rates of dislocation, revision for instability and periprosthetic fracture, and readmission. However, the analysis showed higher risk of revision for aseptic loosening with the direct anterior approach.[45] As the orthopaedic community continues to evolve, evidence such as this has been paramount to understand the benefits and associated risks of new techniques in an attempt to mitigate additional morbidity and improve patient outcomes.

LIMITATIONS OF REGISTRIES

There are several limitations of clinical registries that present ongoing challenges. The accuracy and completeness of data collected starts at the local level and can be applied to the regional and national levels. The goal of national clinical registries to obtain at least 80% compliance of participating units with at least 90% of procedural reporting is a daunting task even for the largest registries. For example, a recent analysis of the Danish Hip Arthroplasty Register identified only two-thirds of primary THAs revised for the diagnosis of PJI were captured by the registry, and that approximately 25% of such cases could not be confirmed to be infected.[46] This represents one of the ongoing challenges imposed on registries in which further progress, such as corroboration and validation with other available databases, may be necessary for improvement.

Orthopaedic clinical registries also differ on definitions that define endpoints under study, as well as the specific type and complexity of data collected. The Norwegian registry does not define component addition as a revision surgery, but rather a reoperation. For example, the Norwegian registry classifies patellar resurfacing of a previously unresurfaced patella simply as a reoperation.[25] The SKAR does not consider the exchange of an insert, as in the case of infection, a revision. The reported implant survivorship of registry studies depends directly on the specific endpoints under study, such as revision; as in the examples provided, such definitions are not universal among registries, with some reoperations considered a revision in some registries but not in others. The inherent differences in the type of data collected subsequently affect analysis, with each registry providing associations between outcomes and patient or implant characteristics. Although attempts have been made to define core datasets, such as the minimum dataset by the ISAR, there is not unanimous adoption among all registries.

As registries continue to make comparisons of results at the local and national levels, risk stratification of cohorts has become exceedingly important. Registries are continuing to collect more data on patient comorbidities and characteristics, as well as a multitude of orthopaedic factors that can influence outcomes; however, risk stratification of cohorts and different end points is an intricate and evolving process. This highlights an apparent limitation of current orthopaedic registries, as the nature of failure is often multivariable and there is a fundamental inability of registries to control for all associated variables. It is important to understand that within any registry, the representative associations identified via analysis do not necessarily arise from causality, as confounding variables are present.[47]

A fundamental requirement of clinical registries is to reliably capture index and revision procedures to effectively evaluate outcomes and survivorship. Loss of patient follow-up or patient migration to hospital systems not captured by the registry can lead to invalid conclusions on outcomes of interest. This is especially important for developing registries such as the AJRR, with data capture rates currently limited by participating healthcare systems; large registries such as the SHAR, SKAR, AOANJRR, and NJR utilize national healthcare systems limiting loss of follow-up. A recent analysis of Medicare fee-for-service beneficiaries undergoing arthroplasty in the United States was performed, given the low rates of loss to follow-up in this population, which identified more than 10% of patients at 5 years and more than 18% of patients at 10 years migrated out of the county or state of index where the procedure was performed, resulting in loss of longitudinal follow-up.[48] Other potential limitations, mostly affecting registries in the United States, include trying to track and follow an extremely large number of joint procedures each year, special issues related to patient privacy laws, the large number of private and public insurance and payer options, and the availability of information and reports from various registries. Because most registries in the United States are not supported by government funding, the organizations that run them require sometimes substantial fees or subscriptions in order to participate, receive reports, and access data.[11,25,49] All of these limitations emphasize that clinical registries are imperfect in complete data collection and patient follow-up but can serve as a rich area for future improvement and direction.

FUTURE OUTCOMES

Advancements in technology have been critical to the success and growth of clinical registries. Electronic applications for data collection and storage, as well as applications for data retrieval, sharing, patient outcome questionnaires, and more robust computerized analysis have expanded the clinical and economic importance of registries. Natural language processing is a recent advancement that allows an electronic automated algorithm to collect data of interest from electronic medical records; this tool has shown promising results in accurate and efficient data extraction, a process that through manual review may require excess cost and time, and be more subject to error.[50,51] Additionally, automated data capture systems and algorithms can serve as additional checkpoints in incoming data acquisition to minimize inherent human and systematic error, decrease erroneous data, and adjust for missing information.[4]

As the impetus continues to change in health care, away from volume-driven fee-for-service reimbursement to value-based models, understanding and utilizing PROMs to incorporate patient input will be critical for advancements in quality and cost of care. The emergence of PROMs to aid in measuring the results of arthroplasty in a manner other than revision is of great interest, with potential use in structural, process, and outcome measures. Efforts to understand the scenarios in which each PROM is most effective is ongoing, as collection grows within registries and applications expand within value-based health care.[52]

The role of clinical registries in understanding care and outcomes in orthopaedics is tightly intertwined in the future development of optimal performance measures. Application of registry data in risk-adjusted models will enhance performance evaluation and have socioeconomic implications in directing preferred clinician networks, as well as overall reimbursement. As clinical registries expand in health care coverage, supplementation with other data sources such as claims data will provide healthcare systems more insight to long-term outcomes and resource utilization, ultimately influencing change to improve patient-centered care.[53]

SUMMARY

Clinical registries currently serve as powerful tools that affect health care professionals and the overarching healthcare system. Registry data analysis can provide input on the identification and implementation of best care practice, with the ability to focus on individual patient attributes. The healthcare system benefits as clinical registries are utilized to improve quality of care from both patient outcome and economic perspectives. As registries increase coverage and completeness, their use will expand to direct healthcare policymaking and reimbursement.

REFERENCES

1. Gliklich RE, Leavy MB, Dreyer NA, eds: *Registries for Evaluating Patient Outcomes: A User's Guide.* [Internet], ed 4. Agency for Healthcare Research and Quality, 2020. Section I, Creating Registries.

2. Gliklich RE, Dreyer NA, Leavy MB, eds: *Registries for Evaluating Patient Outcomes: A User's Guide.* [Internet], ed 3. Agency for Healthcare Research and Quality (US), 2014. Section 2, Planning a Registry.

3. Berry DJ, Kessler M, Morrey BF: Maintaining a hip registry for 25 years: Mayo Clinic experience. *Clin Orthop Relat Res* 1997;344:61-68.

4. Hansen VJ, Greene ME, Bragdon MA, et al: Registries collecting level-I through IV data: Institutional and multicenter use: AAOS exhibit selection. *J Bone Joint Surg Am* 2014;96(18):e160.

5. Malchau H, Garellick G, Berry D, et al: Arthroplasty implant registries over the past five decades: Development, current, and future impact. *J Orthop Res* 2018;36(9):2319-2330.

6. International Society of Arthroplasty Registries: Available at: https://www.isarhome. org/bylaws. Accessed March 15, 2021.

7. American Joint Replacement Registry: Available at: https://www.aaos.org/registries/ registry-program/american-joint-replacement-registry/. Accessed March 15, 2021.

8. Gliklich RE, Leavy MB, Dreyer NA, eds: *Registries for Evaluating Patient Outcomes: A User's Guide* [Internet], ed 4. Agency for Healthcare Research and Quality (US), September 2020. Chapter 3, Registry Design.

9. Fleischmann M, Vaughan B: The challenges and opportunities of using Patient Reported Outcome Measures (PROMs) in clinical practice. *Int J Osteopath Med* 2018;28:56-61.

10. Rolfson O, Eresian Chenok K, Bohm E, et al: Patient-reported outcome measures in arthroplasty registries. *Acta Orthop* 2016;87(suppl 1):3-8.

11. Wilson I, Bohm E, Lübbeke A, et al: Orthopaedic registries with patient-reported outcome measures. *EFORT Open Rev* 2019;4(6):357-367.

12. Swedish Hip Arthroplasty Registry: SHAR 2019 Annual Report. Available at: https://registercentrum.blob.core.windows.net/shpr/r/VGR_Annual-report_ SHAR_2019_EN_Digital-pages_FINAL-ryxaMBUWZ_.pdf. Accessed March 15, 2021.

13. Australian Orthopaedic Association National Joint Replacement Registry: AOANJRR 2020 Annual Report. Available at: https://aoanjrr.sahmri.com/documents/10180/689619/Hip%2C+Knee+%26+Shoulder+Arthroplasty+New/6a07a3b8-8767-06cf-9069-d165dc9baca7. Accessed March 15, 2021.

14. American Joint Replacement Registry: AJRR 2020 Annual Report. Available at: https://connect.ajrr.net/2020-ajrr-annual-report. Accessed March 15, 2021.

15. Vajapey SP, Li M: Medical device recalls in orthopedics: Recent trends and areas for improvement. *J Arthroplasty* 2020;35(8):2259-2266.

16. Smith AJ, Dieppe P, Howard PW, Blom AW: Failure rates of metal-on-metal hip resurfacings: Analysis of data from the National Joint Registry for England and Wales. *Lancet* 2012;380(9855):1759-1766.

17. Australian Orthopaedic Association National Joint Replacement Registry: AOANJRR 2012 Annual Report. Available at: https://aoanjrr.sahmri.com/documents/10180/60142/Annual+Report+2012. Accessed March 15, 2021.

18. Rolfson O, Bohm E, Franklin P, et al: Patient-reported outcome measures in arthroplasty registries Report of the Patient-Reported Outcome Measures Working Group of the International Society of Arthroplasty Registries Part II. Recommendations for selection, administration, and analysis. *Acta Orthop* 2016;87 (suppl 1):9-23.

19. Gray CF, Rizk PA, Parvataneni HK: Leveraging patient reported outcome measures from the American Joint Replacement Registry to predict total joint arthroplasty

patient outcomes at one year. Poster presentation at: American Association of Hip and Knee Surgeons Virtual Meeting; November 5-8, 2020.

20. Kavanagh BF, Ilstrup DM, Fitzgerald RH: Revision total hip arthroplasty. *J Bone Joint Surg Am* 1985;67(4):517-526.

21. Berry DJ, Harmsen WS, Ilstrup D, Lewallen DG, Cabanela ME: Survivorship of uncemented proximally porous-coated femoral components. *Clin Orthop Relat Res* 1995;319:168-177.

22. Abdel MP, Cottino U, Larson DR, Hanssen AD, Lewallen DG, Berry DJ: Modular fluted tapered stems in aseptic revision total hip arthroplasty. *J Bone Joint Surg Am* 2017;99(10):873-881.

23. Kremers HM, Howard JL, Loechler Y, et al: Comparative long-term survivorship of uncemented acetabular components in revision total hip arthroplasty. *J Bone Joint Surg Am* 2012;94(12):e82.

24. Jenkins DR, Odland AN, Sierra RJ, Hanssen AD, Lewallen DG: Minimum five-year outcomes with porous tantalum acetabular cup and augment construct in complex revision total hip arthroplasty. *J Bone Joint Surg Am* 2017;99(10):e49.

25. Delaunay C: Registries in orthopaedics. *Orthop Traumatol Surg Res* 2015;101(1 suppl):S69-S75.

26. Bengtson S, Borgquist L, Lidgren L: Cost analysis of prophylaxis with antibiotics to prevent infected knee arthroplasty. *BMJ* 1989;299(6701):719-720.

27. Malchau H, Herberts P, Eisler T, Garellick G, Söderman P: The Swedish Total Hip Replacement Register. *J Bone Joint Surg Am* 2002;84-A(suppl 2):2-20.

28. Kärrholm J, Mohaddes M, Odin D, et al: The Swedish Hip Arthroplasty Register – Annual Report 2017. Available at: https://registercentrum.blob.core.windows.net/shpr/r/Eng_Arsrapport_2017_Hoftprotes_final-Syx2fJPhMN.pdf. Accessed October 4, 2023.

29. Varnum C, Pedersen AB, Rolfson O, et al: Impact of hip arthroplasty registers on orthopaedic practice and perspectives for the future. *EFORT Open Rev* 2019;4(6):368-376.

30. Australian Orthopaedic Association National Joint Replacement Registry: Available at: https://aoanjrr.sahmri.com/background. Accessed March 15, 2021.

31. de Steiger RN, Hang JR, Miller LN, Graves SE, Davidson DC: Five-year results of the ASR XL acetabular system and the ASR hip resurfacing system: An analysis from the australian orthopaedic association national joint replacement registry. *J Bone Joint Surg Am* 2011;93(24):2287-2293.

32. Porter M, Armstrong R, Howard P, Porteous M, Wilkinson JM: Orthopaedic registries – The UK view (National Joint Registry): Impact on practice. *EFORT Open Rev* 2019;4(6):377-390.

33. Massoud SN, Hunter JB, Holdsworth BJ, Wallace WA, Juliusson R: Early femoral loosening in one design of cemented hip replacement. *J Bone Joint Surg Br* 1997;79(4):603-608.

34. Ayers DC, Franklin PD: Joint replacement registries in the United States: A new paradigm. *J Bone Joint Surg Am* 2014;96(18):1567-1569.

35. Pugely AJ, Martin CT, Harwood J, Ong KL, Bozic KJ, Callaghan JJ: Database and registry research in orthopaedic surgery: Part 2 – Clinical registry data. *J Bone Joint Surg Am* 2015;97(21):1799-1808.

36. Levine BR, Springer BD, Golladay GJ: Highlights of the 2019 American Joint Replacement Registry Annual Report. *Arthroplast Today* 2020;6(4):998-1000.

37. The American Academy of Orthopaedic Surgeons registry program. Available at: https://www.aaos.org/registries/. Accessed July 15, 2021.

38. Quality Payment Program: Centers for Medicare & Medicaid services merit-based incentive payment system quality payment program. Available at: https://qpp.cms.gov/mips/overview. Accessed July 15, 2021.

39. The Michigan arthroplasty registry collaborative quality initiative. Available at: http://marcqi.org/about-marcqi/marcqi-background/. Accessed March 15, 2021.

40. Hallstrom B, Singal B, Cowen ME, Roberts KC, Hughes RE: The Michigan experience with safety and effectiveness of tranexamic acid use in hip and knee arthroplasty. *J Bone Joint Surg Am* 2016;98(19):1646-1655.

41. Hood BR, Cowen ME, Zheng HT, Hughes RE, Singal B, Hallstrom BR: Association of aspirin with prevention of venous thromboembolism in patients after total knee arthroplasty compared with other anticoagulants: A noninferiority analysis. *JAMA Surg* 2019;154(1):65-72.

42. Hughes RE, Cornish E, Hallstrom BR: Why registries are important: The example of the Michigan Arthroplasty Registry Collaborative Quality Initiative (MARCQI). *Arthroplast Today* 2020;6(4):747-748.

43. National Implant Registries Kaiser Permanente: Available at: https://national-implantregistries.kaiserpermanente.org/about. Accessed March 15, 2021.

44. Paxton EW, Kiley ML, Love R, Barber TC, Funahashi TT, Inacio MCS: Kaiser Permanente implant registries benefit patient safety, quality improvement, cost-effectiveness. *Jt Comm J Qual Patient Saf* 2013;39(6):246-252.

45. Charney M, Paxton EW, Stradiotto R, et al: A comparison of risk of dislocation and cause-specific revision between direct anterior and posterior approach following elective cementless total hip arthroplasty. *J Arthroplasty* 2020;35(6):1651-1657.

46. Gundtoft PH, Pedersen AB, Schønheyder HC, Overgaard S: Validation of the diagnosis 'prosthetic joint infection' in the Danish hip arthroplasty register. *Bone Joint J* 2016;98-B(3):320-325.

47. Berry DJ, Lewallen DG, Haddad FS: National joint registries, in Mont MA, Tanzer M, eds: *Orthopaedic Knowledge Update®: Hip and Knee Reconstruction*, ed 6. American Academy of Orthopaedic Surgeons, 2022, pp 109-115.

48. Etkin CD, Lau EC, Watson HN, et al: What are the migration patterns for U.S. primary total joint arthroplasty patients? *Clin Orthop Relat Res* 2019;477(6):1424-1431.

49. Gomes LSM, Roos MV, Takata ET, et al: Advantages and limitations of national arthroplasty registries. The need for multicenter registries: The Rempro-SBQ. *Rev Bras Ortop* 2017;52(suppl 1):3-13.

50. Fu S, Wyles CC, Osmon DR, et al: Automated detection of periprosthetic joint infections and data elements using natural language processing. *J Arthroplasty* 2021;36(2):688-692.

51. Sagheb E, Ramazanian T, Tafti AP, et al: Use of natural language processing algorithms to identify common data elements in operative notes for knee arthroplasty. *J Arthroplasty* 2021;36(3):922-926 .

52. Squitieri L, Bozic KJ, Pusic AL: The role of patient-reported outcome measures in value-based payment reform. *Value Health* 2017;20(6):834-836.

53. Bhatt DL, Drozda JP, Shahian DM, et al: ACC/AHA/STS statement on the future of registries and the performance measurement enterprise: A report of the American College of Cardiology/American Heart Association Task Force on Performance Measures and The Society of Thoracic Surgeons. *J Am Coll Cardiol* 2015;66(20):2230-2245.

Employing Standardized Clinical Care Pathways to Improve Health Outcomes and Lower Costs

Prakash Jayakumar, MD, PhD • Eugenia Lin, MD
Kenoma Anighoro, MD, MBA
Karl Koenig, MD, MS, FAAOS

INTRODUCTION

Standardized care pathways in orthopaedic surgery offer a pragmatic, evidence-based strategy for operationalizing high-value, integrated care for a range of musculoskeletal problems while reducing unwarranted variation and waste, improving outcomes, and lowering costs. This chapter defines and explores concepts behind standardized clinical pathways (SCPs), tools and technologies enabling SCPs, and the evidence to date for SCPs in orthopaedic practice.

BACKGROUND

The transformation of practice and payment models in the United States from volume to value-based health care – defined as care improving health outcomes benefiting patients relative to cost – has been stimulated by an escalation in health care spending (from 7% gross domestic product in 1970 to 17% in 2019[1]) without a commensurate improvement in population health outcomes.[2] Underlying this health care paradox is unwarranted variation, inequity, and poor access to evidence-based treatments and preventive and supportive care, patient harm, and waste.[3,4] Unwarranted variation – the variation in utilization of services that cannot be explained by variations in a patient's condition or preferences – is reflected in widely varying outcomes of care. Inequity and poor access derive from underutilization of evidence-based interventions, especially

Dr. Koenig or an immediate family member serves as a paid consultant to or is an employee of Surgical Directions. None of the following authors or any immediate family member has received anything of value from or has stock or stock options held in a commercial company or institution related directly or indirectly to the subject of this chapter: Dr. Jayakumar, Dr. Lin, and Dr. Anighoro.

for the underserved, the vulnerable, and people of color. Harm relates to under-treatment as well as inappropriate diagnosis, overtreatment, and medical error; and waste involves any factor not enhancing patient outcomes or resources that could provide greater value if applied to another population.[4] To date, payers, clinicians, and policymakers in US health care have used various strategies to overcome these challenges including cost containment, capitation, prior authorization of expensive services, introducing penalties, intensifying resources, and implementing new technologies. Although these efforts offer variable levels of benefit, they often fail to achieve better value for patients, tackle the inappropriate utilization of treatments and low-value interventions, or equitably distribute resources across the wider system. This is mostly because such strategies are applied to the existing health care delivery system without an emphasis on fundamentally changing the structure. Although challenging, these problems also spark opportunities to deliver greater value through improvement in the systems and processes involved in health care delivery.

Advances in the science of process improvement within complex systems have revolutionized the business sector and manufacturing industry.[5] The application of "systems thinking" uses a holistic approach that focuses on the dynamic interplay between the components of various processes within a system to drive function, the changes in system function over time, and their effects on the wider system. This approach has elevated performance in a variety of fields.[6,7] Further, it has been identified that more variation within a system leads to more waste, impeding the ability to consistently deliver better results. Such insights have prompted initiatives to reduce variation and increase standardization.[5] Simply put, if it is assumed that every system and its processes are intentionally and optimally designed to achieve the results they get, then to improve results, the system and its underlying processes need to be changed. But how does this relate to high-value orthopaedic care?

Concepts of systems thinking and the science of process improvement have been incorporated within the field of health care quality improvement.[8] A series of landmark reports in the 1990s and early 2000s, with findings such as 44,000 to 98,000 deaths occurring annually due to medical errors, brought patient safety and systems improvement to the forefront.[9-11] When designing optimal systems, there is a need to differentiate between normal and "special cause" (or unwarranted) variation as a way to eliminate waste, mitigate harm, and achieve improved quality, outcomes, and lower costs. Orthopaedic surgery has a strong legacy in standardizing care practices, in part due to the high prevalence of conditions that often have an assortment of viable treatment options.[12,13] From prophylactic antibiotics prior to total joint arthroplasty (TJA), to enhanced perioperative management of fragility fractures, the field is a rich source of processes and services that can be redesigned, tested, and standardized for improvement.[14]

The readiness to adopt standardized care pathways and practices has been mixed among stakeholders in health care and orthopaedics who may view such efforts as precursors of so-called cookbook or cookie-cutter medicine, where there may be a perceived loss of clinician autonomy, opportunity to exercise professional judgement, and ability to provide individualized, patient-centered care.[15,16] Instead, standardization can function as a vehicle for delivering high-value care for patients through system and process improvements. Systemization of repetitive and broadly applicable tasks and interventions allows the measured application of best evidence and practices to create a standardized pathway that can be tweaked or adjusted to the individual, when necessary, without losing the effectiveness of reproducibility. Although each patient is indeed unique, there are sufficient commonalities and evidence-based, best practices that should be standardized in order to more predictably achieve better outcomes and lower costs.[17,18] This chapter defines and explores concepts behind standardized clinical pathways (SCPs), tools and technologies enabling SCPs, and the evidence to date for SCPs in orthopaedic practice.

STANDARDIZED CLINICAL PATHWAYS
Definition

SCPs (a term used interchangeably with standardized clinical care pathways, evidence-based care pathways, critical pathways, diagnostic therapeutic pathways, integrated care pathways) can be defined as standardized, multidisciplinary, multifaceted care pathways that incorporate evidence-based guidelines and best practices to improve health care quality, outcomes, and costs for patients.[19] An operational definition has also been developed involving four key criteria: (1) structured multidisciplinary plans of care; (2) translation of guidelines or evidence into local structures; (3) detailing of steps in a course of treatment or care within a plan, pathway, algorithm, guideline, or protocol; and (4) standardization for a specific population.[19]

The Concept of Integration

SCPs within complex systems invariably require different levels of care integration.[4,20-22] Integrated care is defined as coordinated care across professionals, facilities, and support systems that is continuous over time and between visits, tailored to patients' needs and preferences and based on shared responsibility between patients and caregivers while systematically measuring outcomes.[22,23] Singer et al[21,23] classified integration into structural, functional, normative, interpersonal, and process integration, which dynamically interacts with contextual factors to affect quality, efficiency, and patient outcomes and experiences (**Figure 1**). Integrated care delivery has also been described as horizontal integration and vertical integration.[24,25] Horizontal integration describes the integration of organizations that provide similar services, such as single specialty group practices, multispecialty group practices, virtual physician networks, independent practice associations, or multihospital systems. Vertical integration describes the integration of organizations offering differing levels of care, services, or functions such as hospital ownership of physician practices, physician-hospital organizations, management services, clinically integrated networks, foundation models, and financially integrated healthcare organizations. Vertically integrated systems make the clinical case for taking complete clinical and

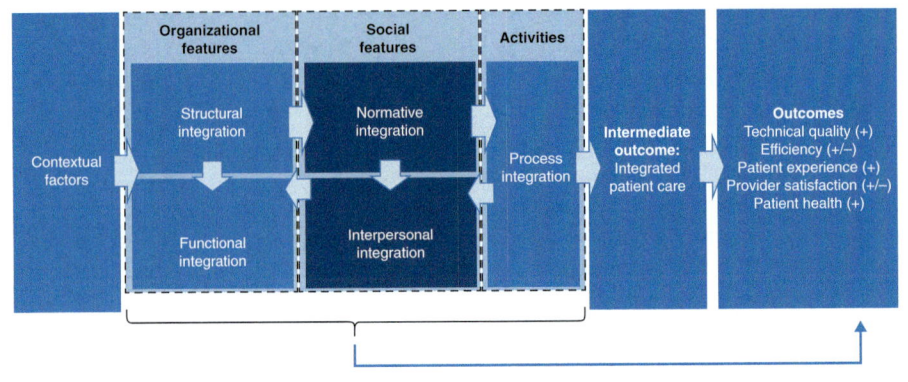

FIGURE 1 A conceptual model of types of integration in health care. Structural integration relates to physical, operational, financial aspects of integration among teams and organizations. Functional integration relates to policies and protocols for enhancing care coordination and decision-making. Normative integration involves culture and the appetite to prioritize integrated patient care across the organization or organizations. Interpersonal integration relates to teamwork among health care professionals from different disciplines and their relationships with patients and caregivers. Process integration represents organizational actions intended to integrate patient care into a single coordinated process across people and units. Organizational features reflect the setup of structures and systems. Activity elements relate to different actions and activities involved in care delivery. Social features involve the experience of integrated care by patients and family members. (Reproduced with permission from Singer SJ, Kerrissey M, Friedberg M, Phillips R: A comprehensive theory of integration. *Med Care Res Rev* 2020;77[2]:196-207.)

financial responsibility for the whole patient while improving patient outcomes and experiences. These systems also make an economic case through economies of scale, broadening patient coverage while simultaneously consolidating delivery and administrative processes (reducing duplication), thereby lowering health care costs resulting from process duplication between organizations.[26] Whichever form of integration, SCPs may offer more effective payer and clinician access to health data, analytics to guide management, coordination, and individualized clinical and administrative consumer experiences.[27] They also serve to bolster the bottom line around meaningful, real-time communication among different clinicians – a feature that must be incentivized, facilitated, and maintained in order to deliver high-value care.

QUALITY IMPROVEMENT

Quality improvement is a framework for systematically improving care delivery to patients through a continuous and cyclical process in order to achieve predictable and sustainable results.[8,28] The landmark article by Donabedian describes the triad of structure, process, and outcome to evaluate the quality of health care alongside seven pillars of quality that aim to inform efforts to improve care.[29] Further, the Model for Improvement framework, developed by the Associates in Process Improvement, provides a powerful tool to accelerate selection, testing, and implementation of changes for improvement[5,8,28] (**Figure 2**). Three core questions are posed prior to testing involving improvement teams (discussed in the next paragraphs). Teams executing improvement projects should include members representing three areas of expertise: clinical system leadership, technical expertise, and day-to-day leadership. Clinical system leadership ensures sufficient authority to support development, testing, implementation, and maintenance of the change. Clinical leaders should anticipate implications and effect on the wider system. Technical expertise affords guidance on what to measure and how to measure using effective tools, data collection, synthesis, and visualization. Technical experts will have a deep understanding of the subject, intended change or intervention, and process(es) involved, with support from implementation scientists and improvement experts as needed. Day-to-day leadership drives the project, ensures adherence to the project plan, implements the changes and tests, and monitors the captured data while maintaining close contact with the clinical champions. The day-to-day leader also needs to have a strong understanding of the system, and how changes can trigger effects in other parts of the system. The working members of the improvement team should also work with a project sponsor – a person or group with executive authority that has access to enterprise-level management, other parts of the network, or strategies to overcome barriers, while maintaining accountability and the overarching goal.

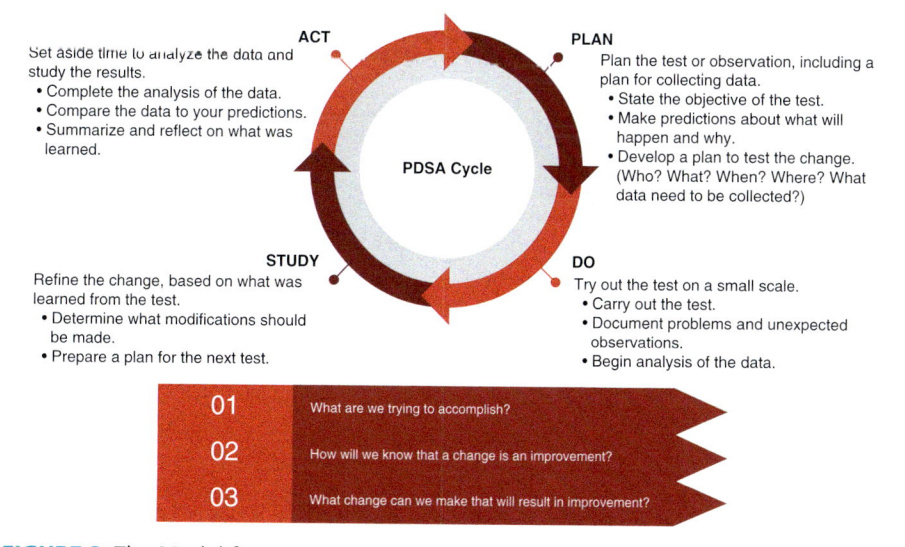

FIGURE 2 The Model for Improvement.

Question 1 (Setting Aims): "What Are You Going to Improve, by How Much, Over What Time, and for Whom?"

The 2001 report, Crossing the Quality Chasm: A New Health System for the 21st Century,[11] outlined six aims for improvement for healthcare systems that continue to form the basis of quality improvement: safety (avoiding injury from care intended to help patients); effectiveness (aligning care with science and avoiding overuse of ineffective care or underuse of effective care); patient-centeredness (respecting patient choices, preferences, values, and needs); timeliness (reducing wait times for patients, caregivers, and clinicians); efficiency (reducing waste); and equity (reducing variation and closing racial and ethnic gaps in health status). Aims can be developed using the SMART criteria (ie, aims that are Specific, Measurable, Achievable, Realistic, Timebound). This question relates to affected patient populations as well as systems.

Question 2 (Choosing Measures): "How Will You Know If Change Is An Improvement?"

Measurement is integral to quality improvement. This question helps define whether initiatives are on track to improve the system via reliable, user-friendly measures.[8,28] Measures for improvement include outcome, process, and balancing measures. Outcome measures reflect how the system affects the patient as well as other health care stakeholders. Process measures relate to the effect on processes or systems behind the aim. Balance measures view the whole system and whether change designed to improve one or more parts of the system triggers unintended consequences elsewhere in the system. Although there are several commonalities between measurement for learning and improvement compared to measurement for research, improvement measures differ in terms of purpose (ie, knowledge to drive daily practice), process (ie, iterative testing with multiple sequential and observable tests), and practicality (ie, controlling biases from test to test and gathering just enough information to swiftly complete test cycles).

Question 3 (Selecting Changes): "What Changes Can You Make That Will Lead to An Improvement?"

Changes leading to improvement relevant to patients, health care professionals, or administrators usually relate to one or more change concepts—approaches that can develop ideas (both creatively and through application of knowledge and evidence) to inform testable interventions.[8]

The elimination of waste concept is defined as the removal of non-value--adding activities within organizations. Orthopaedic practices may draw upon the seven wastes exemplified by the Toyota production system in improving their processes and systems: waste of overproduction, waiting, transportation, processing (redundancy), inventory, motion, and production of defective parts or products.[30] The workflow improvement concept relates to targeting workflow planning and process components that can lead to better pathways, products, and services. Changes involving the optimization of inventory require a comprehensive understanding of relevant inventory, associated capital investment, storage, handling, tracking, access, and maintenance before reducing any surplus to minimize waste. Concepts examining change in the working environment may identify real-world opportunities to develop, test, support, and implement changes more effectively. Change concepts improving the producer/customer interface can enable stakeholders to better understand customer needs and expectations before reaping the benefits of products and services. Although many ideas for improvement can come from suppliers (ie, medical device companies, recruitment agencies), customers (ie, patients, surgeons) often provide the most valuable input. Time management concepts offer opportunities to focus on aspects such as reduction in wait times for services, cycle times for various functions and assets, lead time for obtaining supplies and deliveries, and development time for new products. Enhancing this change concept can provide a competitive advantage for practices. Reducing variation is a critical change concept that fosters improvement through increasing the predictability of quality, outcomes, and costs, related to processes and products. Strategies for handling variations often center on evidence and best practices. Error reduction is an important change concept that recognizes factors causing uncertainty within real-world settings (such as human error through handling of multiple tasks sequentially, simultaneously and/or rapidly in clinical situations). Human error is frequently associated with an individual; however, errors often trace back to failures within the system. The number of opportunities to make errors within a system combined with the probability of making an error culminate in a total error frequency. System redesign and implementing specific changes can reduce the probability of individuals making an error for a given opportunity (known as error proofing). Strategies for error proofing include reducing the number of steps within a process, incorporating safety champions and adverse event response teams, instituting periodic safety briefings and safety reporting, integrating technology to automate repetitive tasks, and implementing checks to limit errors from actions performed almost subconsciously within pathways. Finally, focusing on products and services can promote change for improvement beyond targeting processes alone. The three key questions from the Model for Improvement framework are illustrated in the context of various orthopaedic practice scenarios (**Figure 3**).

PLAN-DO-STUDY-ACT CYCLE

Plan-Do-Study-Act (PDSA) cycles help test change in real-world settings once team members are defined and the aims, measures, and change concepts are established. PDSA frameworks provide a cyclical, iterative, and action-oriented approach to planning, implementing, studying, learning, and acting on changes (**Figure 2**). "Plan" denotes plans for testing, observation, and data collection; "Do" reflects executing the test at a smaller scale while recording issues and commencing data analysis; "Study" focuses on data analysis and synthesis of results; and "Act" pertains to refinement of changes, defining modifications, assimilating learnings from the test, and preparing for the next test. The team and organization conducting the project then decides whether the change is an improvement, and to adapt, adopt, or abandon the change. After testing, learning, refining, and implementing changes at a smaller scale through several PDSA cycles, the organization

Setting	Context	Aim	Measures	Change Concept(s)	Team
Trauma Inpatient	Fragility fracture management	To ensure that elderly patients receive timely access to medical and surgical care by decreasing transfer time from emergency department to an inpatient bed within 1 hr of admission decision full medical review within 2 hours; and surgery within 48 hours as indicated, tracked over 3 months	% patients meeting transfer time target; % patients meeting medical review time target; % patients meeting time to surgery target; Other – inpatient length of stay; immediate postoperative complications / complication rates.	Workflow improvement; Improving patient interface; Time management; Reducing variation	Clinical leader(s): Internal medicine, orthopaedic surgeon, anesthetist; Technical expert(s): nurse manager or coordinator; Day-to-day leader: Clinical nurse specialist; Other: Elderly care team, dietitians, physical therapist, anesthetist (pain management)
Elective outpatient	Osteoarthritis management	To improve outpatient care pathway for hip and knee osteoarthritis by decreasing wait time by 7.5% and improving number of patients on structured exercise program by 10% over 6 months	% patients meeting wait time target; % patients meetings exercise program enrollment target; patient-reported outcome measures; numeric rating scale-satisfaction	Time management; Improving the patient interface; Workflow improvement	Clinical leader(s): Orthopaedic surgeons, senior physical therapist; Technical expert(s): Administrator with Lean /Six Sigma experience; Day-to-day leader: Clinic nurse manager, medical assistants; Other: Physical therapy and orthopedic clinic coordinators, operations manager
Elective inpatient	Postoperative elective surgery protocol	To reduce high-hazard adverse drug events from over-sedation by narcotics and benzodiazepines by 65% within 3 months. To attain over 95% adherence to new drug	Adverse drug events per 1000 doses record review; % adherence to new checklist medication reconciliation measure	Error reduction / error proofing; Improving the clinician interface	Clinical leader(s): Anesthetist, orthopaedic surgeons, PACU nurse manager; Technical expert(s): Clinical pharmacist, patient safety team; Day-to-day leader: Orthopaedic nursing team; Other: Pharmacy technicians, medical assistants

FIGURE 3 The model for improvement applied to various orthopaedic practice scenarios.

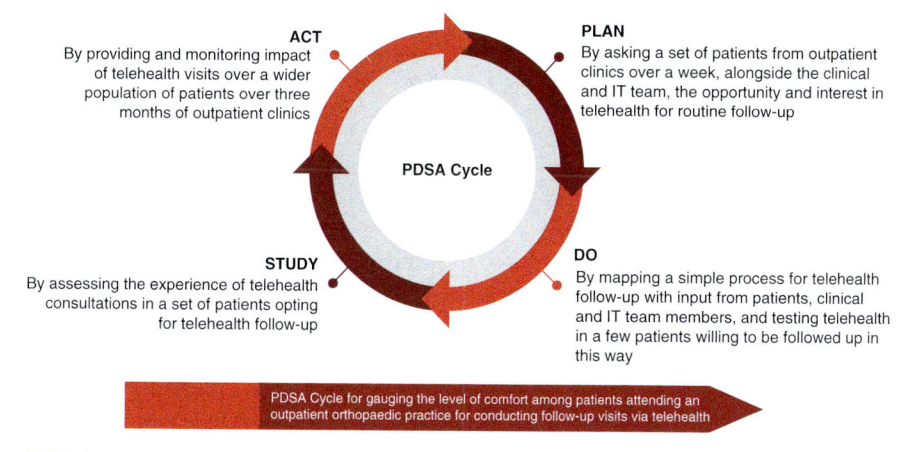

FIGURE 4 A PDSA cycle for gauging the level of comfort among patients attending an outpatient orthopaedic practice for conducting follow-up visits via telehealth.

may then choose to implement changes at scale. A PDSA cycle is illustrated in the context of applying a telehealth service within an orthopaedic practice (**Figure 4**).

Following cycles of testing, learning, and refining changes at a relatively small scale, the change may be ready for wider implementation and spread. Spread is defined as the process of taking effective implementation processes from a pilot population and replicating the change or changes in other areas of the organization or organizational network at a local, regional, or national level. Scaling for an orthopaedic practice may require further adaptations to optimize infrastructure, sequences of tasks, and processes, resources, hiring policies, training, and financial renumeration. A range of techniques including Lean, Six Sigma, and Total Quality Management offer approaches to quality improvement and development of optimal care pathways. Regardless of which techniques are adopted, working rapidly, learning iteratively, and adhering to a systematic process of quality improvement offers the best chances of success.

TOOLS AND TECHNOLOGIES FOR ENABLING SCPs

A variety of quality and process improvement tools and technologies can help enable SCPs in orthopaedic practices. These tools and technologies can be applied to specific phases of the care pathway, to the whole pathway, or to the system in its entirety.[12] Assets can be characterized at the patient, physician, and systems level and orthopaedic surgeons should leverage tools at each level in quality improvement efforts and SCP development.[31,32] Many of these tools and technologies are discussed elsewhere in this book.

Patient-Facing Tools

Tools enabling the capture of patient-generated health data, defined as health-related data created, recorded, and gathered from patients (or caregivers) to help establish a patient's health status, are integral to value-based care and SCPs.[33,34]

Patient-Reported Outcome Measures/Patient-Reported Experience Measures

Patient-reported outcome measures (PROMs) are validated measures of capability, mindset, and circumstances, reported by the patient, enabling quantification of the effect of medical interventions from the patient's perspective.[32,35] Similarly, patient-reported experience measures (PREMs) are subjective measures of patient experiences of healthcare systems ranging from measures of satisfaction with various structural and functional aspects of health care, such as waiting times, access to facilities, and ability to navigate services, to the quality of communication and relationships with health care professionals and teams.[34,36,37] Both PROMs and PREMs have made a shift from research settings to clinical practice and policy making as indicators of patient-centered performance improvement. PROMs, for instance, are fast becoming standardized performance measures, administered at designated time points with an established risk-adjusted scoring methodology.[38] Such tools will play an increasing role in reimbursement as health care shifts from volume-driven care toward outcomes and value-based care. Because reducing variation remains integral to this transformation, longitudinal data generated by PROMs can be a useful component in tracking, monitoring, and decision support within SCPs.[35] Several general health-specific and condition-specific PROMs have been applied across orthopaedic practices, most commonly to measure symptoms and functional outcomes before and after surgical interventions.[39] Professional societies such as the American Academy of Orthopaedic Surgeons (AAOS) and International Consortium for Health Outcome Measurement have compiled standardized outcome measures and measurement sets including PROMs for clinical application.[40,41] National payers such as the Centers for Medicare & Medicaid Services incentivize PROMs collection through standardized processes of quality reporting and bonus payment initiatives.[42] Further, the Consumer Assessment of Healthcare Providers and Systems provide a suite of PREMs developed by the Agency for Healthcare Research and Quality, rating key areas of patient experience related to structural, functional, and interpersonal aspects of care delivery.

Shared Decision Making-Related Outcome Measures and Patient Decision Aids

Shared decision-making (SDM) is a concept that empowers patients to become active participants in developing management plans and selecting appropriate treatments for their condition with clinical teams.[43,44] In SDM, informed treatment decisions, aligned with a patient's preferences, needs and values, are made through expert communication and high-quality patient education. SDM may be incorporated into SCPs to improve patient satisfaction, decision quality, patient outcomes, and appropriate utilization of health care resources. Shared decision making-related outcome measures can be utilized as part of an orthopaedic service's SDM initiative alongside decision aids. In a manner similar to PROMs, shared decision making-related outcome measures provide a measure of the patient's perspective in relation to various elements of the decision-making process, from decision quality, level of collaboration during SDM, preparing for decision making, and decisional conflict, to decision support and satisfaction with the clinical consultation. Patient decision aids (PDAs) are tools designed to facilitate SDM by helping patients better understand evidence-based information, the potential benefits and harms of various treatments, and facilitate communication between patients and clinicians.[45-47] Importantly, these tools are distinct from patient education materials in that they more actively direct patients toward making an informed choice, aligned with their preferences, between multiple treatment options. In orthopaedic practice, PDAs have been studied most frequently in persistently painful preference sensitive conditions (ie, where multiple valid treatment options exist) such as degenerative disease of the spine and osteoarthritis (OA) of the hip and knee.[47-49] Decision aids take multiple forms, including written booklets, videos, and interactive digital tools, provided to patients before, during, or after encounters with orthopaedic surgeons. PDAs may also be effective in empowering patients to make informed decisions at a given point in time as well as providing ongoing guidance along different phases of a care pathway. Payers, clinicians, and policymakers are increasingly encouraging the standardization of these value-adding tools in orthopaedic practice.[43,44,50] Tools and checklists for the development and application of PDAs are also provided by the International Patient Decision Aid Standards initiative.[51]

Physician-Facing Tools

Physician-facing tools enabling clinical decision support provide timely and relevant person-specific information to inform clinically oriented decisions that can also improve efficiency, utilization, quality, outcomes and costs of care.[52,53] Such tools can be divided into clinical risk assessment tools, web-based orthopaedic personalized predictive tools, standardized clinical checklists, clinical practice guidelines (CPGs), and standardized clinical assessment and management plans (SCAMPs).

Clinical risk assessment tools provide validated metrics that can be utilized by surgeons to better assess the risks associated with a given treatment option. In orthopaedic practice, clinical risk assessment tools such as the Risk Assessment and Predictor Tool, predict length of stay and discharge destination following total joint arthroplasty.[54] This function assists patients, clinicians, administrators, and caregivers in taking necessary clinical actions (eg, preparing patient charts and orders), nonclinical actions (eg, preparing for an overnight stay), and allocating resources more effectively. Similar risk assessment tools have been developed for frail, elderly patients with hip fractures to predict postoperative morbidity and mortality.[55]

Web-based orthopaedic personalized predictive tools provide personalized predictions of clinical outcomes based on the analysis of large volumes of data utilizing algorithmic mathematical modeling and predictive analytics.[54,56-59] A recent study identified 31 discrete web-based orthopaedic personalized predictive tools designed to provide personalized prediction in various orthopaedic specialties including trauma and fracture management, spinal surgery, total joint arthroplasty, and musculoskeletal oncology.[60]

Standardized Checklists

Standardized clinical checklists in health care and orthopaedics, analogous to those routinely used in the aviation industry, have now become widely adopted.[61] The World Health Organization Surgical Safety Checklist, since its introduction in 2008, has transformed perioperative patient safety in surgical care.[61] Although this checklist is primarily designed to increase safety awareness and reduce perioperative medical error, it also enhances team communication and consistent execution of procedural steps along the surgical care pathway.[62] The AAOS has developed multiple checklists through their appropriate use criteria initiative, which uses a modified Delphi method to create standardized tools, such as a preoperative checklist to facilitate hip fracture management in elderly patients.[63] Further, in a move to address the social determinants of health and social unmet needs, a set of checklists and screening tools have also been developed, including the Protocol for Responding to and Assessing Patients' Assets, Risks, and Experiences, developed by the National Association of Community Health Centers,[64] and the Accountable Health Communities Health-Related Social Needs Screening Tool developed by Centers for Medicare & Medicaid Services.[65]

CPGs and SCAMPs

CPGs are statements developed by the systematic distillation of high-quality evidence into clinical recommendations to support decision making around specific clinical scenarios.[66] SCAMPs are clinician-driven tools, created by multidisciplinary teams, based on iterative and evolving analyses of internally collected data, emerging evidence, best practices, and sound expert opinion when evidence is limited. CPGs are centered on the best available evidence at a point in time and are less frequently updated compared to SCAMPs. Although CPGs provide a more rigid tool where adherence is key and deviations from guidelines are generally discouraged, their design costs are relatively low and adoption less labor intensive. In contrast, SCAMPs are dynamic entities designed around decision tree frameworks where deviations from the care pathway based on a physician's clinical acumen is encouraged at any stage.[67,68] This flexibility assumes higher design and implementation costs and tends to be more labor intensive.

Both CPGs and SCAMPs can help reduce practice pattern variations, optimize resource utilization, reduce costs, and improve patient health outcomes.[69-71] Professional societies such as the AAOS and American College of Chest Physicians have developed numerous CPGs spanning a range of conditions and interventions[69] from venous thromboembolism and antibiotic prophylaxis, to the prevention of surgical site infections.[66] However, CPGs have also met with some resistance and disengagement from clinicians due to their rigid dependence on the strength of supporting evidence, the need for repeated updates every few years, and questions around their usability in more diverse patient populations.[69,72] In contrast, SCAMPs may serve as a more effective and continuous process improvement tool capable of targeting diverse populations and complex clinical scenarios, as long as resources are sufficient and there is adequate buy-in from the wider healthcare organization alongside any payers or regulatory agencies with a stake in the system.[16,71]

System-Level Tools

Electronic Medical Records and Data Analytic Engines

Robust, interoperable, and user-friendly electronic medical records (EMRs) are foundational tools for SCPs that enable advanced administrative and management capabilities, improved learning, and reduction in variation and waste within health systems. EMRs can also standardize care and provide a more holistic, longitudinal view of patients while improving coordination and continuity of care within multidisciplinary teams. The functions of these platforms now extend beyond basic repositories of health information, toward the administration and collection of detailed clinical metrics, patient outcomes, and other forms of data including social determinants of health. EMRs should ideally be supported by a strong data analytics engine, advanced enterprise-level data warehouse, and/or cloud systems. This will often serve as a foundational asset for most orthopaedic practices and quality improvement projects.

Patient Portals

Patient portals facilitating patient education, enabling channels for communication, and continuity of care may be part of the EMR or stand-alone, enhancing patient engagement in the care delivery process. Such portals are usually secure websites that allow patients to access personal health information online using a secure username and password.[73,74] These platforms can facilitate patient-centered SCPs and quality improvement projects by providing patients with open access to a standardized set of records related to visits, medication lists, and laboratory results, as well as a secure means of communication with clinicians to request prescription refills, ask questions about their care, and schedule appointments.

Outcome Measurement Platforms

Myriad commercial and research-grade patient outcome measurement platforms exist, enabling electronic capture of PROMs and other forms of patient-generated health data. Digitization enables functionalities (eg, data visualization and analysis) and efficiencies (eg, time saving, automation). Most electronic PROM platforms support remote delivery, allowing patients to complete questionnaires by text, email, smartphone, tablet, or their desktop computers at home.[75] In addition, these electronic platforms offer integration into EMRs, enabling the review of information in real time with patients and team members.[39]

Clinical Registries

Local, regional, and national clinical registries and databases capturing various clinical, process, and patient-level metrics may support efforts to standardize aspects of orthopaedic practices and networks.[76] Several registries have been developed in the United States since the Mayo Clinic Total Joint Arthroplasty (TJA) registry in 1969, ranging from those at a regional level, such as the Michigan

---

Arthroplasty Registry Collaborative Quality Initiative, to national initiatives including the Function and Outcomes Research for Comparative Effectiveness in Total Joint Replacement registry and the AAOS/American Joint Replacement Registry.[77-80] These registries variably capture PROMs alongside clinical outcomes, including readmission rates, complications, and implant survivorship.[39] Other registries, including those sponsored by industry, capture data around medical devices, enabling surveillance for safety and performance.[81] The big data housed within many registries offers a powerful source of information for generating substantial clinical insights as well as opportunities for advanced decision support.[77,82,83] The UK National Hip Fracture Database provides evidence to drive SCPs, influencing the development of CPGs to influence the standardized management of these common injuries.[76] The UK National Joint Registry has been utilized extensively for benchmarking, reporting TJA performance in a standardized fashion, and has more recently been used to develop a patient-facing decision support tool for those considering TJA.[84]

SCPs in Orthopaedic Practice

Significant variation in orthopaedic practice patterns have resulted in escalating costs without necessarily achieving a corresponding improvement in patient or clinical outcomes, patient experiences, or patient safety.[72] Those developing SCPs to confront this issue should have a robust understanding around the level of complexity involved in pathways and processes, organizational capacity to implement the SCP and change, and ways to maintain improvement, instead of reverting back to quick fixes such as cost containment without regard to patient outcomes or maximizing value.[17,85] Numerous SCPs have been implemented in orthopaedics to date, targeting improvement across a variety of metrics.[14,86] Systematic reviews examining the implementation of SCPs show that most trials and improvement efforts focus on lowering postoperative length of stay, complications, and costs; improving processes such as clinical documentation; improving adherence to evidence-based guidelines; or exceeding quality and safety benchmarks.[87,88] Orthopaedic practices could also learn from the experiences of other specialties in implementing SCPs. For instance, considerable advances have been made in oncology around multidisciplinary team-based SCPs providing standardized care and utilization of novel pharmaceutical and biologic therapies.[89]

EFFECT OF SCPs FOR MUSCULOSKELETAL CARE IN GENERAL

Systematic reviews and meta-analyses have highlighted the variability and non-linear nature of musculoskeletal care pathways for various conditions, including the management of hip and knee pain.[90] This signals the need for a systems approach to process improvement and standardization, with increased development and access to SCPs, particularly those delivering 360° whole-person care. Although most musculoskeletal SCPs target the surgical pathway, there remain a few important examples that focus on primary care, prevention, and nonsurgical management.[91-93]

Quality improvement involving the primary care of musculoskeletal conditions has focused on quality of triage, referral management processes, and bolstering primary care provider education.[91,94] A multifaceted intervention based on Cochrane reviews involving musculoskeletal educational programs for general practitioners, alongside locally agreed-on clinical pathways, increased transparency and feedback around referral rates, and improved clinical audit and peer review.[91] Underpinned by quality improvement and behavioral change theories, the intervention observed improved quality in referral letter content and pathway adherence, reduced variability in referral rates, higher patient ratings of how well general practitioners explained musculoskeletal conditions, and increased patient satisfaction with the appointment in general.[91]

Comprehensive management of osteoarthritis (OA) in the form of an OA physical activity care pathway has been developed to support patients with OA of the hip and knee.[92] Individuals reporting less than 150 minutes per week of moderate-to-vigorous physical activity at baseline were recruited from primary care clinics and underwent a 3-month OA physical activity care pathway intervention. This included three physical activity goal-setting coaching calls, three check-in emails, and links made to community-based and online physical activity resources (**Figure 5**). The pathway demonstrated improvements in time spent performing physical activities per week (assessed using an accelerometer), PROMs (measured using the Western Ontario and McMaster Universities Arthritis Index), and satisfaction after 4 months.[92] Findings were fed back into modifying the pathway, enhancing patient self-monitoring processes, and generating further impact through positive behavioral change around physical activity.

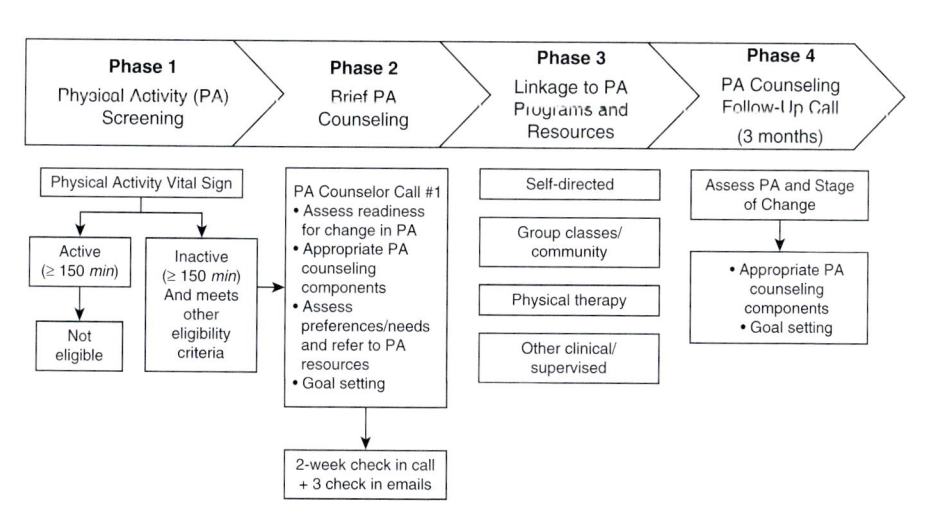

FIGURE 5 Osteoarthritis physical activity care pathway. (Reproduced with permission from Allen K, Vu MB, Callahan LF, et al: Osteoarthritis physical activity care pathway (OA-PCP): Results of a feasibility trial. *BMC Musculoskelet Disord* 2020;21[1]:308.)

SCPs have been developed in primary care management of low back pain using a stratified approach involving best-practice pathways and prognostic screening.[95] The STarT Back program has shown, in randomized controlled trials, both clinical effectiveness with improved disability at 12 months (Roland-Morris Disability Questionnaire) and cost-effectiveness in terms of incremental quality-adjusted life years (QALYs) compared to nonstratified current best practices.[95] SCPs have also been developed in the management of common soft-tissue conditions that can be challenging when there are limited evidence-based treatment options and often longer and more protracted courses of rehabilitation.[93] A standardized, therapist-led Achilles tendon pathway for Achilles tendinopathy, developed and implemented using elements of the Model of Improvement framework and a series of PDSA cycles, showed improvement in patient satisfaction, reduced variation and duplication of treatments, investigations, and consultations, with lower costs.[93]

EFFECT OF SCPs FOR ORTHOPAEDIC SURGICAL CARE

An array of SCPs have been developed in orthopaedic surgery, mostly focused on primary TJA for hip and knee OA – two of the most commonly performed elective surgical procedures.[14,96] There has been growing national interest in improving value and appropriate utilization of total hip and total knee arthroplasty (THA and TKA), with almost 1.3 million THAs and TKAs performed in the United States in 2014 and total hospital costs exceeding $20 billion.[97] TJA has a strong track record in benefiting individuals with advanced hip or knee OA and consistently demonstrates improvements in symptom intensity, level of incapability, and quality of life.[98-100] However, the escalation and variation in utilization of TJA surgery, outcomes (eg, complications, utilization, PROMs), adherence to evidence-based processes (eg, surgical times, length of stay, discharge disposition, and post-acute care) and costs (risk-adjusted episode payments) across the United States has caused concern.[101,102] Further, the rise in revision surgery adds to this burden. Van Citters et al[14] describe a staged process for developing multidisciplinary SCPs that aim to deliver high-value, patient-centered care for those undergoing TJA. In a process involving clinical leaders from high-performing institutions (eg, those with lower inpatient costs, 30-day readmissions, shorter length of stay, improved adherence to quality metrics), and experts in patient safety, patient experience, and improvement science, the investigators applied a combination of quantitative and qualitative methods to design a care pathway extending from presurgical office visits to 12 months post-discharge. Multiple change opportunities were identified, from ways to enhance communication, collaboration, and team and patient engagement, to standardizing care protocols and information flows. A range of SCPs have now been developed to improve the preoperative, perioperative, and postoperative TJA care pathway.[103-106] These include various forms of fast-track, rapid recovery, rapid mobilization, outpatient surgery, and enhanced recovery after surgery protocols. Meta-analysis evaluating SCPs in THA and TKA demonstrate such pathways invariably achieve shorter lengths of stay and fewer complications.[96] These pathways include various combinations of standardized patient selection criteria, preoperative medical risk assessment, testing, and optimization, patient and clinician education and engagement, expectation management and goal setting, multidisciplinary team-based coordination (including role setting, timing of surgeries, operating room on-time starts and utilization, preprinted care plans), opioid-sparing analgesia and multimodal pain management, standardized anesthetic and surgical techniques, standardized postoperative management (catheterization, venous thromboembolism and antibiotic prophylaxis, blood management and fluid resuscitation protocols), accelerated mobilization (including postoperative day 0 mobilization and multiple day inpatient physical therapy sessions), early postdischarge planning, home assessment, and optimization of home self-care over postacute care utilization.[107-111] Large database studies exploring optimal use of process standards (eg, adherence to venous thromboembolism and antibiotic prophylaxis) serve as important predictors of clinical and process level outcomes over surgical volume alone.[112,113]

SCPs in TJA have demonstrated significant reductions in length of stay,[106-111,114-122] earlier mobilization,[109] improved functional outcomes,[123] less pain and confusion,[109,115] reduced postsurgical use of opiates,[120,124] increased rates of discharge directly home over post-acute care facilities (ie, skilled nursing facilities, or inpatient rehabilitation facilities),[121,122,124] reduced total costs of perioperative and postoperative care[105,108-110,112,113,122] without an increase in readmissions or overall complications,[107-110,114-116,120-122,124] improved patient satisfaction,[116,121,124] and greater ease in performing physical therapy during rehabilitation.[115] Such findings have been demonstrated in a range of patient populations including those managed via Veterans Health Administration facilities[115] and those under Medicare or Medicaid insurance programs.[107,124,125] Studies have also shown effective utilization of SCPs to drive down costs and improve postsurgical pain and functional outcomes through enhanced recovery at home and in the community:[126] by incorporating virtual clinics for postoperative follow-up,[127] advanced musculoskeletal physical therapist-led postoperative follow-up,[128,129] management of persistent knee pain post-TKR,[130] and technology-enabled rehabilitation (including exercise programs using tablet devices, health coaching using video calls and motivational text messages, physical activity trackers with goal-setting and motivational reminders using wearable sensors, and smartphone-based knee joint motion self-monitoring via goniometer application).[131] Standardization initiatives claiming cost-effectiveness should quantify development, implementation, and maintenance costs of SCPs.[96]

SCPs for TJA that consistently deliver improved outcomes and/or lower costs of care have been scaled at local, regional, and national levels.[128] The Dartmouth Hitchcock "Green Care" model[14] serves as an exemplar of a SCP for TJA applied across institutions and clinician networks, spanning care from initial referral to the surgeon through to 1 year postsurgery.[96] The development of such models focuses on development of generalizable clinical care pathways for primary TJA using inputs from clinical, academic, and patient stakeholders; and identifying system-level and patient-level processes that may provide safe, effective, efficient, patient-centered care for patients undergoing TJA.

In the United States, alternative payment models such as the Centers for Medicare & Medicaid Services Bundled Payment for Care Improvement Initiative and Comprehensive Care for Joint Replacement model have also been developed to standardize payments for all services related to the TJA episode of care in an effort to reduce procedural variation and incentivize clinicians to administer effective care at lower cost compared to fee-for-service reimbursement.[132-134] Such models have shown moderate savings through reduced utilization and operational efficiency (eg, decreased utilization of post-acute care and hospital readmissions) without negatively affecting clinical outcomes.[133-138] However, these procedure-based bundles do not address the potential for overuse of TJA and the risk of "cherry-picking" (choosing healthier or more adherent patients and referring more complex, time-consuming patients to others) and "lemon-dropping" (rejecting complex or less adherent patients, especially those who might use a lot of resources) within environments (and payment systems) that incentivize clinicians based on procedural volume.[139,140] Widespread improvement and financial alignment toward better value for patients is only likely to stem from a shift toward standardized condition-based models of payment and practice incentivizing cost-effective management of patient populations using a range of evidence-based nonsurgical and surgical strategies.[18,140-146] SCPs further lend themselves to the development of episode-based pricing and selecting high-value services, including nontraditional strategies, for example, nutritional guidance and behavioral therapies, in developing effective condition-based episodic payment models.

Integrated practice units are one way to organize and standardize care pathways to generate improved outcomes and lower costs while centering care around the patient's condition. The delivery of greater value for populations across healthcare systems may also depend on effective and standardized integration of primary and secondary care pathways.[147] Several value-adding and evidence-based components of advanced TJA pathways described earlier could serve as drivers for success in operating under such alternative payment models.[113,147]

Integrated practice units have been developed at Dell Medical School at the University of Texas at Austin to provide high-value, coordinated, multidisciplinary care for patients with a range of musculoskeletal conditions, financed by condition-based bundled episode payments[148] (**Figure 6**). All patients attending these integrated practice units have access to a team of health professionals (orthopaedic surgeon, associate clinician [eg, advance practitioner, chiropractor, or nurse practitioner], physical therapist, a dietician, and a behavioral health-trained social worker and medical assistants) throughout the full cycle of care. The standardized episode of care from initial referral up to 1 year includes a range of services from physical therapy and exercise, imaging, intra-articular injections, lifestyle modification (including dietary advice and weight loss counselling), and social support (case management, smoking and alcohol cessation, behavioral health, and psychotherapy – including cognitive behavioral therapy and pain coping skills training). A technology-enabled shared decision-making approach has been integrated into the pathway for patients considering surgery. The care pathway also incorporates the longitudinal collection of PROMs measuring physical and psychosocial outcomes as an integral component of care delivery and requisite for the condition-based alternative payment model.[149,150] For surgical patients, a

IPU clinic process: patient-facing (1/2)

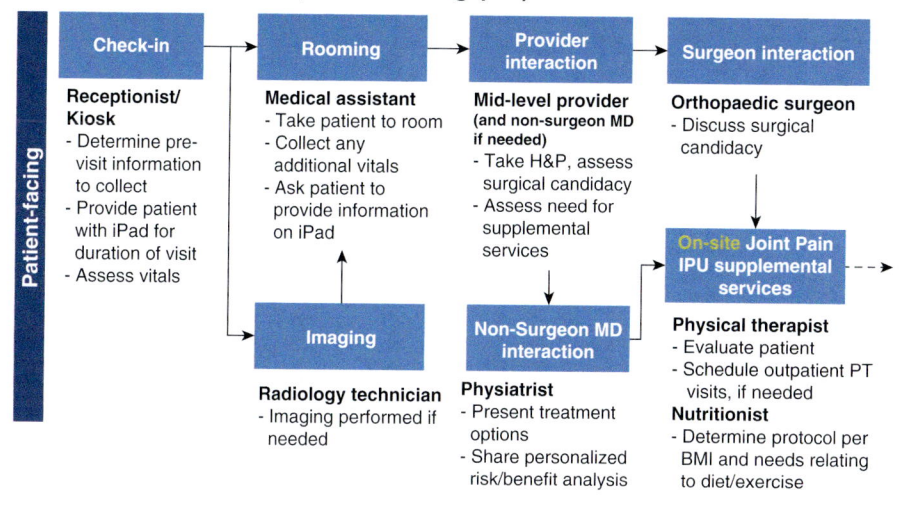

IPU clinic process: patient-facing (2/2)

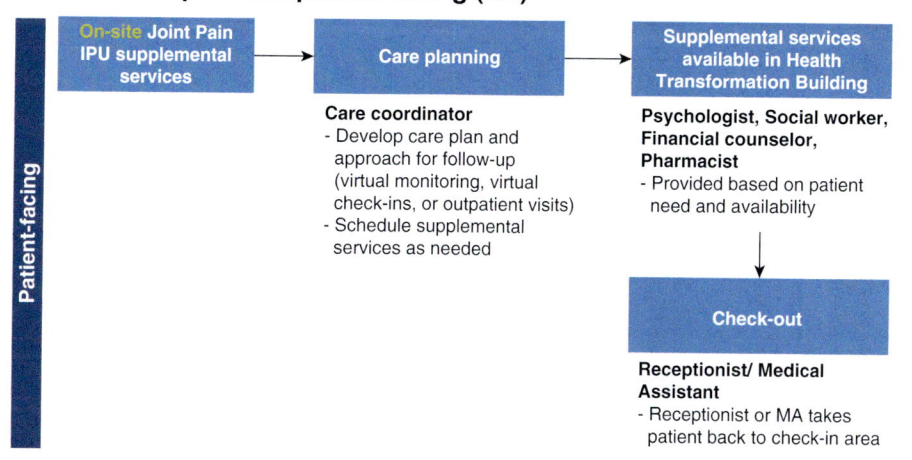

FIGURE 6 Process flow map of the joint pain integrated practice unit (IPU). BMI = body mass index, H&P = history and physical examination, MA = medical assistant, PT = physical therapist. (Reproduced with permission from Morrice DJ, Bard JF, Koenig KM: Designing and scheduling a multi-disciplinary integrated practice unit for patient-centred care. *Health Syst (Basingstoke)* 2019;9[4]:293-316.)

mandatory component of perioperative management includes the Preoperative Assessment and Global Optimization program[151] (**Figure 7**). This program covers the entire perioperative phase and includes design features to guide not only patients, but family members and caregivers. The Preoperative Assessment and Global Optimization process begins following the decision to pursue TJA. A registered nurse conducts telephone interviews, coordinates and registers activities

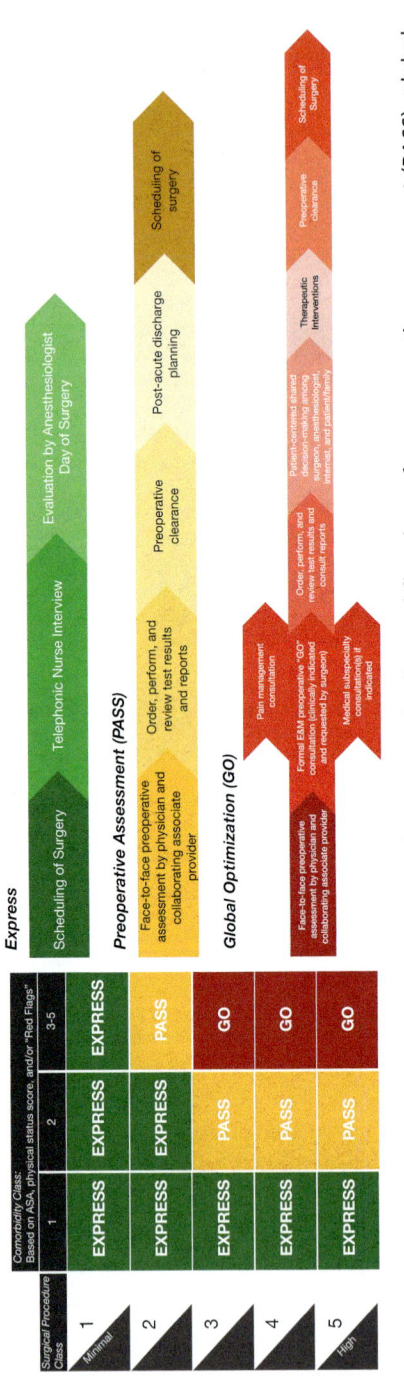

FIGURE 7 Perioperative management matrix, patient categorization and flow lanes for preoperative assessment (PASS), global optimization (GO), or direct to surgery (express). (Reproduced with permission from Vetter TR, Uhler LM, Bozic KJ: Value-based healthcare: Preoperative assessment and global optimization (PASS-GO) – Improving value in total joint replacement care. *Clin Orthop Relat Res* 2017;475[8]:1958-1962.)

with the patient's EMR, and updates a preoperative dashboard, accessible by all relevant clinicians, that tracks the patient's progress. The patient is then risk-stratified and directed to various preoperative optimization activities or channeled directly toward surgery. This model and the alignment achieved between financial and clinical incentives have improved patient flow, outcomes, costs, and system performance and decreased perioperative variability.[152]

SCPs have also been developed using evidence-based protocols to improve outcomes, costs, and practice variation in spinal surgery.[153] Demographic factors (eg, being female), surgical factors (eg, longer surgical times, increased number of fusion levels, greater volumes of crystalloid administration), and patient factors (eg, higher average pain scores on the first postoperative day, and higher cumulative morphine use) are shown to influence procedural outcomes.[154] Similar to TJA, SCPs in spinal surgery incorporate different elements of rapid or enhanced recovery. SCPs for posterior spinal fusion in patients with adolescent idiopathic scoliosis have shown reduced length of stay,[153,155,156] lower perioperative transfusion requirements,[153] reduced time to ambulation,[156] reduced use of patient-controlled analgesia,[154,157] lower postoperative pain scores, earlier return to regular diet, and improved quality of life without an increase in complications rates.[155,156]

The complexity and duration of SCPs designed around surgical procedures can range from those focused on the in-hospital surgical pathway to those spanning several weeks before and after the surgical intervention within models such as anesthetic perioperative care services and perioperative surgical homes.[108,124] Whatever the configuration, SCPs should have the right fit for the organization to enable sustainable change – something that can be evaluated using health technology assessments.[118,157] Undertaking comprehensive evaluations may also elucidate wider effects on other service lines secondary to planned process and pathway changes. For instance, physical therapists providing accelerated rehabilitation for patients following TJA may have reduced capacity to deliver therapy to other patients; and performing enhanced recovery after surgery protocols on a subset of patients can complicate broader surgical scheduling and burden staff caring for patients not under enhanced recovery after surgery protocols.

EFFECT OF SCPs FOR ORTHOPAEDIC TRAUMA CARE

SCPs in orthopaedic trauma have predominantly focused on fracture management in outpatient and ambulatory surgical settings.[158,159] Strategies entailing changes to booking protocols for outpatient surgery and clinician education have demonstrated a reduction in unnecessary hospitalizations for stable, healthier patients awaiting surgical treatment of a fracture by focusing on timely, efficient, and coordinated care.[86,158] Shifting toward preoperative optimization at home, other SCPs have demonstrated lower complication rates, improved patient satisfaction, and lower costs of prehabilitation and coordination of outpatient–inpatient services compared to standard inpatient admission for select patients.[86] Aside from the benefits of performing safe fracture fixation with reduced tissue swelling and maintaining safe movement of other joints to prevent stiffness, there are systemwide benefits in increasing bed capacity.[159] Virtual fracture clinics

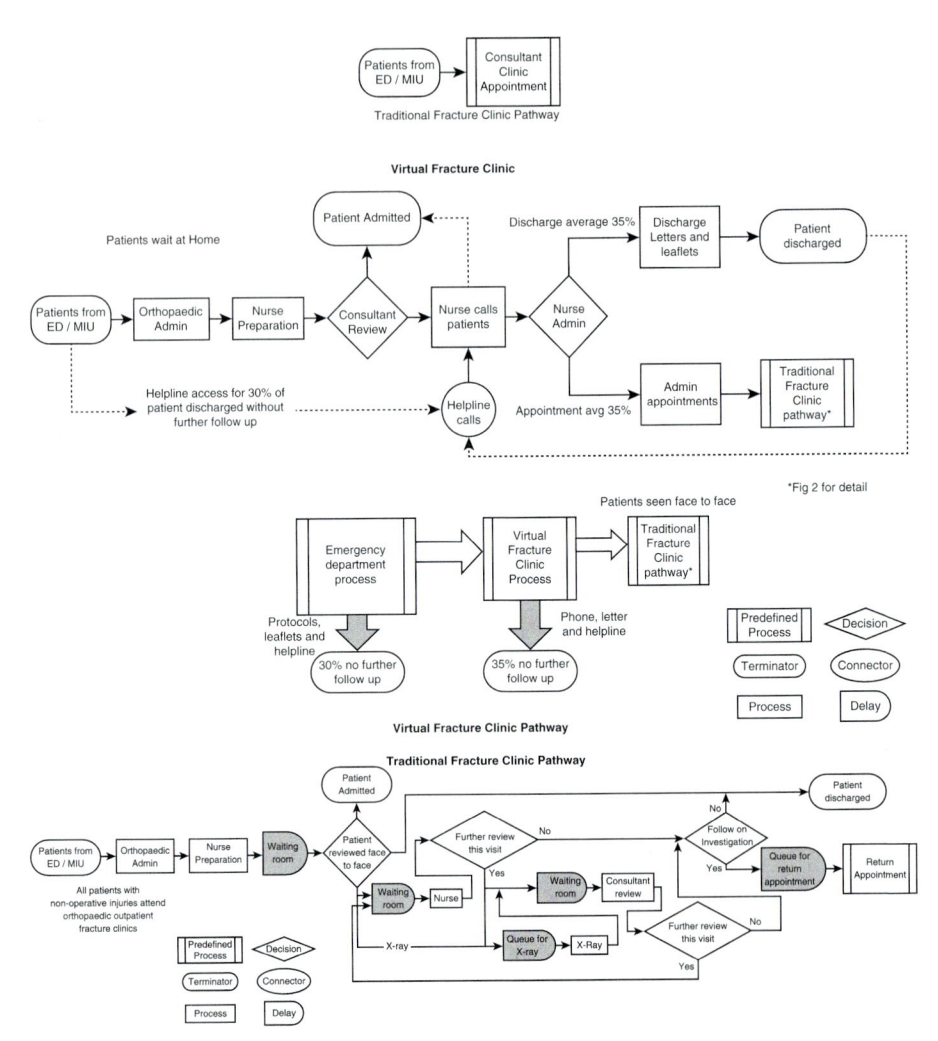

FIGURE 8 Virtual fracture pathway process flow model using the symbols shown to define individual steps in the process. This defines the flow of information and the review process where patients are reviewed without being present. It also includes a predefined process where some patients are seen face to face in a traditional fracture clinic. ED = emergency department, MIU = minor injuries unit

have been developed to improve waiting times,[159] patient experience,[159] costs of care through reducing standard face-to-face, outpatient, and inpatient care[159,160] and reducing the burden on emergency departments without an increase in reattendance rates[161] (**Figure 8**). Discrete event simulation and modeling of such pathways using an activity-based costing approach demonstrates the feasibility of this approach with significant reductions in initial in-person outpatient attendances, daily resource costs for all staff groups, reduction in duplicative testing, and overall cost per patient[160] Systematic reviews show virtual fracture clinics for the management of fifth metatarsal fractures and radial head and neck fractures as highly effective, with opportunities to translate such models to other more stable fracture patterns in appropriate patients. SCPs have also been developed for prehospital and trauma care involving standardized resuscitation parameters for the severely injured patient, improving care coordination and expediting definitive fracture fixation, resulting in reduced complications, hospital length of stay, and costs of care.[162]

A range of SCPs have also been developed for the management of fragility fractures of the hip in elderly patients – a common injury with high morbidity and mortality and traditionally long wait times for emergent surgery, leading to the increased risk of complications. Elderly patients with these injuries are prone to pneumonia, deep vein thrombosis/pulmonary embolus, delirium, pressure sores, and malnutrition, among other complications.[129] Cognitive impairment and poor balance control are strongly associated with delayed recovery of ambulatory function in these patients.[163] Several comprehensive hip fracture SCPs have been developed collaboratively between orthopaedic surgeons, specialists in care of the elderly, anesthesiologists, therapists (physical therapists, occupational therapists), nurses, emergency medicine and internal medicine physicians, and hospital management with variable guidance from professional societies.[129] Recommendations have targeted earlier intensive medical and surgical management, individualized and accelerated rehabilitation, patient engagement and education around falls prevention, earlier consideration of home support, discharge planning, and stratified rehabilitation. Such pathways have demonstrated improvements in early access to specialist medical care,[164] targeted medical optimization (improved fluid resuscitation),[164,165] and management of physiological parameters using clinical decision support tools (eg, modified early warning scores), improved utilization of diagnostic tests and physician consultations,[166,167] earlier surgical intervention or increased surgical intervention within 48 hours of admission,[129,165-170,] improved utilization of medical products (eg, blood products[165]), reduced length of stay,[166,168] reduced complications,[166] greater uptake of secondary prevention such as antiosteoporosis treatments in-hospital,[169] discharge home over transfer to skilled nursing facilities,[129,170] improved medium to longer-term functional outcomes (including balance and physical activity)[170] and mental health outcomes,[129,163] and reduced morbidity[171] and mortality rates.[129,168] Benefits of multidisciplinary SCPs for fragility hip fractures include more expedient timing from the emergency room admission to the operating room, lower length of stay and lower complications rates even in more medically complex patients,[151,152] accounting for fracture configuration and severity. SCPs demonstrating positive effects in many of these outcomes have been scaled across hospital networks as regional and national hip fracture management programs.[170]

SUMMARY

Development of SCPs should involve a systematic process utilizing the best available evidence, principles and practices of quality improvement, and "systems thinking" alongside tools and frameworks for improvement. The ability to develop, test, and implement changes is essential for any individual, group, practice, organization, or network involved in orthopaedic care that wants to continuously improve. Thus, the benefits of care pathway standardization within a framework of value-based, personalized medicine can be achieved at the level of the clinical pathway as well as the entire system. Ongoing efforts are needed to develop, test, and implement innovative SCPs within value-oriented condition-based models of care, while actively involving patients as part of an interdisciplinary team in the SCP development process and evaluating their impact on patient outcomes and costs.

REFERENCES

1. McGough M, Telesford I, Rakshit S, Wager E, Amin K, Cox C: How does health spending in the U.S. compare to other countries? Peterson-KFF Health System Tracker. Available at: https://www.healthsystemtracker.org/chart-collection/health-spending-u-s-compare-countries/. Accessed April 16, 2023.

2. Papanicolas I, Woskie LR, Jha AK: Health care spending in the United States and other high-income countries. *J Am Med Assoc* 2018;319(10):1024-1039.

3. Porter ME, Teisberg EO: *Redefining Health Care: Creating Value-Based Competition on Results.* Harvard Business Review Press, 2006.

4. Dartmouth Atlas of health care. Available at: http://www.dartmouthatlas.org/. Accessed April 16, 2023.

5. Deming WE: *The New Economics for Industry, Government, Education*, ed 3. MIT Press, 2018.

6. Augustsson H, Churruca K, Braithwaite J: Re-energising the way we manage change in healthcare: The case for soft systems methodology and its application to evidence-based practice. *BMC Health Serv Res* 2019;19(1):666.

7. Lobb R, Colditz GA: Implementation science and its application to population health. *Annu Rev Public Health* 2013;34:235-251.

8. Institute for Healthcare Improvement: How to improve. Available at: http://www.ihi.org:80/resources/Pages/HowtoImprove/default.aspx. Accessed October 4, 2023.

9. Brennan TA, Leape LL, Laird NM, et al: Incidence of adverse events and negligence in hospitalized patients. Results of the Harvard Medical Practice Study I. *N Engl J Med* 1991;324(6):370-376.

10. Kohn LT, Corrigan JM, Donaldson MS, eds: Institute of Medicine (US) Committee on Quality of Health Care in America: *To Err is Human: Building a Safer Health System* [Internet]. National Academies Press (US), 2000 [cited February 21, 2021].

11. Institute of Medicine (US) Committee on Quality of Health Care in America: *Crossing the Quality Chasm: A New Health System for the 21st Century.* National Academies Press, 2001. Available at: http://www.ncbi.nlm.nih.gov/books/NBK222274/.

12. Pinney SJ, Page AE, Jevsevar DS, Bozic KJ: Current concept review: Quality and process improvement in orthopedics. *Orthop Res Rev* 2016;8:1-11.

13. McEachern S: Orthopedics one of easiest product lines to integrate. *Health Care Strateg Manage* 1996;14(2):1, 20-23.

14. Van Citters AD, Fahlman C, Goldmann DA, et al: Developing a pathway for high-value, patient-centered total joint arthroplasty. *Clin Orthop Relat Res* 2014;472(5):1619-1635.

15. Martin GP, Kocman D, Stephens T, Peden CJ, Pearse RM: Pathways to professionalism? Quality improvement, care pathways, and the interplay of standardisation and clinical autonomy. *Sociol Health Illn* 2017;39(8):1314-1329.

16. Timmermans S: From autonomy to accountability: The role of clinical practice guidelines in professional power. *Perspect Biol Med* 2005;48(4):490-501.

17. Vanhaecht K, Panella M, van Zelm R, Sermeus W: An overview on the history and concept of care pathways as complex interventions. *Int J Care Pathways* 2010;14(3):117-123.

18. Koenig KM, Bozic KJ: Orthopaedic healthcare worldwide: The role of standardization in improving outcomes. *Clin Orthop Relat Res* 2015;473(11):3360-3363.

19. Lawal AK, Rotter T, Kinsman L, et al: What is a clinical pathway? Refinement of an operational definition to identify clinical pathway studies for a Cochrane systematic review. *BMC Med* 2016;14(1):35.

20. The Burden of Musculoskeletal Diseases in the United States: Prevalence, Societal and Economic Cost. American Academy of Orthopaedic Surgeons, 2008. Available at: https://journals.lww.com/journalacs/Citation/2009/01000/The_Burden_of_Musculoskeletal_Diseases_in_the.31.aspx

21. Singer SJ, Kerrissey M, Friedberg M, Phillips R: A comprehensive theory of integration. *Med Care Res Rev* 2020;77(2):196-207.

22. Porter M: What is value in health care? *N Engl J Med* 2010;363(26):2477-2481.

23. Singer SJ, Burgers J, Friedberg M, Rosenthal MB, Leape L, Schneider E: Defining and measuring integrated patient care: Promoting the next frontier in health care delivery. *Med Care Res Rev* 2011;68(1):112-127.

24. Heeringa J, Mutti A, Furukawa MF, Lechner A, Maurer KA, Rich E: Horizontal and vertical integration of health care providers: A framework for understanding various provider organizational structures. *Int J Integr Care* 2020;20(1):2.

25. Laugesen MJ, France G: Integration: The firm and the health care sector. *Health Econ Policy Law* 2014;9(3):295-312.

26. Orszag P, Rekhi R: The economic case for vertical at in health care. *NEJM Catalyst* 2020;1(3).

27. Evans JM, Baker GR, Berta W, Barnsley J: The evolution of integrated health care strategies. *Adv Health Care Manag* 2013;15:125-161.

28. Langley GL, Moen R, Nolan KM, Nolan TW, Norman CL, Provost LP: *The Improvement Guide: A Practical Approach to Enhancing Organizational Performance*, ed 2. IHI - Institute for Healthcare Improvement. Available at: http://www.ihi.org:80/resources/Pages/Publications/

ImprovementGuidePracticalApproachEnhancingOrganizationalPerformance.aspx. Accessed October 4, 2023.

29. Donabedian A: Evaluating the quality of medical care. *Milbank Mem Fund Q* 1966;44(3-2):166-203.

30. Spear SJ, Bowen K: *Decoding the DNA of the Toyota Production System.* Harvard Business Review. HBR publication, 2006. Available at: https://hbsp.harvard.edu/product/2904-PDF-ENG?Ntt=toyota. Accessed May 5, 2023.

31. Kaplan RS, Jehi L, Ko CY, Pusic A, Witkowski M: Health care measurements that improve patient outcomes. *NEJM Catal Innov Care Deliv* 2021;2(2).

32. Damman OC, Jani A, de Jong BA, et al: The use of PROMs and shared decision-making in medical encounters with patients: An opportunity to deliver value-based health care to patients. *J Eval Clin Pract* 2020;26(2):524-540.

33. SooHoo NF, Lieberman JR, Farng E, Park S, Jain S, Ko CY: Development of quality of care indicators for patients undergoing total hip or total knee replacement. *BMJ Qual Saf* 2011;20(2):153-157.

34. Austin E, Lee JR, Amtmann D, et al: Use of patient-generated health data across healthcare settings: Implications for health systems. *JAMIA Open* 2020;3(1):70-76.

35. Basch E, Torda P, Adams K: Standards for patient-reported outcome-based performance measures. *J Am Med Assoc* 2013;310(2):139-140.

36. Kingsley C, Patel S: Patient-reported outcome measures and patient-reported experience measures. *BJA Education* 2017;17(4):137-144.

37. Weldring T, Smith SMS: Patient-reported outcomes (PROs) and patient-reported outcome measures (PROMs). *Health Serv Insights* 2013;6:61-68.

38. Safran DG: Feasibility and value of patient-reported outcome measures for value-based payment. *Med Care* 2019;57(3):177-179.

39. Makhni EC: Meaningful clinical applications of patient-reported outcome measures in orthopaedics. *J Bone Joint Surg Am* 2021;103(1):84-91.

40. American Academy of Orthopaedic Surgeons: Patient reported outcome measures. Available at: https://www.aaos.org/quality/research-resources/patient-reported-outcome-measures/. Accessed April 16, 2023.

41. Patient-reported outcome measures–International consortium for health outcomes measurement. Available at: https://www.ichom.org/. Accessed April 16, 2023.

42. Centers for Medicare & Medicaid Services: Comprehensive care for joint replacement model. Available at: https://innovation.cms.gov. Accessed April 16, 2023.

43. Barry MJ, Edgman-Levitan S: Shared decision making – Pinnacle of patient-centered care. *N Engl J Med* 2012;366(9):780-781.

44. Bernstein J, Kupperman E, Kandel LA, Ahn J: Shared decision making, fast and slow: Implications for informed consent, resource utilization, and patient satisfaction in orthopaedic surgery. *J Am Acad Orthop Surg* 2016;24(7):495-502.

45. National Quality Forum: National standards for the certification of patient decision aids. Available at: http://www.qualityforum.org/Publications/2016/12/National_Standards_for_the_Certification_of_Patient_Decision_Aids.aspx. Accessed April 20, 2023.

46. Drug and Therapeutics Bulletin: An introduction to patient decision aids. *BMJ* 2013;347:f4147.

47. Adam JA, Khaw FM, Thomson RG, Gregg PJ, Llewellyn-Thomas HA: Patient decision aids in joint replacement surgery: A literature review and an opinion survey of consultant orthopaedic surgeons. *Ann R Coll Surg Engl* 2008;90(3):198-207.

48. Stacey D, Légaré F, Lewis K, et al: Decision aids for people facing health treatment or screening decisions. *Cochrane Database Syst Rev* 2017;4:CD001431.

49. Jayadev C, Khan T, Coulter A, Beard DJ, Price AJ: Patient decision aids in knee replacement surgery. *Knee* 2012;19(6):746-750.

50. Slover J, Shue J, Koenig K: Shared decision-making in orthopaedic surgery. *Clin Orthop Relat Res* 2012;470(4):1046-1053.

51. Holmes-Rovner M, Nelson WL, Pignone M, et al: Are patient decision aids the best way to improve clinical decision making? Report of the IPDAS Symposium. *Med Decis Making* 2007;27(5):599-608.

52. Osheroff JA, Teich JM, Middleton B, Steen EB, Wright A, Detmer DE: A roadmap for national action on clinical decision support. *J Am Med Inform Assoc* 2007;14(2):141-145.

53. Agency for Healthcare Research and Quality: Clinical decision support. Available at: http://www.ahrq.gov/cpi/about/otherwebsites/clinical-decision-support/index.html. Accessed April 16, 2023.

54. Tan C, Loo G, Pua YH, et al: Predicting discharge outcomes after total knee replacement using the risk assessment and predictor tool. *Physiotherapy* 2014;100(2):176-181.

55. Bernstein J, Weintraub S, Hume E, Neuman MD, Kates SL, Ahn J: The new APGAR SCORE: A checklist to enhance quality of life in geriatric patients with hip fracture. *J Bone Joint Surg Am* 2017;99(14):e77.

56. Christensen DL, Dickens JF, Freedman B, et al: Patient-reported outcomes in orthopaedics. *J Bone Joint Surg Am* 2018;100(5):436-442.

57. Sepucha KR, Atlas SJ, Chang Y, et al: Informed, patient-centered decisions associated with better health outcomes in orthopedics: Prospective cohort study. *Med Decis Making* 2018;38(8):1018-1026.

58. Bernstein DN, Fear K, Mesfin A, et al: Patient-reported outcomes use during orthopaedic surgery clinic visits improves the patient experience. *Musculoskeletal Care* 2019;17(1):120-125.

59. Gagnier JJ: Patient reported outcomes in orthopaedics. *J Orthop Res* 2017;35(10):2098-2108.

60. Curtin P, Conway A, Martin L, Lin E, Jayakumar P, Swart E: Compilation and analysis of web-based orthopedic personalized predictive tools: A scoping review. *J Pers Med* 2020;10(4):223.

61. Haynes AB, Weiser TG, Berry WR, et al: A surgical safety checklist to reduce morbidity and mortality in a global population. *N Engl J Med* 2009;360(5):491-499.

62. Grigg E: Smarter clinical checklists: How to minimize checklist fatigue and maximize clinician performance. *Anesth Analg* 2015;121(2):570-573.

63. American Academy of Orthopaedic Surgeons: Appropriate use criteria. Available at: https://www.orthoguidelines.org/go/auc/. Accessed February 21, 2021.

64. NACHC: PRAPARE Implementation and Action Toolkit [Internet]. [cited February 24, 2021]. Available at: https://www.nachc.org/research-and-data/prapare/toolkit/. Accessed October 4, 2023.

65. Hager ER, Quigg AM, Black MM, et al: Development and validity of a 2-item screen to identify families at risk for food insecurity. *Pediatrics* 2010;126(1):e26-e32.

66. American Academy of Orthopaedic Surgeons: Quality Programs & Guidelines (CPGs), [Internet]. [cited February 21, 2021]. Available at: https://aaos.org/quality/quality-programs/. Accessed October 4, 2023.

67. Cabana MD, Rand CS, Powe NR, et al: Why don't physicians follow clinical practice guidelines? A framework for improvement. *J Am Med Assoc* 1999;282(15):1458-1465.

68. Shekelle PG, Ortiz E, Rhodes S, et al: Validity of the Agency for Healthcare Research and Quality clinical practice guidelines: How quickly do guidelines become outdated? *J Am Med Assoc* 2001;286(12):1461-1467.

69. Sanders JO, Bozic KJ, Glassman SD, Jevsevar DS, Weber KL: Clinical practice guidelines: Their use, misuse, and future directions. *J Am Acad Orthop Surg* 2014;22(3):135-144.

70. Grimshaw JM, Russell IT: Effect of clinical guidelines on medical practice: A systematic review of rigorous evaluations. *Lancet* 1993;342(8883):1317-1322.

71. Farias M, Jenkins K, Lock J, et al: Standardized Clinical Assessment and Management Plans (SCAMPs) provide a better alternative to clinical practice guidelines. *Health Aff (Millwood)* 2013;32(5):911-920.

72. Shah AS, Waters PM, Bozic KJ: Orthopaedic healthcare worldwide: Standardized clinical assessment and management plans – An adjunct to clinical practice guidelines. *Clin Orthop Relat Res* 2015;473(6):1868-1872.

73. Dendere R, Slade C, Burton-Jones A, Sullivan C, Staib A, Janda M: Patient portals facilitating engagement with inpatient electronic medical records: A systematic review. *J Med Internet Res* 2019;21(4):e12779.

74. HealthIT.gov: What is a patient portal? [Internet]. [cited February 25, 2021]. Available at: https://www.healthit.gov/faq/what-patient-portal. Accessed October 4, 2023.

75. Borowsky PA, Kadri OM, Meldau JE, Blanchett J, Makhni EC: The remote completion rate of electronic patient-reported outcome forms before scheduled clinic visits-A proof-of-concept study using patient-reported outcome measurement information system computer adaptive test questionnaires. *J Am Acad Orthop Surg Glob Res Rev* 2019;3(10):e19.00038.

76. Patel NK, Sarraf KM, Joseph S, Lee C, Middleton FR: Implementing the national hip fracture database: An audit of care. *Injury* 2013;44(12):1934-1939.

77. Delaunay C: Registries in orthopaedics. *Orthop Traumatol Surg Res* 2015;101(1 suppl):S69-S75.

78. Hallstrom B, Singal B, Cowen ME, Roberts KC, Hughes RE: The Michigan experience with safety and effectiveness of tranexamic acid use in hip and knee arthroplasty. *J Bone Joint Surg Am* 2016;98(19):1646-1655.

79. Ayers DC: Implementation of patient-reported outcome measures in total knee arthroplasty. *J Am Acad Orthop Surg* 2017;25(suppl 1):S48-S50.

80. Ayers DC, Fehring TK, Odum SM, Franklin PD: Using joint registry data from FORCE-TJR to improve the accuracy of risk-adjustment prediction models for thirty-day readmission after total hip replacement and total knee replacement. *J Bone Joint Surg Am* 2015;97(8):668-671.

81. Orthopaedic Data Evaluation Panel (ODEP): [Internet]. [cited February 21, 2021]. Available at: https://www.odep.org.uk/. Accessed October 4, 2023.

82. Porter M, Armstrong R, Howard P, Porteous M, Wilkinson JM: Orthopaedic registries - the UK view (National Joint Registry): Impact on practice. *EFORT Open Rev* 2019;4(6):377-390.

83. Wilson I, Bohm E, Lübbeke A, et al: Orthopaedic registries with patient-reported outcome measures. *EFORT Open Rev* 2019;4(6):357-367.

84. Patient Decision Support Tool: [Internet]. [cited February 25, 2021]. Available at: https://jointcalc.shef.ac.uk. Accessed May 4, 2023.

85. Vanhaecht K, De Witte K, Panella M, Sermeus W: Do pathways lead to better organized care processes? *J Eval Clin Pract* 2009;15(5):782-788.

86. Wolfstadt JI, Wayment L, Koyle MA, Backstein DJ, Ward SE: The development of a standardized pathway for outpatient ambulatory fracture surgery: To admit or not to admit. *J Bone Joint Surg Am* 2020;102(2):110-118.

87. Rotter T, Kugler J, Koch R, et al: A systematic review and meta-analysis of the effects of clinical pathways on length of stay, hospital costs and patient outcomes. *BMC Health Serv Res* 2008;8:265.

88. Rotter T, Kinsman L, James E, et al: The effects of clinical pathways on professional practice, patient outcomes, length of stay, and hospital costs: Cochrane systematic review and meta-analysis. *Eval Health Prof* 2012;35(1):3-27.

89. Brufsky A, Lokay K, McDonald M: Driving evidence-based standardization of care within a framework of personalized medicine. *Am Soc Clin Oncol Educ Book* 2012:e62-e65.

90. Button K, Morgan F, Weightman AL, Jones S: Musculoskeletal care pathways for adults with hip and knee pain referred for specialist opinion: A systematic review. *BMJ Open* 2019;9(9):e027874.

91. Tzortziou Brown V, Underwood M, Westwood OM, Morrissey D: Improving the management of musculoskeletal conditions: Can an alternative approach to referral management underpinned by quality improvement and behavioural change theories offer a solution and a better patient experience? A mixed-methods study. *BMJ Open* 2019;9(2):e024710.

92. Allen K, Vu MB, Callahan LF, et al: Osteoarthritis physical activity care pathway (OA-PCP): Results of a feasibility trial. *BMC Musculoskelet Disord* 2020;21(1):308.

93. Hutchison A-M, Laing H, Williams P, Bodger O, Topliss C: The effects of a new Tendo-Achilles Pathway (TAP) on an orthopaedic department – A quality improvement study. *Musculoskelet Sci Pract* 2019;39:67-72.

94. Joseph C, Morrissey D, Abdur-Rahman M, Hussenbux A, Barton C: Musculoskeletal triage: A mixed methods study, integrating systematic review with expert and patient perspectives. *Physiotherapy* 2014;100(4):277-289.

95. Hill JC, Whitehurst DG, Lewis M, et al: Comparison of stratified primary care management for low back pain with current best practice (STarT Back): A randomised controlled trial. *Lancet* 2011;378(9802):1560-1571.

96. Barbieri A, Vanhaecht K, Van Herck P, et al: Effects of clinical pathways in the joint replacement: A meta-analysis. *BMC Med* 2009;7:32.

97. McDermott KW, Freeman WJ, Elixhauser A: Overview of operating room procedures during inpatient stays in U.S. Hospitals, 2014, in Healthcare Cost and Utilization Project (HCUP) Statistical Brief #233. Agency for Healthcare Research and Quality, December 2017. Available at: https://hcup-us.ahrq.gov/reports/statbriefs/sb233-Operating-Room-Procedures-United-States-2014.pdf. Accessed May 4, 2023.

98. Bumpass DB, Nunley RM: Assessing the value of a total joint replacement. *Curr Rev Musculoskelet Med* 2012;5(4):274-282.

99. Ackerman IN, Bohensky MA, de Steiger R, et al: Substantial rise in the lifetime risk of primary total knee replacement surgery for osteoarthritis from 2003 to 2013: An international, population-level analysis. *Osteoarthritis Cartilage* 2017;25(4):455-461.

100. Barbour KE, Helmick CG, Boring M, Brady TJ: Vital signs: Prevalence of doctor-diagnosed arthritis and arthritis-attributable activity limitation – United States, 2013-2015. *MMWR Morb Mortal Wkly Rep* 2017;66(9):246-253.

101. Schilling PL, He J, Chen S, Placzek H, Bini SA: Risk-adjusted cost performance for 90-day total hip arthroplasty episodes: Comparing US hospitals nationwide Before CJR. *J Arthroplasty* 2020;35(12):3452-3463.

102. Schilling PL, He J, Chen S, Placzek H, Bini S: Risk-adjusted cost performance for 90-day total knee arthroplasty episodes: Data and methods for comparing U.S. hospitals nationwide. *J Bone Joint Surg Am* 2020;102(11):971-982.

103. Spath P: Pathways can improve perioperative process. *Hosp Case Manag* 1998;6(5):90-94, 99-100.

104. Wainwright TW: Consensus statement for perioperative care in total hip replacement and total knee replacement surgery: Enhanced Recovery After Surgery (ERAS®) Society recommendations. *Acta Orthop* 2020;91(3):363.

105. Wainwright T, Middleton R: An orthopaedic enhanced recovery pathway. *Curr Anaesth Crit Care* 2010;21(3):114-120.

106. Kaye AD, Urman RD, Cornett EM, et al: Enhanced recovery pathways in orthopedic surgery. *J Anaesthesiol Clin Pharmacol* 2019;35(suppl 1):S35-S39.

107. Li J, Rubin LE, Mariano ER: Essential elements of an outpatient total joint replacement programme. *Curr Opin Anaesthesiol* 2019;32(5):643-648.

108. Schubert A, Patterson M, Sumrall WD, et al: Perioperative population management for primary hip arthroplasty reduces hospital and postacute care utilization while maintaining or improving care quality. *J Clin Anesth* 2021;68:110072.

109. Chua H, Brady B, Farrugia M, et al: Implementing early mobilisation after knee or hip arthroplasty to reduce length of stay: A quality improvement study with embedded qualitative component. *BMC Musculoskelet Disord* 2020;21(1):765.

110. Gregor C, Pope S, Werry D, Dodek P: Reduced length of stay and improved appropriateness of care with a clinical path for total knee or hip arthroplasty. *Jt Comm J Qual Improv* 1996;22(9):617-628.

111. Ho DM, Huo MH: Are critical pathways and implant standardization programs effective in reducing costs in total knee replacement operations? *J Am Coll Surg* 2007;205(1):97-100.

112. Bozic KJ, Maselli J, Pekow PS, Lindenauer PK, Vail TP, Auerbach AD: The influence of procedure volumes and standardization of care on quality and efficiency in total joint replacement surgery. *J Bone Joint Surg Am* 2010;92(16):2643-2652.

113. Kim K, Iorio R: The 5 clinical pillars of value for total joint arthroplasty in a bundled payment paradigm. *J Arthroplasty* 2017;32(6):1712-1716.

114. Yanik JM, Bedard NA, Hanley JM, Otero JE, Callaghan JJ, Marsh JL: Rapid recovery total joint arthroplasty is safe, efficient, and cost-effective in the veterans administration setting. *J Arthroplasty* 2018;33(10):3138-3142.

115. Duncan CM, Moeschler SM, Horlocker TT, Hanssen AD, Hebl JR: A self-paired comparison of perioperative outcomes before and after implementation of a clinical pathway in patients undergoing total knee arthroplasty. *Reg Anesth Pain Med* 2013;38(6):533-538.

116. Healy WL, Ayers ME, Iorio R, Patch DA, Appleby D, Pfeifer BA: Impact of a clinical pathway and implant standardization on total hip arthroplasty: A clinical and economic study of short-term patient outcome. *J Arthroplasty* 1998;13(3):266-276.

117. Provider overhauls pathway procedures to improve outcomes analysis, care efficiency. *Health Care Cost Reengineering Rep* 1998;3(2):25-29.

118. Vanni F, Foglia E, Pennestrì F, Ferrario L, Banfi G: Introducing enhanced recovery after surgery in a high-volume orthopaedic hospital: A health technology assessment. *BMC Health Serv Res* 2020;20(1):773.

119. Vendittoli PA, Pellei K, Williams C, Laflamme C: Combining enhanced recovery and short-stay protocols for hip and knee joint replacements: The ideal solution. *Can J Surg* 2021;64(1):E66-E68.

120. Alvis BD, Amsler RG, Leisy PJ, et al: Effects of an anesthesia perioperative surgical home for total knee and hip arthroplasty at a Veterans Affairs Hospital: A quality improvement before-and-after cohort study. *Can J Anaesth* 2021;68(3):367-375.

121. Frassanito L, Vergari A, Nestorini R, et al: Enhanced recovery after surgery (ERAS) in hip and knee replacement surgery: Description of a multidisciplinary program to improve management of the patients undergoing major orthopedic surgery. *Musculoskelet Surg* 2020;104(1):87-92.

122. Kee JR, Edwards PK, Barnes CL: Effect of risk acceptance for bundled care payments on clinical outcomes in a high-volume total joint arthroplasty practice after implementation of a standardized clinical pathway. *J Arthroplasty* 2017;32(8):2332-2338.

123. Schotanus MGM, Bemelmans YFL, Grimm B, Heyligers IC, Kort NP: Physical activity after outpatient surgery and enhanced recovery for total knee arthroplasty. *Knee Surg Sports Traumatol Arthrosc* 2017;25(11):3366-3371.

124. Van Horne A, Van Horne J: Patient-optimizing enhanced recovery pathways for total knee and hip arthroplasty in Medicare patients: Implication for transition to ambulatory surgery centers. *Arthroplast Today* 2019;5(4):497-502.

125. Tessier JE, Rupp G, Gera JT, DeHart ML, Kowalik TD, Duwelius PJ: Physicians with defined clear care pathways have better discharge disposition and lower cost. *J Arthroplasty* 2016;31(9 suppl):54-58.

126. Yang H, Dervin G, Madden S, et al: Postoperative home monitoring after joint replacement: Retrospective outcome study comparing cases with matched historical controls. *JMIR Perioper Med* 2018;1(2):e10169.

127. Preston N, McHugh GA, Hensor EMA, et al: Developing a standardized approach to virtual clinic follow-up of hip and knee arthroplasty. *Bone Joint J* 2019;101-B(8):951-959.

128. Harding P, Burge A, Walter K, et al: Advanced musculoskeletal physiotherapists in post arthroplasty review clinics: A state wide implementation program evaluation. *Physiotherapy* 2018;104(1):98-106.

129. Lamb LC, Montgomery SC, Wong Won B, Harder S, Meter J, Feeney JM: A multidisciplinary approach to improve the quality of care for patients with fragility fractures. *J Orthop* 2017;14(2):247-251.

130. Wylde V, Bertram W, Beswick AD, et al: Clinical- and cost-effectiveness of the STAR care pathway compared to usual care for patients with chronic pain after total knee replacement: Study protocol for a UK randomised controlled trial. *Trials* 2018;19(1):132.

131. Wang X, Hunter DJ, Robbins S, et al: Participatory health through behavioural engagement and disruptive digital technology for postoperative rehabilitation: Protocol of the PATHway trial. *BMJ Open* 2021;11(1):e041328.

132. Health Affairs Blog: Expanding payment reforms to better incentivize chronic care for degenerative joint disease. April 23, 2018. Available at: https://www.healthaffairs.org/do/10.1377/hblog20180416.346268/full/. Accessed April 17, 2023.

133. Press MJ, Rajkumar R, Conway PH: Medicare's new bundled payments: Design, strategy, and evolution. *J Am Med Assoc* 2016;315(2):131-132.

134. Navathe AS, Song Z, Emanuel EJ: The next generation of episode-based payments. *J Am Med Assoc* 2017;317(23):2371-2372.

135. Navathe AS, Liao JM, Polsky D, et al: Comparison of hospitals participating in Medicare's voluntary and mandatory orthopedic bundle programs. *Health Aff (Millwood)* 2018;37(6):854-863.

136. Navathe AS, Troxel AB, Liao JM, et al: Cost of joint replacement using bundled payment models. *JAMA Intern Med* 2017;177(2):214-222.

137. Barnett ML, Wilcock A, McWilliams JM, et al: Two-year evaluation of mandatory bundled payments for joint replacement. *N Engl J Med* 2019;380(3):252-262.

138. Navathe AS, Liao JM, Emanuel EJ: Potential unintended effects of Medicare's bundled payments for care improvement program-reply. *J Am Med Assoc* 2019;321(1):107-108.

139. Navathe AS, Liao JM, Dykstra SE, et al: Association of hospital participation in a Medicare Bundled Payment Program with volume and case mix of lower extremity joint replacement episodes. *J Am Med Assoc* 2018;320(9):901-910.

140. Nelson AE, Allen KD, Golightly YM, Goode AP, Jordan JM: A systematic review of recommendations and guidelines for the management of osteoarthritis: The chronic osteoarthritis management initiative of the U.S. bone and joint initiative. *Semin Arthritis Rheum* 2014;43(6):701-712.

141. Bedard NA, Dowdle SB, Anthony CA, et al: The AAHKS clinical research award: What are the costs of knee osteoarthritis in the year prior to total knee arthroplasty? *J Arthroplasty* 2017;32(9 suppl):S8-S10.e1.

142. American Academy of Orthopaedic Surgeons: Clinical Practice Guidelines: Osteoarthritis of the knee. Available at: https://www.aaos.org/quality/quality-programs/lower-extremity-programs/osteoarthritis-of-the-knee/. Accessed May 4, 2023.

143. Lam V, Teutsch S, Fielding J: Hip and knee replacements: A neglected potential savings opportunity. *J Am Med Assoc* 2018;319(10):977-978.

144. Allen KD, Choong PF, Davis AM, et al: Osteoarthritis: Models for appropriate care across the disease continuum. *Best Pract Res Clin Rheumatol* 2016;30(3):503-535.

145. Meiyappan KP, Cote MP, Bozic KJ, Halawi MJ: Adherence to the American Academy of Orthopaedic Surgeons Clinical Practice Guidelines for Nonoperative Management of Knee Osteoarthritis. *J Arthroplasty* 2020;35(2):347-352.

146. Skou ST, Roos EM, Laursen MB, et al: Total knee replacement and non-surgical treatment of knee osteoarthritis: 2-year outcome from two parallel randomized controlled trials. *Osteoarthritis Cartilage* 2018;26(9):1170-1180.

147. Bains M, Warriner D, Behrendt K: Primary and secondary care integration in delivery of value-based health-care systems. *Br J Hosp Med (Lond)* 2018;79(6):312-315.

148. Jayakumar P, Moore MLG, Bozic KJ: Team approach: A multidisciplinary approach to the management of hip and knee osteoarthritis. *JBJS Rev* 2019;7(6):e10.

149. Porter ME, Larsson S, Lee TH: Standardizing patient outcomes measurement. *N Engl J Med* 2016;374(6):504-506.

150. Lee VS, Kawamoto K, Hess R, et al: Implementation of a value-driven outcomes program to identify high variability in clinical costs and outcomes and association with reduced cost and improved quality. *J Am Med Assoc* 2016;316(10):1061-1072.

151. Vetter TR, Uhler LM, Bozic KJ: Value-based healthcare: Preoperative assessment and global optimization (PASS-GO) – Improving value in total joint replacement care. *Clin Orthop Relat Res* 2017;475(8):1958-1962.

152. Morrice DJ, Bard JF, Koenig KM: Designing and scheduling a multi-disciplinary integrated practice unit for patient-centred care. *Health Syst (Basingstoke)* 2019;9(4):293-316.

153. Oetgen ME, Martin BD, Gordish-Dressman H, Cronin J, Pestieau SR: Effectiveness and sustainability of a standardized care pathway developed with use of lean process mapping for the treatment of patients undergoing posterior spinal fusion for adolescent idiopathic scoliosis. *J Bone Joint Surg Am* 2018;100(21):1864-1870.

154. Martin BD, Pestieau SR, Cronin J, Gordish-Dressman H, Thomson K, Oetgen ME: Factors affecting length of stay after posterior spinal fusion for adolescent idiopathic scoliosis. *Spine Deform* 2020;8(1):51-56.

155. Fletcher ND, Murphy JS, Austin TM, et al: Short term outcomes of an enhanced recovery after surgery (ERAS) pathway versus a traditional discharge pathway after posterior spinal fusion for adolescent idiopathic scoliosis. *Spine Deform* 2021;9(4):1013-1019.

156. Nelson KL, Locke LL, Rhodes LN, et al: Evaluation of outcomes before and after implementation of a standardized postoperative care pathway in pediatric posterior spinal fusion patients. *Orthop Nurs* 2020;39(4):257-263.

157. Gooch KL, Smith D, Wasylak T, et al: The Alberta hip and knee replacement project: A model for health technology assessment based on comparative effectiveness of clinical pathways. *Int J Technol Assess Health Care* 2009;25(2):113-123.

158. Ahluwalia R, Cook J, Raheman F, et al: Improving the efficiency of ankle fracture care through home care and day-surgery units: Delivering safe surgery on a value-based healthcare model. *Surgeon* 2021;19(5):e95-e102.

159. Davey MS, Coveney E, Rowan F, Cassidy JT, Cleary MS: Virtual fracture clinics in orthopaedic surgery – A systematic review of current evidence. *Injury* 2020;51(12): 2757-2762.

160. Anderson GH, Jenkins PJ, McDonald DA, et al: Cost comparison of orthopaedic fracture pathways using discrete event simulation in a Glasgow hospital. *BMJ Open* 2017;7(9):e014509.

161. Vardy J, Jenkins PJ, Clark K, et al: Effect of a redesigned fracture management pathway and "virtual" fracture clinic on ED performance. *BMJ Open* 2014;4(6):e005282.

162. Childs BR, Vallier HA: Cost savings associated with a multidisciplinary protocol that expedites definitive fracture care. *Am J Orthop (Belle Mead NJ)* 2014;43(7):309-315.

163. Kang JH, Lee G, Kim KE, Lee YK, Lim JY: Determinants of functional outcomes using clinical pathways for rehabilitation after hip fracture surgery. *Ann Geriatr Med Res* 2018;22(1):26-32.

164. Ollivere B, Rollins K, Brankin R, Wood M, Brammar TJ, Wimhurst J: Optimising fast track care for proximal femoral fracture patients using modified early warning score. *Ann R Coll Surg Engl* 2012;94(4):267-271.

165. Anighoro K, Bridges C, Graf A, et al: From ER to OR: Results after implementation of multidisciplinary pathway for fragility hip fractures at a level I trauma center. *Geriatr Orthop Surg Rehabil* 2020;11:2151459320927383.

166. Loizzo M, Gallo F, Caruso D: Reducing complications and overall healthcare costs of hip fracture management: A retrospective study on the application of a Diagnostic Therapeutic Pathway in the Cosenza General Hospital. *Ann Ig* 2018;30(3):191-199.

167. Swart E, Kates S, McGee S, Ayers DC: The case for comanagement and care pathways for osteoporotic patients with a hip fracture. *J Bone Joint Surg Am* 2018;100(15):1343-1350.

168. Middleton M, Wan B, da Assunçao R: Improving hip fracture outcomes with integrated orthogeriatric care: A comparison between two accepted orthogeriatric models. *Age Ageing* 2017;46(3):465-470.

169. Svenøy S, Watne LO, Hestnes I, Westberg M, Madsen JE, Frihagen F: Results after introduction of a hip fracture care pathway: Comparison with usual care. *Acta Orthop* 2020;91(2):139-145.

170. Jackson K, Bachhuber M, Bowden D, Etter K, Tong C: Comprehensive hip fracture care program: Successive implementation in 3 hospitals. *Geriatr Orthop Surg Rehabil* 2019;10:2151459319846057.

171. Beaupre LA, Cinats JG, Senthilselvan A, et al: Reduced morbidity for elderly patients with a hip fracture after implementation of a perioperative evidence-based clinical pathway. *Qual Saf Health Care* 2006;15(5):375-379.

Historical Payment Models

Kevin A. Lawson, MD • Jessica M. Hooper, MD
James I. Huddleston III, MD, FAAOS

INTRODUCTION

Currently, the predominant method of payment for health care services in the United States has been on a fee-for-service (FFS) basis, meaning that each service is paid for separately and individually. Payment is made for the quantity of procedures performed, without accounting for the quality or efficiency of the care provided. It is important to understand this current iteration of health care delivery before improvements can be made.

HISTORY OF PHYSICIAN PAYMENT/MEDICARE

The history of physician payment in the United States and FFS[1] is closely tied to the history of Medicare. In 1965, Title XVIII of the Social Security Act, called the Health Insurance for the Aged Act, was signed into law, codifying Medicare. At the time, the program comprised a hospital insurance plan (Part A) and supplementary medical insurance for physicians' fees and other health services (Part B) for persons age 65 years and older.[2] Medicare was initially under the control of the Social Security Administration, and the Bureau of Health Insurance was established to administer the program. This bureau was responsible for the development of health insurance policy. In 1977 Medicare was moved from the Social Security Administration to the Health Care Financing Administration, which was established to administer the Medicare and Medicaid programs. In 2001, the Health Care Financing Administration was renamed the Centers for Medicare & Medicaid Services (CMS).[2] Medicare traditionally was an FFS model and set the payment standard for commercial and private insurance programs.

Dr. Hooper or an immediate family member is a member of a speakers' bureau or has made paid presentations on behalf of Smith & Nephew and serves as a paid consultant to or is an employee of Smith & Nephew. Dr. Huddleston or an immediate family member has received royalties from DePuy, a Johnson & Johnson Company, Exactech, Inc., and Wolters Kluwer; serves as a paid consultant to or is an employee of CMS/Yale CORE, DePuy, a Johnson & Johnson Company, and Exactech, Inc.; has stock or stock options held in Corin U.S.A. and Porosteon; has received research or institutional support from Apple, Biomet, and Zimmer; and serves as a board member, owner, officer, or committee member of American Academy of Orthopaedic Surgeons, American Association of Hip and Knee Surgeons, Hip Society, and Knee Society. Neither Dr. Lawson nor any immediate family member has received anything of value from or has stock or stock options held in a commercial company or institution related directly or indirectly to the subject of this chapter.

National health care spending as a percentage of gross domestic product (GDP) was 5.1% in 1960. Over time, this percentage grew steadily, reaching 13.4% in 1992.[3] It became apparent early in Medicare implementation that the cost of the program was growing significantly without any clear method to predict or restrain it. Physician services were reimbursed by the "usual, customary, and reasonable" method, which resulted in variations in payment for similar services by various specialties, differences in geographic payments for similar services, and increasing growth in the cost and utilization of physician services.[4] In an attempt to gain the cooperation of physicians and hospitals, the Social Security Administration's approach to running Medicare was committed to remaining primarily a distributor of popular entitlement benefits, with little focus on cost containment.[5] With no legislative restraint, Medicare tax funds flowed into hospitals, more than doubling between 1970 and 1975, and doubling again by 1980.[6] By 2012, the average annual cost per Medicare beneficiary had risen to $12,210.[7]

At the outset, Medicare reimbursed hospitals and physicians on a cost basis. Because of considerable increases in Medicare spending, the cost basis for reimbursing hospitals was abandoned in 1983, when Congress passed the inpatient prospective payment system (IPPS). The IPPS established diagnosis-related groups (DRGs), which assigned payment amount based on the conditions treated (CMS episode payment models). Other cost-saving programs included the Medicare Economic Index, introduced in 1975, to predict how much the costs of practicing physicians grow annually so that spending increases could be limited (CMS episode payment models). However, the Medicare Economic Index did little to stop the growth in Medicare spending.

RESOURCE-BASED FEE

Relative value scales were in use for many years before the implementation of the specific Medicare physician payment fee schedule. The California Medical Committee on Fees developed a relative value scale, first published in 1956, called the California Relative Value Studies. The values published were based on existing median charges of California physicians. The California Relative Value Studies were updated periodically from 1957 until 1974, when the Federal Trade Commission decided that the studies might constitute a price-fixing scheme, and updates were no longer provided.

In the late 1970s, a team of researchers headed by William C. Hsiao, PhD, of the Harvard School of Public Health, began to study the relationship of medical services and physician work, with the aim of determining the resources consumed in delivery of those services.[8] The economic theory behind a resource-based fee scale is that if fees for medical services are based on the cost (resources) of providing those services, then medical decision making will not be influenced by the price of medical services. The Harvard group determined that physician work could be grouped into three components: preservice work, intraservice work, and postservice work. With minor variations over time, these service period definitions have been used as guidelines to describe time elements of physician work that were considered in developing modern physician payment scales such as the resource-based relative value scale (RBRVS) later introduced by Medicare. The results of the Harvard studies were then published in three separate phases.[9-11]

In 1980, the New Jersey Health Commission, with the support of the Health Care Financing Administration, began a 3-year experiment to introduce the DRG system, to alter the incentives offered to hospitals in order to improve efficiency and, thus reduce growth in health care expenditures.[12] This reimbursement system was designed to constrain hospitals and oblige their administrators to alter the behavior of the physicians and surgeons.[13] Soon after the DRG system was implemented as part of the Medicare program, Congress responded in 1982 with the Tax Equity and Fiscal Responsibility Act, which led to the development of the office of the Secretary of Health and Human Services, and, with the Senate Finance Committee and the House Ways and Means Committee, a proposal for prospective reimbursement by December 31, 1982.[14] DRGs were assigned to be homogenous units of hospital activity to which binding prices could be attached. DRGs set forth a system of payments for the operating costs of hospital inpatient stays under Medicare Part A based on prospectively set rates. This payment system is known as the inpatient prospective payment system (IPPS).[15] The IPPS reimburses inpatient hospital costs (Medicare Part A services) under a single price. Although hospitals received a single prospective per-discharge payment that included all the facility costs, such as room and board, nursing, and costs associated with specialized care and ancillary services, orthopaedic surgeons and other medical professionals continued to receive separate fees for surgery and other services.

Overall, the initiation of IPPS slowed the rate of increase in Medicare spending and hospital resource utilization, and reduced incentives to keep patients in-house, in turn decreasing lengths of stay.[16-18] This was one of the first examples of bundling payments for health care services, which was a change from the traditional FFS model. The DRG system was subsequently adopted by many states' Medicaid programs and private insurance looking for similar cost-saving benefits.[19]

In 2009, CMS expanded IPPS by adding physician professional fees through the Acute Care Episode demonstration program, in which physician-hospital organizations negotiated a prospective payment to cover both the inpatient facility (Part A) and inpatient physician (Part B) costs for patients undergoing 9 orthopaedic and 28 cardiovascular services and procedures.[20,21] This adoption lowered costs of care for CMS.

COMMON PROCEDURAL TERMINOLOGY CODES

The Common Procedural Terminology (CPT®) code set was created by the American Medical Association in 1966 to standardize procedural coding for record keeping, billing, and insurance claims. It has evolved and expanded extensively since that time and is now the most used method of coding for procedures and services. In 1983, CMS adopted the CPT code set as part of their Healthcare Common Procedure Coding System.[2] CMS first required state Medicaid programs to use the CPT code system in 1986. In 1996, The Health Insurance Portability and Accountability Act designated the Healthcare Common Procedure Coding System, and therefore CPT codes, as the standard for electronic transmission of healthcare information.[22] CPT codes are currently used by physicians when documenting services rendered in each episode of patient care.

MEDICARE PHYSICIAN FEE SCALE

The Medicare Physician Fee Schedule (MPFS) is an RBRVS and has been the basis for payment for the care of Medicare beneficiaries since January 1, 1992. Prior to the implementation of the MPFS, physicians submitted claims for payment to CMS, and payment was determined by the usual, customary, and reasonable rate of prevailing charges in a geographic area for the same or similar services.[23] Due to the progressive rise in payments for physicians' services across America, the congressional mandates contained in the Consolidated Omnibus Budget Reconciliation Act of 1985 directed the appointment of a Physician Payment Review Commission that would annually make recommendations to Congress regarding adjustments to the reasonable charge levels for physicians' services, and changes in the methodology for determining the rates of payment for physicians' services under Medicare Part B.

In a 1988 congressional report, the Physician Payment Review Commission recommended that the usual, customary, and reasonable payment system should be replaced with a physician fee schedule based primarily on the resource costs incurred in an efficient medical practice.[24] Soon after the submission of these reports, the 101st Congress delivered a major change to how Medicare would reimburse physicians and other clinicians by passage of 1989 bill HR3299.[25] Section 6102 amended title XVIII of the Social Security Act to require CMS to develop a resource-based payment methodology for reimbursement of physician services. These elements became the legislative basis for development of an RBRVS. The RBRVS fractionated payment for a physician service into three components: physician work, practice expense, and practice liability insurance. This system introduced many important elements including the relative value unit (RVU) and a payment conversion factor, among others. The RVU developed national uniform relative values for all physicians' services with the relative value of each service equal to the sum of RVUs. RVUs represented physician work, practice expenses (PE), and the cost of professional liability insurance (MP). Nationally uniform conversion factors were established to convert RVUs into dollar payment amounts. Payments based on RVUs are calculated by adjusting the RVUs by the geographic practice cost indices (GPCI) to reflect variations in the costs of furnishing the services. The conversion factor (CF) is calculated based on a statutory formula by CMS Office of the Actuary.[26] The formula used for calculation is:

$$\text{Payment} = \left[\begin{array}{l} (\text{RVU work} \times \text{GPCI work}) + (\text{RVU PE} \times \text{GPCI PE}) \\ + (\text{RVU MP} \times \text{GPCI MP}) \end{array}\right] \times \text{CF}$$

This model is currently in use.

Section 6102 of HR3299 also required the Secretary to transmit to Congress and make available to the public a model fee schedule by September 1, 1990, in order to provide an early opportunity for public review of the fee schedule methodology. When published, the addenda to the model fee schedule provided preliminary estimates of the RVUs associated with the approximately 1,400 services studied as part of the Harvard RBRVS study. This led to the creation of the MPFS, which was first published in 1991. Additionally, a Medicare Volume Performance Standard (MVPS) was established to target expenditures and adjust the physician fee schedule as needed. When the spending target was exceeded, the update was adjusted to establish the rate of increased or decreased spending for the next year. The use of the MVPS worked well to identify the rate of growth of spending on physician services on an annual basis and adjust the update accordingly but did not meet the desired objective of controlling the costs of spending on physician services.[27]

RELATIVE UPDATE COMMITTEE

In 1991, in response to the introduction of the MPFS, the American Medical Association formed the Specialty Society Relative Update Committee (RUC) to act as an expert panel advising CMS on relative values for new and revised CPT codes.[28] It is a voluntary organization composed of representatives from 32 medical specialty societies. The American Academy of Orthopaedic Surgeons is represented at the RUC; as of 2023, the American Association of Hip and Knee Surgeons does not have unique representation in the RUC. The RUC has submitted more than 5,800 relative value recommendations over its 23-year history. These recommendations are approved by CMS in 90% of the cases.[29]

GLOBAL PERIOD

In 1992, as a result of the Harvard studies, the concept of a global period for procedures emerged. The global period allowed for a total work value to be calculated for the surgeon's services, including resources utilized, labor, and risk. The time utilized to perform the service and the intensity with which that time is expended are evaluated and periodically updated to reflect evolution in delivery of care. The technical expertise required to perform a procedure skillfully is also taken into account relative to other comparable procedures. Specifically, the individual components of the global surgical package, the preservice, intraservice, and postservice elements, are derived from surgeons who perform the procedure in question. The duration of the global period varies by type of surgery, but 90 days is the standard for most orthopaedic procedures. The 90-day global payment scheme is a payment bundle at the level of physician reimbursement, which was a change from the standard FFS model as part of earlier Medicare reimbursement models.

SUSTAINABLE GROWTH MODEL

The Balanced Budget Act of 1997 was enacted to replace the MVPS with a sustainable growth rate (SGR) standard, and control the actual growth in Medicare spending for physician services. The fundamental concept of the SGR tied the growth of US health care expenses to the US GDP. The formula required an annual adjustment of FFS payments to maintain budget neutrality.[30] The fee schedule was adjusted positively or negatively each year based on whether expenditures were above or below the SGR targets. The annual SGR was established by estimations of available data at the beginning of the fiscal year, and there was no legislative mechanism that allowed adjustment as more refined data from prior fiscal years became available, thus reducing the accuracy of the SGR estimate. This process created difficulty in the ability to accurately forecast upward or downward adjustments for the SGR calculation.

The Balanced Budget Reduction Act of 1999 required development of aggregate spending criteria to create expenditure targets that would allow comparisons to growth targets. The Balanced Budget Reduction Act also incorporated the rate of GDP growth into the SGR calculation. The GDP grew faster than Part B Medicare expenditures from 1997 to 2000, resulting in positive updates at a rate of at least 4% each year. As the economy began to slow in the early 2000s, the rate of Part B expenditures far exceeded the rate of economic growth. From 2002 to 2013, actual spending far exceeded the projected spending targets, resulting in a negative update for each calendar year. Beginning in 2003, Congress passed legislation each year, called the "doc fix," to avert significant cuts to physician payment.[31] The SGR system was amended in 2003 by the Medicare Modernization Act, which required the per capita GDP rate to be measured on a 10-year average as opposed to an annual rate. Utilization of the MVPS and SGR methodologies has been largely unsuccessful in controlling or affecting the increasing costs and utilization of health care services over the past 25 years.[32]

CASH PAY

A less commonly employed alternative payment model is the cash-pay practice. Under this model, the third-party payer is removed from the equation entirely and the patient pays the physician's professional fees directly out of pocket. Hospital fees and post-acute care charges are variable and depend mostly on prenegotiated rates and the financial structure of the care delivery team. Under some arrangements, the physician's professional fees are paid directly, and the acute care episode remains covered by negotiated private insurance rates. In other settings, the patient's out-of-pocket payment covers the entire episode of care.

It is important to note that under this model, the surgeon cannot continue to bill CMS for care provided to Medicare beneficiaries, as it is illegal for a clinician to charge a separate fee in addition to allowed Part B payments. Instead, the surgeon must opt out of Medicare, which does not mean that they cannot continue to care for Medicare patients, only that the clinician will not submit Part B claims to Medicare for the care provided during cash-pay care. As of January 1, 1998, an amendment to the Social Security Act permits surgeons and their Medicare patients to enter into private written financial contracts.

PROBLEMS WITH FFS

As the US healthcare system continues to grow more rapidly relative to other segments of the economy, multiple problems associated with the FFS system have been recognized by policymakers.[33,34] Traditional FFS reimbursement models incentivize clinicians based on volume and intensity of services, rather than value of care delivered, potentially leading to excessive use of services and increased expenditures.[35] The FFS model does little to incentivize resource stewardship or coordination across clinicians, because separate and unique payment systems exist for hospitals (medical severity-adjusted DRG), physicians (CPT), and clinicians providing postacute care, even when related to a single episode of care. Additionally, the FFS model is blind to patient health outcomes, as payment is rendered for provision of services regardless of the outcome. Consequently, the quality and cost of care for common orthopaedic procedures varies greatly among clinicians under FFS models.[36]

Opponents of FFS models argue that a system based on volume of services provided rather than value delivered to patients provides no incentives for clinicians to reduce or eliminate wasteful spending and/or strive for optimal patient outcomes. Moreover, an FFS system may paradoxically reward poor outcomes, as clinicians caring for patients experiencing adverse events or complications continue to bill for these episodes independently and in addition to the initial treatment. Finally, a system of separate payments for health care encourages the fragmentation of care delivery whereby independent clinicians have little regard for redundant or additional payments to other clinicians for related services.

Given the growing concern that US health care costs are spiraling out of control, the political and economic conditions from 2007 to 2010 encouraged and, in some respects, facilitated the most extensive health care reform in the United States since the enactment of Medicare.[37] On March 23, 2010, President Barack Obama signed the Patient Protection and Affordable Care Act (ACA) into law, with the aims of increasing access to care, reducing the cost of care, and improving the quality of care delivered.[38] Section 3021 of the ACA established the Centers for Medicare & Medicaid Services Innovation Center, charged with developing and studying alternative payment models for physician reimbursement.[39]

SUMMARY

The changes that have taken place in physician reimbursement and payment structures since the beginning of Medicare are reflective of the country's financial priorities. The FFS system is limping along, helped by temporary "doc fixes" that protect physician reimbursement without balancing the budget. Since the passage of the ACA in 2010, the focus of the healthcare system has shifted to value-based care, incentivizing positive outcomes and limiting expenses. Many practices functioning under a pure FFS model have struggled to adapt, as value-based care is fundamentally at odds with an FFS model. As long as the ACA remains the national health care policy, alternative payment models will continue to evolve and will eventually become the status quo, changing the way physicians provide patient care and are compensated for their services.

REFERENCES

1. Porter ME, Kaplan RS: How to pay for health care. *Harv Bus Rev* 2016;94(7-8):88-98, 100, 134.

2. Centers for Medicare & Medicaid Services: History: CMS' program history [Internet]. 2015 [cited November 26, 2016]. Available at: http://www.cms.gov/About-CMS/Agency-Information/History/index.html?redirect=/History. Accessed November 1, 2020.

3. Gornick ME, Warren JL, Eggers PW, et al: Thirty years of Medicare: Impact on the covered population. *Health Care Financ Rev* 1996;18(2):179-237.

4. Chassin MR, Kosecoff J, Park RE, et al: Does inappropriate use explain geographic variations in the use of health care services? A study of three procedures. *J Am Med Assoc* 1987;258(18):2533-2537.

5. Marmour T: *Political Analysis and American Medical Care.* Cambridge University Press, 1983.

6. Stevens R: *In Sickness and in Wealth: American Hospitals in the Twentieth Century.* Johns Hopkins University Press, 1999, p 284.

7. Blumenthal D, Davis K, Guterman S: Medicare at 50 – Origins and evolution. *N Engl J Med* 2015;372(5):479-486.

8. Hsiao WC, Stason WB: Toward developing a relative value scale for medical and surgical services. *Health Care Financ Rev* 1979;1(2):23-38.

9. Hsiao WC, Braun P, Becker ER, et al: *A National Study of Resource-Based Relative Value Scales for Physician Services: Phase I Final Report to the Health Care Financing Administration.* Harvard School of Public Health, 1988.

10. Hsiao WC, Braun P, Becker ER, et al: *A National Study of Resource-Based Relative Value Scales for Physician Services: Phase II Final Report to the Health Care Financing Administration.* Harvard School of Public Health, 1990.

11. Hsiao WC, Braun P, Becker ER, et al: *A National Study of Resource-Based Relative Value Scales for Physician Services: Phase III Final Report to the Health Care Financing Administration.* Harvard School of Public Health, 1992.

12. Kimberly J, de Pouvourville G, d'Aunno T, eds: Origins of DRGs in the United States: A technical, political, and cultural story, in *The Globalization of Managerial Innovation in Health Care.* Cambridge University Press, 2008.

13. Eastaugh SR: Managing risk in a risky world. *J Health Care Finance* 1999;25(3):10-16.

14. Gray WM, Metwalli AM: Tax Equity and Fiscal Responsibility Act of 1982: An incentive to improve productivity in health care. *Health Care Manage Rev* 1987;12(2):31-35.

15. Shih T, Chen LM, Nallamothu BK: Will bundled payments change health care? Examining the evidence thus far in cardiovascular care. *Circulation* 2015;131(24):2151-2158.

16. Chulis GS: Assessing Medicare's prospective payment system for hospitals. *Med Care Rev* 1991;48(2):167-206.

17. White C: Why did Medicare spending growth slow down? *Health Aff (Millwood)* 2008;27(3):793-802.

18. Feinglass J, Holloway JJ: The initial impact of the Medicare prospective payment system on US health care: A review of the literature. *Med Care Rev* 1991;48(1):91-115.

19. Carter GM, Jacobson PD, Kominski GF, Perry MJ: Use of diagnosis-related groups by non-Medicare payers. *Health Care Financ Rev* 1994;16(2):127-158.

20. Centers for Medicare & Medicaid Services: Medicare Acute Care Episode (ACE) Demonstration, 2017. Available at: http://innovation.cms.gov/initiatives/ACE. Accessed February 7, 2023.

21. The Centers for Medicare & Medicaid Services: Medicare program; advancing care coordination through episode payment models (EPMs); cardiac rehabilitation

incentive payment model; and changes to the comprehensive care for joint replacement model (CJR) [Internet]. Available at: https://www.federalregister.gov/documents/2016/08/02/2016-17733/medicare-program-advancing-care-coordinationthrough-episode-paymentmodels-epms-cardiac. Accessed November 1, 2020.

22. Grider DJ: *Coding With Modifiers: A Guide to Correct CPT and HCPCS Level II Modifier Usage*, ed 5. American Medical Association, 2014, xv, p 497.

23. Healthcare.gov: Usual, Customary, and Reasonable (UCR). Available at: https://www.healthcare.gov/glossary/ucr-usual-customary-and-reasonable/#:~:text=The%20amount%20paid%20for%20a,to%20determine%20the%20allowed%20amount. Accessed November 1, 2020.

24. Physician Payment Review Commission: Annual Report to Congress. PPRC, 1988. Available at: https://archive.org/stream/physicianpayment00phys/physicianpayment00phys_djvu.txt. Accessed November 1, 2020.

25. Text of H.R. 3299 (101st): Omnibus Budget Reconciliation Act of 1989. Available at: https://www.govtrack.us/congress/bills/101/hr3299/text. Accessed November 1, 2020.

26. Medicare Program; CY 2022 Payment Policies Under the Physician Fee Schedule and Other Changes to Part B Payment Policies; Medicare Shared Savings Program Requirements; Provider Enrollment Regulation Updates; and Provider and Supplier Prepayment and Post-Payment Medical Review Requirements [Internet]. Available at: https://www.federalregister.gov/documents/2021/11/19/2021-23972/medicare-program-cy-2022-payment-policies-under-the-physician-fee-schedule-and-other-changes-to-part. Accessed April 28, 2023.

27. Hahn J, Mulvey J: *Medicare Physician Payment Updates and the Sustainable Growth Rate (SGR) System*. Congressional Research Service, 2012.

28. Urwin JW, Emanuel EJ: The relative value scale update committee: Time for an update. *J Am Med Assoc* 2019;322(12):1137-1138.

29. The American Medical Association: RBRVS Overview, 2020. Available at: http://www.ama-assn.org/go/rbrvs. Accessed November 1, 2020.

30. Hirsch JA, Rosenkrantz AB, Ansari SA, Manchikanti L, Nicola GN: MACRA 2.0: Are you ready for MIPS? *J Neurointerv Surg* 2017;9(7):714-716.

31. National Council for Behavioral Health: Medicare sustainable growth rate formula and doc fix explained, 2014. Available at: https://www.thenationalcouncil.org/capitol-connector/2014/03/sustainable-growth-rate-formula/. Accessed November 1, 2020.

32. Aaron HJ: Three cheers for logrolling – The demise of the SGR. *N Engl J Med* 2015;372(21):1977-1979.

33. McLawhorn AS, Buller LT: Bundled payments in total joint replacement: Keeping our care affordable and high in quality. *Curr Rev Musculoskelet Med* 2017;10(3):370-377.

34. James BC, Poulsen GP: The case for capitation. *Harv Bus Rev* 2016;94(7-8):102-111, 134.

35. Miller HD: From volume to value: Better ways to pay for healthcare. *Health Aff (Millwood)* 2009;28(5):1418-1428.

36. Tomek IM, Sabel AL, Froimson MI, et al: A collaborative of leading health systems finds wide variations in total knee replacement delivery and takes steps to improve value. *Health Aff (Millwood)* 2012;31(6):1329-1338.

37. Chambers MC, El-Othmani MM, Saleh KJ: Health care reform: Impact on total joint replacement. *Orthop Clin North Am* 2016;47(4):645-652.

38. Gwam CU, Mohamed NS, Etcheson JI, et al: Changes in total knee arthroplasty utilization since the implementation of ACA: An analysis of patient-hospital demographics, costs, and charges. *J Knee Surg* 2020;33(7):636-645.

39. Siddiqi A, White PB, Mistry JB, et al: Effect of bundled payments and health care reform as alternative payment models in total joint arthroplasty: A clinical review. *J Arthroplasty* 2017;32(8):2590-2597.

Pay for Performance

Kevin Wang, MHA • Raquel Mayne, MPH, MS, RN, CPHQ
Catherine H. MacLean, MD, PhD

INTRODUCTION

The purpose of a healthcare system should be to improve the health and functioning of its population;[1] therefore, it makes sense that health care quality has been described by the Institute of Medicine (IOM) as "the degree to which health care services for individuals and populations increase the likelihood of desired health outcomes and are consistent with current professional knowledge."[2] The standard framework for understanding how quality of care can be measured was proposed by Donabedian[3] more than 30 years ago (**Figure 1**). Within this framework, care structures influence care processes, which in turn affect health outcomes. Foundational to the framework is the definition of high-quality medical care as that which is expected to achieve the best balance of health benefits and risks; or medical care that best improves health or prevents health decline. It is important to note that in both definitions, quality is defined not by absolute health outcomes, but rather in terms of the probability of achieving maximal health benefit as a result of the medical care provided. Within the context of these definitions, the IOM has defined six aims for the US healthcare system, which are often used to guide the development and implementation of quality programs.[4] Specifically, health care should be safe, effective, patient-centered, timely, efficient, and equitable (**Table 1**).

RATIONALE FOR INCENTIVIZING QUALITY

The goal of pay-for-performance (P4P) programs is to promote performance improvement and in some cases to also decrease costs. Development of these programs was galvanized by reports demonstrating that health care delivery in the United States can be unsafe and inefficient. In 1999, the IOM published *To Err Is Human*, which estimated that medical errors due to misuse, overuse, or underuse contributed to approximately 100,000 deaths per year.[5] This ranked medical errors as the fifth leading cause of death in the United States after heart disease, cancer, stroke, and chronic lower respiratory disease.[6] In more recent reports, the United

Dr. MacLean or an immediate family member serves as a board member, owner, officer, or committee member of American College of Physicians. Neither of the following authors nor any immediate family member has received anything of value from or has stock or stock options held in a commercial company or institution related directly or indirectly to the subject of this chapter: Kevin Wang and Raquel Mayne.

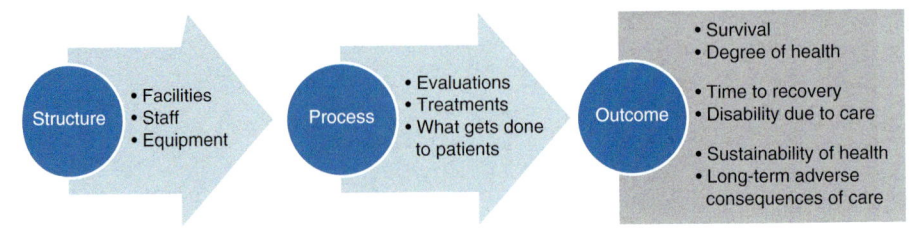

FIGURE 1 Donabedian framework for healthcare quality.

States has been shown to have significantly worse health outcomes than other developed nations.[7] Consistent with these outcomes, as many as 55% of Americans do not receive appropriate evidence-based care from their clinicians.[8] Some reimbursement models may compete against quality improvement goals; for example, capitation may encourage underuse of effective methodologies and fee-for-service (FFS) may encourage overuse of ineffective treatments.[4]

Measuring care quality is important in orthopaedics, for which perioperative and overall complication rates for high-risk surgeries can be as high as 19% and 55%, respectively.[9] Significant variation in orthopaedic outcomes exists across geographic areas.[10,11] Likewise, there is variation in the performance of care processes. For example, the Dartmouth Atlas demonstrates significant geographic variation in hospital discharges for total hip arthroplasty, total knee arthroplasty, and back surgery across the United States.[12] Likewise, the length of time for which patients are prescribed narcotics after surgery can vary by up to 25%.[13] Although some variation can be explained by inconclusive evidence about the efficacy of care

TABLE 1 Institute of Medicine Aims for the US Healthcare System
Safe care: Avoiding harm to patients from the care that is intended to help them
Effective care: Providing services based on scientific knowledge to all who could benefit and refraining from providing services to those not likely to benefit (avoiding underuse and misuse, respectively)
Patient-centered care: Providing care that is respectful of and responsive to individual patient preferences, needs, and values and ensuring that patient values guide all clinical decisions
Timely care: Reducing waits and sometimes harmful delays for both those who receive and those who give care
Efficient care: Avoiding waste, including waste of equipment, supplies, ideas, and energy
Equitable care: Providing care that does not vary in quality because of personal characteristics such as sex, ethnicity, geographic location, and socioeconomic status

processes generally, or for certain populations, there is also variation when the evidence is clear. Approximately 50% of patients with low back pain receive care in accordance with imaging guidelines and best practices,[14] and certain procedures such as knee arthroscopy for osteoarthritis continue to be overutilized despite evidence supporting nonsurgical management.[15]

In 2001, IOM published *Crossing the Quality Chasm*, a 10-year strategy to address the six aims of health care improvement[4] (**Table 1**). Inherent to the strategy was a need for system redesign to ensure that: (1) clinical decision making is aligned with a patient's individual values and the local care delivery level; (2) the most up-to-date science is used in care delivery, and guaranteeing efficient and coordinated care at the healthcare organization level; (3) effective care is delivered across services and settings; and (4) financial, regulatory, and health policy mechanisms would advance the improvement aims.[16]

RATIONALE FOR P4P

For decades, mechanisms to incentivize quality have been used in attempts to improve the quality of patient care. The first movement came from developing quality metrics of outcomes and evidence-based processes to allow for clinician and hospital-level measurement and reporting. The goal of measurement and reporting was to raise awareness of performance, determine baseline performance metrics, and create targets for improvement. However, measurement and reporting alone produced only modest effects and, although necessary, were not sufficient to improve quality.[17]

Financial incentives were introduced as another lever to align clinicians with payers and policymakers to improve the quality of care. P4P programs work by tying financial bonuses and/or penalties to quality measures that are, ideally, meaningful to clinicians and payers or policymakers. These measures are typically based on performing evidence-based processes or achieving an outcome of interest such as decreased complication rates, readmissions, or mortality. One of the benefits of P4P programs is that they offer a way to track measurement and payments. The economic theory of tying financial incentives to clinical care is the hope that clinicians will focus more resources on quality improvement to achieve those bonuses or avoid penalties. By focusing on quality improvement, the care that patients receive will improve and payers will reduce the amount of health care expenditures related to poor-quality care. In the words of a previous administrator for the Centers for Medicare & Medicaid Services (CMS), "You get what you pay for. And we ought to be paying for better quality."[18]

FACTORS THAT AFFECT P4P

The effects of P4P programs on improving quality of care have been mixed. Program design, the size of the incentives and/or penalties, the type of care affected, and the validity of the measures used all can affect program results.

In an international systematic review, P4P was shown to improve compliance with care processes in the short term but did not show substantial effect beyond 3 years.[19] Greater improvement was observed when baseline performance was poor.

The observed effect on patient outcomes was mixed, partially because of the limited availability of rigorous studies.[19]

Many factors may limit the measurable effect of P4P programs. At the most basic level, a paucity of meaningful, validated, and reliable quality measures relevant to a particular program limits how well a program can be assessed. Although improving patient outcomes is the ultimate goal of any quality program, using outcomes to assess the efficacy of a P4P program requires risk adjustment using variables that may not be collected routinely in clinical practice. Additionally, most P4P programs run over a 1-year period, which may not be long enough to achieve optimal outcomes for certain diseases or procedures. Process measures are more easily measured and actionable by physicians, especially over a short time period. However, utilization of measures that physicians do not view as a meaningful representation of the quality of the care they provide can affect not only collection, but also performance on those measures. Additionally, because some measures require volume thresholds, many physicians may not qualify for many metrics.

As a result of the fragmented nature of payments in the United States, physicians may be enrolled in multiple P4P programs using different metrics. This creates administrative complexity for the physician, which can be costly, requiring up to 11 hours a week per orthopaedic surgeon.[20] Some programs also assign accountability to the physician group level, which can diffuse responsibility for overall performance among individual physicians or create frustration with inappropriate attribution.[21]

Programs have a higher chance of success when the outcomes and metrics of focus are clinically meaningful to both patients and clinicians and tap into both extrinsic and intrinsic motivation. In addition, programs should have leadership and organizational support to provide meaningful resources for improvement, including regular, individualized feedback and workflows that facilitate adherence to processes.[22] Practices that lack this support, including many so-called safety net institutions, which have limited financial resources, will be challenged to improve. Because safety net institutions treat a disproportionate share of disadvantaged patients, tying reimbursement to P4P funds that may not be attainable could inadvertently worsen health disparities.

TYPES OF P4P PROGRAMS

P4P refers to a payment model in which financial incentives or penalties are tied to the performance of an individual clinician, clinical group, hospital, or integrated health system. P4P is considered a form of alternative payment model designed to incentivize greater quality of care for patients or an opportunity to reduce overall health care expenditures by promoting appropriate utilization of care.

The Health Care Payment Learning & Action Network (LAN) was established by CMS in 2015 to advance value-based payment models by establishing a forum through which clinicians, consumers, employers, payers, and other stakeholders could engage to accelerate the transition to alternative payment models (APMs). In addition to developing a framework for APMs, the LAN has developed resources to help stakeholders engage successfully in APMs.[23]

The LAN framework categorizes health care payments into four categories (**Figure 2**):

- Category 1: FFS payments for individual encounters and procedures that have no link to quality or value.
- Category 2: FFS linked to quality and value, including pay-for-performance.
- Category 3: APMs with shared savings or downside risk, such as episode-based bundled payments.
- Category 4: Population-based payments, in which an accountable entity manages conditions such as musculoskeletal care for entire populations or provides comprehensive management of an entire population's health such as through global budgets.

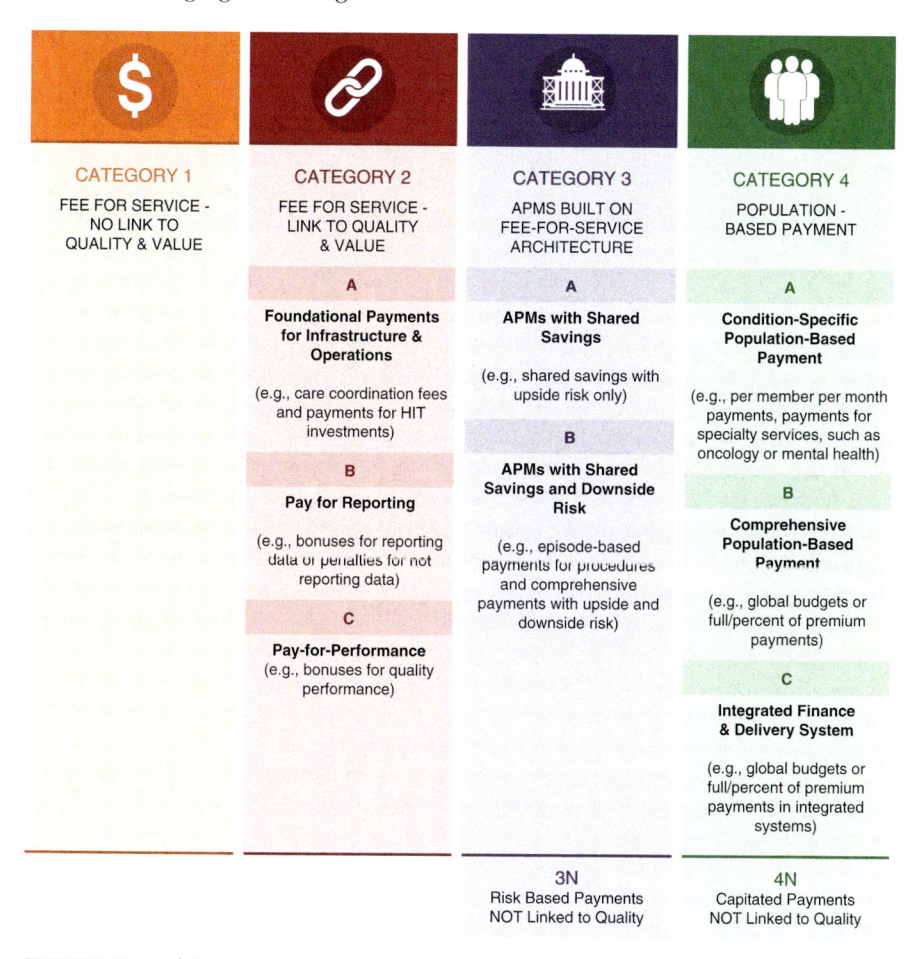

FIGURE 2 Health care payment learning and action network alternative payment model framework. (Reproduced with permission from McCarron D: *Alternative Payment Model (APM) Framework*. Health Care Payment Learning & Action Network, 2017. Available at: https://hcp-lan.org/workproducts/apm-refresh-whitepaper-final.pdf.)

Category 1

Traditional FFS models are those in which there is no relationship between payment and quality. In these models, volume is incentivized and there is no penalty for poor quality. The LAN seeks to develop alternative models to move away from Category 1.

Category 2

In this category, payments remain FFS, but are linked to quality and/or value. Payments in this category span a spectrum from foundational payments to build the infrastructure and operations needed to deliver high value care; to paying for reporting; to P4P on quality metrics. Sequential implementation across this spectrum can ready clinicians for success at each subsequent Category 1 model and eventually for more advanced payment models in Categories 3 and 4.

Foundational incentives might be used to help health systems to acquire electronic medical records or to support the hiring of care managers for chronic disease management programs. Pay-for-reporting requires that clinicians submit quality data to a payer, especially if data are not appropriate for collection via insurance billing claims. Because collecting, processing, and submitting these data may be tedious and involve extra effort, payers can incentivize clinicians by offering a positive or negative incentive for reporting. Examples of this include the inpatient quality program for hospitals, which include submitting data such as chart-abstracted measures for sepsis management or for electronic clinical quality measures for processes such as deep vein thrombosis prophylaxis.

P4P programs build on FFS payments with the addition of payments based on performance on specified quality measures. In some cases, the payment might come in the form of a bonus payment; in others performance might adjust up or down the rates of FFS payments for a group of services. Programs can include multiple types of performance measures, such as clinical outcomes (for example, the rate of infections or readmissions) or include process measures such as delivering antibiotics or adherence to best practices.

Category 3

Although these models are built on a standard FFS payment model, they also include an 'alternative' payment mechanism that is fundamentally different from FFS. These models promote cost-of-care savings, generally offering clinicians an opportunity to share in savings that are achieved. Most programs in this model have a quality gate that must be met to be eligible for the shared savings (models 3A and 3B), although some are based entirely on savings without a quality component (3N). Programs in this model are focused on discrete services (eg, advanced imaging or emergency department visits), procedures (eg, total joint replacement), or care episodes (eg, all care provided from the time of admission for a procedure until 30, 60 or 90 days afterward). Generally, care provided is paid at the usual FFS rate with a retrospective determination of the shared savings based on comparison with a preset baseline. In upside risk-only models (3A), clinicians share the savings with the payer, without risk of penalty if there are no savings or there are excess costs relative to the baseline. Other models (3B) include both upside and downside risk. In these models clinicians are at risk for any excess costs relative to baseline. Models with downside risks are classified as advanced APMs. The original CMS Bundled Payment for Care Improvement (BPCI) model for lower extremity joint replacement was an upside-only model with a quality gate (3A). Bundled Payment for Care Improvement-Advanced and the Comprehensive Care for Joint Replacement Model both have downside risk and a quality gate (3B). Some health plans have advanced imaging management programs with the goal to reduce advanced imaging in certain populations (eg, all patients treated by the clinician or patients with low back pain). There is no quality gate, but clinicians can share in the savings from reduced utilization of advanced imaging (model 3N).

Category 4

Payment in these models is population-based rather than service-based or procedure-based. Clinicians are paid a flat amount of money, typically on a per patient per time period basis, to provide all needed health services for defined populations. The value opportunity for population as opposed to service-based payment is in prevention, avoidance of unnecessary care, and efficiencies from care coordination. In some models the population is defined by conditions (4A). Common examples include so-called specialty carveouts for mental health or oncology. When the population is broad, (eg, all members of a health plan or all employees at a company), the payment model is considered comprehensive (4B). In these models, clinicians are paid either on a per patient per time period basis or are given a global budget, both of which are used to cover all health care costs for that population. Large multispecialty groups such as Optum or Village MD may participate in these models. A further level of efficiency can be obtained when there is integration across the finance and care delivery systems (4C), such as with Kaiser Permanente. These models have some type of quality performance standards, though they vary. For example, a plan paying for a specialty carveout or comprehensive population management may define some minimal level of quality to obtain or retain the contract. Likewise, an employer could require some level of quality from entities that are integrated across finance and care delivery. Population payment models that have no quality requirements would be classified as a 4N model.

Ideally, performance measures for P4P programs should be mutually agreed on by both the payer and the clinician within the program. Likewise, measures should meet criteria for being valid, reliable, and meaningful and be validated by consensus-based entities such as the National Quality Forum. Transparency about how quality is defined in relation to payment incentives could allow clinicians and payers to emphasize which funds should be used to achieve the best possible health outcomes and encouraging accountability. These payment models are typically easier to administer because they build on existing FFS payment infrastructure, allowing both the clinicians and the payers to determine the overall incentives owed.

SURVEY OF US P4P PROGRAMS

A 2019 report on the state of alternate payment models found that 25.1% of US insurance payments were linked to Category 2, P4P programs, whereas 35.8% of US insurance payments were linked to Category 3, shared savings, bundled payment, or population-based payments.[24]

Some of the most widely known P4P programs are administered via CMS. As the country's largest payer, CMS has developed hospital-focused and physician-focused P4P programs: Hospital Value-Based Purchasing, Hospital Readmissions Reduction Program, Hospital-Acquired Conditions Reduction Program, and Merit-based Incentive Payment System (MIPS).

Hospital Value-Based Purchasing was created in 2010 as part of the Affordable Care Act. Hospitals are held accountable for composite performance across several domains, each receiving an even weight including the patient experience, mortality, safety, and efficiency. Measures related to orthopaedic surgery include total hip/knee complication rates, patient satisfaction, hospital-acquired infections, and Medicare spending per beneficiary, an aggregate cost-efficiency measure. Hospital performance is measured relative to peers based on a hospital's relative improvement from prior years or absolute performance against other hospitals, with CMS using whichever score is generally higher. Incentive payments or penalties are generated by withholding 2% of a hospital's total Medicare payments in 1 year. This creates a total pool in which hospitals can be paid or receive penalties, a process known as a budget-neutral approach in which CMS does not need to create additional funds for incentives. Hospitals that score above a relative threshold will receive additional payments on top of the 2% of payments that were withheld, whereas hospitals that score below the threshold will not receive the entire 2% of payments back from CMS. The threshold changes depending on the performance scores for all hospitals in a specific year. One study showed that hospitals did not have significant improvement, except for reduction in mortality for patients admitted with pneumonia.[25]

MIPS was enacted in 2017 as part of the CMS Quality Payment Program. It is one of the only P4P programs that specifically focuses on physicians or physician groups. In this program, physicians are held accountable for performance across four domains, including quality, improvement activities, promoting interoperability, and cost. Physicians are given significant flexibility to choose their specific quality measures, with up to 40 measures applicable to orthopaedic surgery, ranging from documentation of advance care planning to patient-reported outcomes after surgery, to the use of prophylactic antibiotics. Physicians must report on at least six quality measures, many of which can be collected from the electronic health record. Improvement activities require physicians to attest to performing specific actions with the goal of improving quality or outcomes. Promoting interoperability require physicians to use the electronic health record in meaningful ways with a patient or their other clinicians. Cost is measured by CMS directly as a way of improving cost efficiency for care, which can be procedure specific. Scores for all four domains are aggregated to an overall physician performance score. Each year,

CMS sets a performance threshold. Physicians with performance scores above the threshold will receive financial incentives in the form of a positive payment adjustment for Medicare professional fees. Physicians with scores below the threshold receive a penalty in the form of a negative payment adjustment. CMS designed this program to be budget-neutral, as is value-based purchasing, so that any penalties are redistributed as financial incentives for those who score above the threshold. In a 2018 review of quality measures used in MIPS, the American College of Physicians' Performance Measures Committee found that up to one-third of quality measures were not valid.[26] A significant criticism of the MIPS program has been that the flexibility in choosing measures has created some confusion and significant burden on clinicians. Physicians who are part of large health systems have significantly higher performance scores than independent clinicians,[27] perhaps due to systemwide infrastructures designed to maximize performance on MIPS. At the same time, physicians with a greater proportion of socially disadvantaged patients also had lower MIPS scores.[28]

Many commercial health care plans have made a commitment to value-based care and APMs, though they lag behind those of CMS. In 2019, 14.2% of commercial payments were tied to Category 2 P4P models.[24] Many commercial health plans have instead focused on the shared savings model, either with primary care physicians as part of patient-centered medical homes or accountable care organizations, where clinicians help to reduce spending while maintaining or improving quality. Many surgical or procedural specialists may be engaged through bundled payments, where shared savings can be generated by specialists overseeing a patient's entire episode of care, or through placement in tiered networks or via a hospital's designation as a center of excellence with preferential rates or the potential for increased volume.

Commercial insurers typically will organize P4P programs around quality measures that are either externally validated or internally developed. Performance measures may include in-hospital adverse events, 30-day readmission rates, or length of stay. Regional markets may also have the capability to independently add additional measures that can be discussed between the insurer and clinical groups. For example, United Healthcare has a P4P program called the Quality-Based Physician Incentive Program that focuses on quality metrics as well as performing clinically appropriate procedures at designated facilities.[29] Quality metrics include the incidence of wrong site/side/procedure/patient/implants, incidence of patient burns, proportion of patients with appropriate prophylactic antibiotic timing, surgical site infection rates, rate of unplanned transfers, and unplanned rates of return to the operating room.

However, most commercial plan-sponsored physician-based P4P programs focus on care delivered by primary care physicians. This is in part driven by the interest of plans to perform well on population-level Healthcare Effectiveness Data and Information Set (HEDIS) measures, which are heavily skewed toward primary care. Developed and administered through the National Committee for Quality Assurance, performance on HEDIS measures are used by employers to inform health plan purchasing.[30] For example, Aetna's physician P4P programs[31] such as its Better Health P4P program, include a combination of HEDIS measures and customized measures defined by clinicians.[32] Aetna plans provides detailed information on individual physician performance for each agreed-on measure. Measures may be retired and replaced after several periods of top-level performance. Likewise, the Blue Cross Blue Shield Physician Group Incentive Program rewards physicians, generally primary care physicians, for achieving improvements in multiple areas including process, efficiency, clinical quality outcomes, infrastructure, and patient safety performance measures.[33]

P4P programs can also exist as part of a physician's compensation or via gain-sharing programs within hospitals or medical groups. Bundled payment programs such as the CMS Comprehensive Care for Joint Replacement or Bundled Payments for Care Improvement-Advanced programs have allowed for exceptions to traditional anti-kickback and Stark law restrictions to allow hospitals to share in financial rewards with hospitals. Hospitals are required to ensure that physicians meet quality measures or annual goals are met before disbursing any potential incentive awards.

PRINCIPLES FOR SUCCESSFUL PROGRAMS

From the start, clinicians should have a meaningful role in designing P4P programs. The financial incentives should be consequential enough to have an effect, and historically have ranged from 1% to 3% of payments. Penalties may be included, although clinicians should carefully work with actuarial firms such as Milliman to model the impact. These actuarial firms can help to determine whether participation is warranted based on historical performance and finances.

To be successful, orthopaedic surgeons should agree on clearly defined and clinically meaningful quality measures. Unlike clinical guidelines, quality measures must leave no room for interpretation and allow exclusions from denominators for cases where care patterns warrant variation. These quality measures must also be fair and accurate. It is also important to ensure that any outcome measures, such as complication or readmission rates, be risk-adjusted to prevent adverse selection of patients. Doing so can help ensure equity of care. Many agreements also allow for programs to be 3 to 5 years in duration. A longer time range with annual goals being discussed at each point allows for incremental improvement over time, especially if measures have a significant data lag. Finally, clinicians should carefully monitor how measures and patients are attributed. Some measures may only have been validated and endorsed for reporting at an institutional level. Shifting accountability to an individual surgeon, such as in the case of infection rates, may be inappropriate, as prevention of infection may be the responsibility of an entire care team. It is also important to determine how patients are attributed, especially in some measures that monitor cost efficiency, which many times are assigned to the physician who has the plurality of claims for an individual patient.

Clinicians must also have the infrastructure available to understand historical patterns of performance and have up-to-date information on their current performance. Many quality measures are calculated using administrative data such as insurance claims. Because of any potential time lag, it may not always be possible to receive real-time feedback. Insurers will typically provide annual feedback reports. For example, CMS will send hospitals annual reports on performance as well as individual case information to verify any patient complications. These data are important to review and identify any opportunities for quality improvement or to confirm as a complication. In some cases, insurers may share claims data. Using a data aggregator, such as a Datagen, to process this information is helpful in gaining insights into performance. Many new quality measures also use data directly from the electronic health record. Analysts can use the specifications for these quality measures to create reports that will be more meaningful to monitor performance and identify areas for improvement. One difficulty that orthopaedic surgeons may have is prioritizing the development and feedback of these reports, especially in larger health systems that have competing demands for analytical staff and infrastructure. Ensuring consistent and accurate reporting is important, especially if specific measures are self-reported to an insurer at the end of a reporting period.

SUMMARY

Given the poor health outcomes experienced by Americans along with known care gaps, improving the care quality is of urgent importance. Despite decades of effort, progress has been slow in preventing patient harm and reducing unnecessary variation in care delivery. If properly deployed, P4P could accelerate quality improvement by linking financial incentives or penalties to physician and hospital payments. In 2019, up to one-fourth of all payments were tied to some form of P4P programs, although many of these programs have shown little improvement in patient outcomes. For success, clinicians should have meaningful engagement in the design and execution of P4P programs understanding the financial consequences and opportunities; selecting meaningful quality measures; and participating in the design and monitoring of quality improvement programs.

REFERENCES

1. President's Advisory Commission on Consumer Protection and Quality in the Health Care Industry. Available at: https://govinfo.library.unt.edu/hcquality/. Accessed May 5, 2023.

2. Lohr KN, Schroeder SA: A strategy for quality assurance in medicare. *N Engl J Med* 1990;322(10):707-712.

3. Donabedian A: *Explorations in Quality Assessment and Monitoring. The Definition of Quality and Approaches to Its Assessment*. Health Administration Press, 1980, vol 1.

4. Institute of Medicine (US) Committee on Quality of Health Care in America: *Crossing the Quality Chasm: A New Health System for the 21st Century*. National Academies Press (US), 2001. Available at: http://www.ncbi.nlm.nih.gov/books/NBK222274/. Accessed May 5, 2023.

5. Institute of Medicine (US) Committee on Quality of Health Care in America; Kohn LT, Corrigan JM, Donaldson MS, eds: *To Err Is Human: Building a Safer Health System*. National Academies Press, 2000. Available at: http://www.ncbi.nlm.nih.gov/books/NBK225182/. Accessed May 5, 2023.

6. NCHS Data Visualization Gallery - Leading Causes of Death in the United States, 2020. Available at: https://www.cdc.gov/nchs/data-visualization/mortality-leading-causes/index.htm. Accessed May 5, 2023.

7. U.S. Health Care from a Global Perspective. Commonwealth Fund, 2022. Available at: https://www.commonwealthfund.org/publications/issue-briefs/2023/jan/us-health-care-global-perspective-2022. Accessed May 5, 2023.

8. McGlynn EA, Asch SM, Adams J, et al: The quality of health care delivered to adults in the United States. *N Engl J Med* 2003;348(26):2635-2645.

9. Sciubba DM, Yurter A, Smith JS, et al: A comprehensive review of complication rates after surgery for adult deformity: A reference for informed consent. *Spine Deform* 2015;3(6):575-594.

10. Garriga C, Leal J, Sánchez-Santos MT, et al: Geographical variation in outcomes of primary hip and knee replacement. *JAMA Netw Open* 2019;2(10):e1914325.

11. Desai A, Bekelis K, Ball PA, et al: Variation in outcomes across centers after surgery for lumbar stenosis and degenerative spondylolisthesis in the spine patient outcomes research trial. *Spine (Phila Pa 1976)* 2013;38(8):678-691.

12. Surgical Discharges. Dartmouth Atlas of Health Care. Available at: https://www.dartmouthatlas.org/interactive-apps/surgical-discharges/. Accessed May 5, 2023.

13. Boylan MR, Suchman KI, Slover JD, Bosco JA: Patterns of narcotic prescribing by orthopedic surgeons for Medicare patients. *Am J Med Qual* 2018;33(6):637-641.

14. Chou R, Qaseem A, Owens DK, Shekelle P; Clinical Guidelines Committee of the American College of Physicians: Diagnostic imaging for low back pain: Advice for high-value health care from the American College of Physicians. *Ann Intern Med* 2011;154(3):181-189.

15. Adelani MA, Harris AHS, Bowe TR, Giori NJ: Arthroscopy for knee osteoarthritis has not decreased after a clinical trial. *Clin Orthop Relat Res* 2016;474(2):489-494.

16. Berwick DM: A user's manual for the IOM's "Quality Chasm" report. *Health Aff (Millwood)* 2002;21(3):80-90.

17. McGlynn EA: Improving the quality of U.S. health care—What will it take? *N Engl J Med* 2020;383(9):801-803.

18. Why Doctors so Often Get It Wrong. *The New York Times*. Available at: https://www.nytimes.com/2006/02/22/business/why-doctors-so-often-get-it-wrong.html. Accessed May 5, 2023.

19. Mendelson A, Kondo K, Damberg C, et al: The effects of pay-for-performance programs on health, health care use, and processes of care: A systematic review. *Ann Intern Med* 2017;166(5):341-353.

20. Casalino LP, Gans D, Weber R, et al: US physician practices spend more than $15.4 billion annually to report quality measures. *Health Aff (Millwood)* 2016;35(3):401-406.

21. Christianson JB, Knutson DJ, Mazze RS: Physician pay-for-performance. Implementation and research issues. *J Gen Intern Med* 2006;21(suppl 2):S9-S13.

22. Michtalik HJ, Carolan HT, Haut ER, et al: Use of provider-level dashboards and pay-for-performance in venous thromboembolism prophylaxis. *J Hosp Med* 2015;10(3):172-178.

23. McCarron D: *Alternative Payment Model (APM) Framework*. Health Care Payment Learning & Action Network, 2017. Available at: https://hcp-lan.org/workproducts/apm-refresh-whitepaper-final.pdf. Accessed May 8, 2023.

24. APM Measurement Progress of Alternative Payment Models. Available at: https://hcp-lan.org/workproducts/apm-methodology-2019.pdf. Accessed May 5, 2023.

25. Ryan AM, Krinsky S, Maurer KA, Dimick JB: Changes in hospital quality associated with hospital value-based purchasing. *N Engl J Med* 2017;376(24):2358-2366.

26. MacLean CH, Kerr EA, Qaseem A: Time out – Charting a path for improving performance measurement. *N Engl J Med* 2018;378(19):1757-1761.

27. Johnston KJ, Wiemken TL, Hockenberry JM, Figueroa JF, Joynt Maddox KE: Association of clinician health system affiliation with outpatient performance ratings in the Medicare merit-based incentive payment system. *J Am Med Assoc* 2020;324(10):984-992.

28. Khullar D, Schpero WL, Bond AM, Qian Y, Casalino LP: Association between patient social risk and physician performance scores in the first year of the merit-based incentive payment system. *J Am Med Assoc* 2020;324(10):975-983.

29. Quality-Based Physician Incentive Program (QPIP). Available at: https://www.uhcprovider.com/en/reports-quality-programs/qpip-reports.html. Accessed May 5, 2023.

30. HEDIS and Performance Measurement. National Committee for Quality Assurance. Available at: https://www.ncqa.org/hedis/. Accessed May 5, 2023.

31. Provider manual: Resources, policies and procedures at your fingertips. Available at: https://www.aetna.com/content/dam/aetna/pdfs/aetnacom/health-care-professionals/office_manual_hcp.pdf. Accessed May 5, 2023.

32. 2022 Aetna Better Health Provider Pay-for-Performance (P4P) Proposal Template. https://www.aetnabetterhealth.com/content/dam/aetna/medicaid/pennsylvania/provider/pdf/abhpa_provider_pay-for-performance_letter.pdf. Accessed January 1, 2022.

33. Physician Group Incentive Program. Available at: https://www.bcbsm.com/amslibs/content/dam/public/providers/documents/value/physician-group-incentive-program-basics.pdf. Accessed May 4, 2023.

Episodic Bundled Payment Models

Christopher Doria Skeehan, MD, FAAOS
James D. Slover, MD, MS, FAAOS
Ran Schwarzkopf, MD, MSc, FAAOS

INTRODUCTION

Currently, total joint arthroplasty (TJA) is one of the most successful surgical procedures performed, generating 2.07 and 1.85 lifetime quality-adjusted life years per patient for total hip arthroplasty (THA) and total knee arthroplasty (TKA), respectively.[1] Although extremely effective at improving the lives of patients, the annual combined cost of these procedures accounts for more than $7 billion from the Centers for Medicare & Medicaid Services (CMS). This represents 1% to 2% of the entire CMS annual payouts to physicians and hospitals and is the single greatest procedural cost to the agency.[2] In 2014, approximately 1 million primary TKAs and THAs were performed in the United States, with nearly 2 million annual procedures anticipated by 2030.[3,4] Although orthopaedic surgeons' Part B payments represent only 12% of the total reimbursement for THA and TKA, surgeons control approximately 90% of the cost of care through clinical decision making and orders.[5] In an attempt to encourage surgeons and hospitals to become better financial stewards of patient care, the US Congress empowered CMS with new legislation to create novel alternative payment models (APMs) for the delivery of TJA.

THE DEVELOPMENT OF BUNDLED CARE IN THE UNITED STATES

In an effort to contain the cost of surgical care, CMS developed the concept of APMs through the Affordable Care Act of 2010. In 2015, the Sustained Growth Rate was repealed and replaced by the Medicare and CHIP Reauthorization Act

Dr. Slover or an immediate family member is a member of a speakers' bureau or has made paid presentations on behalf of Pacira; serves as a paid consultant to or is an employee of Horizon Pharma; has received research or institutional support from Biomet and Smith & Nephew; and serves as a board member, owner, officer, or committee member of American Academy of Orthopaedic Surgeons, AJRR Hip Society Steering Comm Member, American Association of Hip and Knee Surgeons, Hip Society, and PCORI Advisor Board Shared Decsion Making. Dr. Schwarzkopf or an immediate family member has received royalties from Smith & Nephew; serves as a paid consultant to or is an employee of Intelijoint, Smith & Nephew, and Zimmer; has stock or stock options held in Gauss surgical, Intelijoint, and PSI; has received research or institutional support from Smith & Nephew; and serves as a board member, owner, officer, or committee member of American Academy of Orthopaedic Surgeons and American Association of Hip and Knee Surgeons. Neither Dr. Skeehan nor any immediate family member has received anything of value from or has stock or stock options held in a commercial company or institution related directly or indirectly to the subject of this chapter.

(MACRA) which replaced the Sustained Growth Rate with Quality Payment Programs. Two pathways within the framework of Quality Payment Programs were the Merit-Based Incentive Payment System (MIPS) and APMs.

MIPS consolidated three already existing value-based fee-for-service programs into one. The program created four performance categories that would generate a final score that was used to adjust hospital or clinician reimbursement. MIPS was developed to be budget neutral, so both negative and positive adjustments to reimbursement were limited to 4% of the original rate. In contrast, APMs are a payment approach that gives added incentive payments to provide high-value care. APMs can provide structure that can apply a specific clinical condition, a care episode, or a population.[6]

What is Episodic Bundled Care?

Episodic bundled care is an APM where a triggered episode of care (EOC) is the basis for the treatment of a patient condition. All costs of care during the episode are tallied and any savings below a predetermined target price are shared with clinicians. Additionally, any expenses over the target price are assessed as penalties to the clinician. Therefore, the clinician or organization assumes risk, with responsibility for both the cost and outcomes of the care delivered during the EOC. Spending below the preset target price can establish eligibility for incentive payments, while spending above the target price will result in the clinician or organization being found financially accountable for the difference. APMs include the Bundled Payments for Care Improvement (BPCI), the Comprehensive Care for Joint Replacement (CJR), and the Advanced Bundled Payments for Care Improvement (BPCI Advanced).

Bundled Payments for Care Improvement

The CMS BPCI was established in 2011. This was a voluntary episodic bundled care program created "to improve patient care through payment innovation that fosters improved coordination and quality through a patient-centered approach."[7] It was considered an introduction to value-based payment systems in which hospitals or clinicians could pick the type of procedure or medical treatment to be included in the bundle. BPCI provided a flat target price that included all services rendered 72 hours prior to admission, any acute care services, and any services during the 90-day postacute period. This postadmission period included all postacute care services, such as rehabilitation and readmission costs that were related to the initial Medicare severity diagnosis-related group (MS-DRG) that triggered the episode. Most readmissions were considered related, with some studies demonstrating 92% of all readmissions were considered related.[8] A few separate unrelated procedures were excluded from the bundle. As part of the program, CMS also audited charges that occurred between 90 and 120 days to ensure services were not being delayed to avoid the bundle.

Participants in BPCI could choose from one of four models for reimbursement:

- Model 1: Retrospective payments for acute care hospital stays only, where a hospital was paid a discounted amount based on the inpatient prospective

payment system rates for specific MS-DRGs while physicians were paid separately under the Medicare physician fee schedule (PFS).
- Model 2/3: A retrospective bundled payment arrangement where expenditures were quarterly reconciled against an EOC's target price.
  - Model 2: Acute and postacute care
  - Model 3: Postacute care only
- Model 4: A prospective bundled payment that encompassed all services performed by the hospital and clinicians during an EOC that lasted the entire patient stay.[7]

Model 2 was the most popular model utilized for lower extremity joint replacement (LEJR). BPCI for LEJR was initiated in two phases. Phase 1 commenced on January 1, 2013, which allowed participants to develop patient care pathways and cost savings measures prior to assuming full financial risk in phase 2. Phase 2 commenced on July 1, 2015, with phase 1 ending on September 30, 2015. Phase 2 was extended and completed on September 20, 2018.

Comprehensive Care for Joint Replacement

On April 1, 2016, the next iteration of bundled care, the CJR commenced. This was an involuntary program for those hospitals already enrolled in BPCI as well as other hospitals in 67 different metropolitan service areas. The program was proposed to end on December 31, 2020, but was extended for an additional 3 years in June 2020. On December 1, 2017, CMS excluded involuntary enrollment for rural hospitals and hospitals in 33 of the 67 metropolitan service areas, allowing clinicians to opt out of the program. Unlike BPCI, CJR included only MS-DRG 469 and 470 (Major Joint Replacement or Reattachment of Lower Extremity with or without major complications or comorbidities) with incorporation of ICD10 diagnosis codes for hip fracture into the target price. Similar to BPCI, participating hospitals were financially accountable for the quality and cost of the care rendered during the bundled period. Payments were made to the hospital following the standard fee-for-service model. Target prices for years 1 through 3 were established based on the hospital's historic standardized spending and regional historical standardized spending. Target prices incorporated a 3% discount to create initial savings. Years 4 and 5 target prices were entirely based on regional pricing. CMS would perform an annual audit of the total expenditures for services rendered under Parts A and B, compare those against the target price, and based on the cost award the hospital additional payments or penalize them for overpayment. Quality metrics were used to alter the 3% discount rate and increase the savings for hospitals that performed well to ensure quality was maintained. This was accomplished by using a CMS CJR composite quality score. Those hospitals with higher quality scores would see a reduction in the discount rate from 3% to 1.5%. These quality bonuses were provided if the score was in the top 70th percentile in years 1 to 3 and top 60th percentile years 4 to 5 against the regional standard. Fifty percent of the quality score represented the NQF#1550 for hospital-level risk standardized complication rate following elective THA/TKA, 40% the NQF#0166

HCAHPS (Hospital Consumer Assessment of Healthcare Providers and Systems) survey, and 10% the voluntary THA/TKA patient-reported outcomes (PROs). In 2015, stakeholders recognized Hip dysfunction and Osteoarthritis Outcome Score for Joint Replacement/Knee dysfunction and Osteoarthritis Outcome Score for Joint Replacement and PROMIS Global Health or the Veterans RAND 12-Item Health Survey as acceptable PRO scores for reporting.[5] From 2016 to 2020, the target price for an uncomplicated LEJR without femoral neck fracture in the CJR program decreased by 2.9% to 6.6%, depending on the region. Although this decrease in target price demonstrates that increases in efficiency can result in decreases in the regional cost per EOC for LEJR, continued decreases in target prices each year are quickly approaching a floor where participating institutions are no longer able to earn a net income from participation in bundled payments programs.

CJR did not initially include outpatient LEJR in bundles. The removal of TKA and THA from the inpatient-only list in 2018 and 2020 allowed clinicians to bill CMS using the outpatient prospective payment system instead of the inpatient prospective payment system. This avoided triggering a bundle with an anchor MS-DRG 469/470 hospitalization. With healthier, younger patients having procedures being performed as outpatients, this meant that those patients entering into bundles would be more infirm, medically complex, surgically complex, and/or older. Recently CMS released proposed rule CMS-5529-P, which extends CJR for an additional 3 years beyond the earlier end date of December 31, 2020. In addition to extending the program, the new rule will establish a blended rate MS-DRG 470 without hip fracture combining both outpatient and inpatient TKA/THA.

Although most patients who were enrolled in BPCI and CJR underwent LEJR for primary or secondary osteoarthritis, bundles could also include LEJR for patients with hip fractures, musculoskeletal tumors, and revision LEJR. Althausen and Mead[9] demonstrated that hip fractures were more costly to treat in the bundle and therefore represented a greater financial liability in the bundled payment model for participating hospitals. Lott et al[10,11] demonstrated that despite decreases in length of stay, readmission, cost of care per episode, and increased discharges to home, hip fracture patients still had a total cost of care while utilizing an established BPCI pathway of $49,993 per EOC. CJR accounted for this by separating the fractures from the nonfractures and creating a different target price, allowing institutions to successfully treat these patients using the bundled payment system. Gammal et al[12] reviewed an administrative claims database within their hospital system for the oncologic and nononcologic cost of an EOC. They found the average cost of an oncologic EOC necessitating THA was $43,771 versus $23,779 for a nononcologic EOC. THA performed for oncologic reasons was also found to be an independent risk factor for greater EOC costs. Although not commonplace, some institutions opted to include revision LEJR in their bundled care arrangement. Courtney et al[13] examined the appropriateness of bundles for revision LEJR. Although revision LEJR performed in a bundle did demonstrate a reduced length of stay compared to the prebundled cohort, the LEJR revision bundled group received less reimbursement from CMS for the index hospitalization with equivalent costs of care.

BPCI Advanced

The third CMS iteration of episodic bundled care in the United States is BPCI Advanced. This program started accepting its first cohorts on October 1, 2018, and its second cohorts on January 1, 2020. CMS made BPCI Advanced a voluntary program. Participation would exempt physicians from MIPS, but those hospitals already enrolled in CJR were not allowed to switch to BPCI Advanced. Enrollment criteria included an electronic medical record system, payments based on MIPS comparable quality measures, and entities willing to bear more than nominal financial risk. Similar to CJR, BPCI Advanced was a single retrospective bundled payment system with a 90-day EOC duration. Target pricing was calculated from the regional cost average, then a 3% cost savings discount was applied by CMS to set the price. Instead of just including MS-DRG 469/470 as does CJR, BPCI Advanced included 31 inpatient and 4 outpatient clinical episodes starting at model year 3. The clinical episodes included were back and neck except spinal fusion, double joint replacement of the lower extremity, fractures of the femur and hip or pelvis, hip and femur procedures except major joint, lower extremity/humerus procedure except hip, foot, femur, major joint replacement of the lower extremity, major joint replacement of the upper extremity, and spinal fusion. The program exempted hospitals from the reporting requirements associated with MIPS and qualified them for incentive payments. Payments would ultimately be tied to quality metrics. For years 1 through 3, those included all-cause hospital readmissions, hospital-level complication rates, hospital 30-day all-cause mortality rates, advanced care plans, and some perioperative care metrics, including selection of prophylactic antibiotic, excess days in acute care, and CMS patient safety indicators. During year 4, alternative quality measures would be available to use instead of the administrative quality measures, including five claims-based and registry-based measures as well as all-cause readmission and advanced care plan. Preliminary target prices were provided prior to each model year.

OUTCOMES OF EPISODIC BUNDLED CARE FOR HIP AND KNEE REPLACEMENT

The Bundled Payments Care Initiative and the follow-up program CJR were successful in achieving their goals of containing the cost of TJA, seeing significant reductions in the cost per EOC while maintaining or improving outcomes[13-16] and improving hospital efficiency. In a systematic review by Agarwal et al,[15] the authors noted that the bundled care programs were effective at maintaining quality while reducing cost of LEJR EOCs, but not other conditions. Most notably, Dummit et al[17] who reported that those hospitals performing in BPCI relative to control hospitals reduced their EOC cost for TJA by $3,286 versus $2,119 in the control hospitals. After the first 2 years of CJR, Barnett et al[18] found a 3.1% decrease in the cost to perform LEJR relative to those performed immediately prior to the implementation of the program.

Early participants in the program developed strategies to reduce costs to less than the initial target episode price set by CMS, were better positioned to retain financial solvency when performing LEJRs on the Medicare population in future iterations of the program and in other bundled payment plans. For example, at a single, large urban, academic, tertiary care hospital, reforms were targeted at reducing readmissions, reducing the length of stay, reducing implant/supply/drug costs, reducing the time spent in the operating room, changing the discharge disposition of patients to more cost-efficient alternatives, and decreasing the use of unnecessary testing or consultations.[8] These goals were achieved by developing standardized clinical pathways that directed the care of more than 90% of patients with LEJR, with exclusion from the pathways directed by set criteria rather than physician preference. Clinical care coordinators were hired to oversee patient involvement and facilitate adherence to the pathways, facilitate care at transition points, and provide a communication pathway from patients to clinicians.[8] At the same institution, those interventions resulted in the average length of stay decreasing from 4.27 to 3.58 days, discharges to inpatient facilities decreased from 65% in 2012 to 44% in 2013, and readmissions decreased from 17% in 2011 to 11% in 2013.[19] Furthermore, from 2013 to 2016, during that same institution's involvement in BPCI, the length of stay decreased from 3.58 to 2.96 days. Discharges to an inpatient rehabilitation facility decreased from 44% to 28%, the 90-day all-cause readmission rate decreased from 13% to 8% and the cost per EOC decreased by 20%, demonstrating continued improvement is possible.[20] As a result, in February 2020, CMS issued proposed rule CMS-5529-P, which extended the program for an additional 3 years. It also proposed reforms to the process of target price reconciliation, risk adjustment for hip fractures by proposing the creation of a new MS-DRG for LEJR for hip fractures, and the inclusion of outpatient LEJR into bundles.[21]

FACTORS THAT CAN INFLUENCE PATIENT OUTCOMES IN EPISODIC BUNDLED CARE

One of the challenges for success in bundled payment models has been the lack of risk adjustment of target payments for the diversity of patients that enter into bundles. BPCI and CJR provide two risk-adjusted categories, LEJR with and without major comorbidities. CJR added additional risk adjustment by including a third pathway for hip fractures that was also implemented in BPCI Advanced.

To maximize quality and minimize complications, clinicians are incentivized to consider patient risk profiles carefully and to optimize their condition where they can in order to have success in the bundle. The effect of chronic medical conditions on length of stay, risk of readmission, and the cost for an EOC can be significant. Rozell et al[22] found that preoperative narcotic use, heart failure, stroke, chronic kidney disease, chronic obstructive pulmonary disease, Charlton Comorbidity Index greater than 5, and liver disease were more likely to require hospitalization of greater than 3 days, whereas chronic kidney disease and chronic obstructive pulmonary disease were independent risk factors for a length of stay longer than 3 days. Similarly, Phillips et al[23] examined the cost and risk factors for readmission after primary LEJR. They found a mean readmission rate of 6.1%, of which 79.7% were medically related. Independent risk factors for readmission were age older than 75 years, body mass index greater than 35 kg/m^2, history of congestive heart failure, diabetes mellitus, and renal disease. Urish et al[24] examined the national readmission database for the effect on the 30-day EOC cost of readmission after primary TKA. They found a readmission rate of 4%, with the median cost of readmission being $6,753. Risk factors for readmission were congestive heart failure, chronic kidney disease, and length of stay longer than 4 midnights. In addition, readmissions that required revision surgery resulted in an overall cost of care of $52,162 versus $18,514 for those that did not require revision surgery, highlighting the need to reduce complications that require additional surgery. Clair et al[25] were also able to quantify the cost of readmissions for THA and TKA patients involved in the BPCI bundle. Surgical complications that required readmission, excluding a single outlier, had a mean cost of $36,038 for THA and $27,979 for TKA. Medical complications requiring readmissions were $22,775 for THA and $24,283 for TKA. In addition, when examining the treatment of osteoarthritis of the knee and hip with LEJR, Bernstein et al[26] looked at the cost of a 90-day EOC for TKA versus THA. The study found that the mean 90-day EOC cost for TKA was $1,998 more than that of a THA EOC. Patients of lower socioeconomic status can also consume more hospital resources than those patients on private insurance. Courtney et al[27,28] found that patients of lower socioeconomic status with Medicaid insurance had more medical comorbidities, needed a longer acute care length of stay, were more likely to be discharged to a rehabilitation facility, and were at greater risk of 90-day readmission versus privately insured patients. Medicaid insurance was a significant independent risk factor for increased hospital costs with an odds ratio of 3.64.

Optimization of preoperative comorbidities is critical to controlling the cost of an EOC by reducing the number of complications and readmissions. For example, Karas et al[29] examined the preoperative profile of medical comorbidities and subsequent 90-day global Medicare payments for TJA prior to the patient's hospital enrolling into CJR to examine anticipated cost of an EOC. On average, alcoholism, anemia, diabetes, and obesity increased the cost of a 90-day EOC from between $1,425 to $9,308.

As a result of these factors, there has been some concern that performance incentives could cause clinicians to preferentially treat younger, healthier patients and to minimize treatment for older, more complex, and more infirm patients.[30] This could threaten access to these procedures to certain patient populations. Cairns et al[31] thought that better risk stratification is needed based not only on diagnosis, but also on socioeconomic status and general health. Increased risk stratification could be used to adequately compensate physicians and hospitals for more difficult cases and help prevent restriction in access to care of these procedures that substantially improve quality of life. Currently, there is limited evidence to suggest this actually occurs. Two studies on the delivery of care during CJR performed at a single large tertiary academic medical center noted no change in differential/biased patient selection after CJR bundle implementation.[32,33] Both studies also noted that the cost for care remained the same despite cost savings and efficiency metrics imposed.

MAKING EPISODIC BUNDLED CARE WORK FOR YOUR PRACTICE

Based on the cost savings success of BPCI and CJR, episodic bundled care will likely be a payment model for TJA expanded by CMS and other payers in the future. Continued decreasing target prices compounded with limited risk adjustment for sicker and more complex patients means that practice and patient optimization are paramount for the success of any group or hospital participating in a bundled payment program.

Reducing Costs and Time in the Operating Room

Being wise financial stewards of the surgical theater is fast becoming a requirement for the modern orthopaedic surgeon. Implants, operating room supplies, and drug costs can vary widely among hospitals[34] and implant prices can often represent a large percentage of the intraoperative cost to an EOC. Using a single preferred vendor for most primary implants can save up to 23% per implant.[35] Collins et al[36] showed that establishing a reference price for vendors can save up to 16% of the cost of revision TKA implants at some centers. In addition, standardizing draping among surgeons streamlines the purchasing of equipment and storage and can save significant amounts of money when compounded over the number of surgeries performed annually.[37] Closely examining the cost of individual drapes and whether evidence supports their use can continue to decrease the disposable cost per case.[37] An additional source of cost savings in the operating room can be found by minimizing the number of trays required to be processed and sterilized during a procedure. The mean cost to processing and sterilization is estimated to be $75 per tray.[38] In addition, reducing the number of trays can decrease the time spent setting up and turning over a room, reducing operating room use per surgical case.[38,39] Intra-articular injections have been shown to improve postoperative pain control. This has included various "injection cocktails" and more recently developed liposomal bupivacaine. Although significantly more expensive, no clear evidence exists that this drug offers any benefit over ropivacaine for multimodal periarticular injections for TJA.[40,41]

Reducing the Length of Stay

Reducing the length of stay for patients undergoing TJA can be a major source of cost savings during an EOC. Strategies that reduce the length of stay include setting patient expectations early during the preoperative encounter for how long they will remain in the hospital. Addressing postoperative placement issues preoperatively prevents extended inpatient stays while awaiting insurance authorization or for a bed to become available.[8] Evidence-based postoperative pain management pathways to include maximizing regional anesthesia, intraoperative blocks, and periarticular injections[42] as well as structured multimodal postoperative pain protocols[43] help keep the patient's pain under control and allows shorter lengths of stay. Utilization of the Enhanced Recovery After Surgery pathway has been shown in THA and TKA to reduce the length of stay without increased rates of readmission.[44,45] However, length of stay is less important than ensuring discharge and avoiding readmissson, as discussed in the next paragraphs.[46]

Postacute Care

Postacute care can be a significant cost during the EOC. Examining the cost difference between four different postacute care discharge dispositions, an EOC cost with only self-care was $19,027, home with home health assistance $22,358, skilled nursing facility $41,115, and inpatient rehabilitation $41,234.[8] Keeping patients in the hospital longer if it facilitates a discharge to home instead of an inpatient rehabilitation facility can be cost saving. It has been shown that keeping patients up to 5.2 days in the hospital to allow for a discharge to home was less expensive than discharging those patients to a postacute inpatient rehabilitation facility.[46] Optimizing the use of postacute services through strategies such as avoiding unnecessary follow-up appointments during the global period allows for better postoperative resource use. In addition, routine follow-up with primary care physicians during the global period should be used only when needed in medically complex patients. Clinical care coordinators can help reduce resource utilization until the patient is out of the 90-day global period.[8]

Reducing Readmissions

Hospital readmissions during the 90-day global period for either medical or surgical complications related to LEJR can result in large cost increases to the EOC. Early experience with BPCI demonstrated that Medicare considered a readmission as "related" approximately 92% of the time.[8] Therefore, reducing readmission is one of the most important and effective cost containment strategies. Pathways developed to prevent readmission after LEJR included utilizing clinical care coordinators as gatekeepers and facilitating communication between clinical staff and the patient prior to issues necessitating a visit to the emergency room that can result in a readmission. Establishing a formal communication channel between visiting nurse services and clinicians to have patients evaluated in the office or a hospital-owned urgent care center instead of an outside emergency department can save costs while maintaining the quality of care. This can also be accomplished by leveraging technology such as smartphone applications or telemedicine to evaluate patients as needed. For common postoperative complications such as minor wound issues or deep vein thrombosis, creating strict readmission guidelines helps standardize the process and removing variation in treatment can reduce costs, while maintaining quality for patients.[8,19,20]

Optimizing Use of Patient Testing and Consultations

In bundled payments, all tests and consultations performed during the global period come out of the target price set by CMS. Therefore, it is critical to order only what is clinically necessary for patient care. For example, frequent routine postoperative plain radiographs of primary TKA have been shown to be medically unnecessary while also increasing the cost of care.[47] Additionally, the routine sending of femoral heads for pathologic evaluation during primary uncomplicated THA adds a mean cost of $100 to $200 per case without adding significant clinical benefit.[48]

Postoperative blood transfusion can be one of the most expensive postoperative interventions performed after TJA. Evidence-based, cost-effective blood management strategies to prevent transfusion include routine use of tranexamic acid,[49-52] utilizing acetylsalicylic acid[53] and sequential pneumatic compression devices for postoperative deep vein thrombosis prophylaxis, avoiding reinfusion drains,[54] and establishing evidence-based triggers for postoperative transfusion.

Evidence-based management of urinary tract conditions in the perioperative period can help avoid unnecessary testing and interventions in patients undergoing TJA. Whether or not to treat asymptomatic preoperative bacteriuria prior to TJA is a controversial topic. Asymptomatic bacteriuria can result in a higher postoperative rate of infection after TJA, but the infection is typically not the same bacteria isolated from urine, and preoperative antibiotic therapy does not influence risk of periprosthetic joint infection.[55,56] Symptomatic bacteriuria also has a much clearer association with postoperative periprosthetic joint infection and should be treated prior to patients undergoing TJA.[56] Similarly, intervention for urinary retention should take on a minimalist approach, with no routine catheter placement,[57] routine postoperative bladder scans, and intermittent catheterization if needed.[58] Failure of intermittent catheterization may result in an indwelling catheter, but this should be discontinued as soon as possible.

THE FUTURE OF EPISODIC BUNDLED CARE

Programs such as bundled payment plans were designed to curb the increasing national cost of LEJR by transitioning from a fee-for-service model to a shared risk model where the financial liability of the procedure, hospital stay, and 90-day global period is shifted onto the institutions and physicians performing the procedures. Ultimately, bundled care for LEJR has been successful at achieving this goal, demonstrating significant decreases in EOC spending since the program inception without a decrease in quality of care.[14-18]

Given the success of BPCI and CJR to drive quality and value in LEJR, there has been significant interest in private payer and self-insured bundles to replicate these successes. Key differences between CMS bundles and private bundles are the individual institution's ability to negotiate every aspect of the agreement. EOC length (including start and stop time), target price, built-in risk stratification based on diagnosis, inclusion criteria, and exclusion criteria can all be negotiated when establishing a private bundle.[59]

CMS has used bundled care for multiple non-LEJR conditions and procedures as well. Agarwal et al[15] reported in a systematic review of the results of BPCI and CJR that although these programs were effective at reducing the cost and maintaining the quality of care for LEJR, they were less successful for non-LEJR conditions and procedures (spine fusion, shoulder arthroplasty, cardiac surgery, medical conditions). When comparing LEJR, cardiac valve procedures, and spinal surgery against nonbundled care conditions, there was an increase in EOC costs of $8,291 for spinal fusion, no change in EOC cost for cardiac valve procedures, and a $3,017 decrease in EOC for LEJR.[60] Joynt Maddox et al[61] investigated congestive heart failure, pneumonia, chronic obstructive pulmonary disease, sepsis, and acute myocardial infarction for the effect of BPCI on EOC cost. The authors found that involvement in bundles did not change the EOC cost, length of stay, readmission rate, or mortality when compared with control groups.

SUMMARY

Given the success of bundled care for LEJR for reducing costs for delivering care for CMS, they will likely continue to be an important program for supporting TJA. Episodic bundled payments for LEJR will continue to evolve, and likely will be applied to other orthopaedic procedures and conditions, with both surgical and nonsurgical bundle payment programs possible, due to the demonstrated positive effect on the value of care in LEJR.

REFERENCES

1. Elmallah RK, Chughtai M, Khlopas A, et al: Determining cost-effectiveness of total hip and knee arthroplasty using the short form-6D utility measure. *J Arthroplasty* 2017;32(2):351-354.

2. Comprehensive Care for Joint Replacement Model. Available at: https://innovation. cms.gov/innovation-models/cjr. Accessed October 13, 2020.

3. Sloan M, Premkumar A, Sheth NP: Projected volume of primary total joint arthroplasty in the U.S., 2014 to 2030. *J Bone Joint Surg Am* 2018;100(17):1455-1460.

4. Kurtz S, Ong K, Lau E, Mowat F, Halpern M: Projections of primary and revision hip and knee arthroplasty in the United States from 2005 to 2030. *J Bone Joint Surg Am* 2007;89(4):780-785.

5. Iorio R, Yates A Jr, Huddleston JI III: Bundled Payments, Advocacy, and Changes of the BPCI. Video presentation at 2020 Focal Committee Webinars. Focal Committee Webinars, American Association of Hip and Knee Surgeons, April 16, 2020. Available at: https://www.aahks.org/focal/focal-recordings/. Accessed April 27, 2023.

6. The Quality Payment Program. Available at: https://qpp.cms.gov/. Accessed October 13, 2020.

7. Bundled Payments for Care Improvement: General Information. Available at: https://innovation.cms.gov/innovation-models/bundled-payments. Accessed October 13, 2020.

8. Iorio R: The Center for Quality and Patient Safety NYULMC Hospital for Joint Diseases Bundled Payment, CCJR, Risk Factor Stratification, and the Ethics of Risk Factor Modification prior to TJA. Oral presentation. American Association of Hip and Knee Surgeons Fall Meeting, November 2019, Dallas, TX.

9. Althausen PL, Mead L: Bundled payments for care improvement: Lessons learned in the first year. *J Orthop Trauma* 2016;30(suppl 5):S50–S53.

10. Lott A, Haglin JM, Belayneh R, Konda S, Egol KA: Bundled payment initiative for hip fracture arthroplasty patients: One institution's experience. *J Orthop Trauma* 2019;33(3):e89-e92.

11. Lott A, Belayneh R, Haglin J, Konda S, Egol KA: Effectiveness of a model bundle payment initiative for femur fracture patients. *J Orthop Trauma* 2018;32(9):439-444.

12. Gammal ID, Matuszak SJ, Kenan S, Larsen CG, Kiridly DN, Goodman HJ: To bundle or not to bundle? The financial impact of pathologic hip disease on hip arthroplasty episodes of care. *J Arthroplasty* 2020;35(6):1480-1483.

13. Courtney PM, Ashley BS, Hume EL, Kamath AF: Are bundled payments a viable reimbursement model for revision total joint arthroplasty? *Clin Orthop Relat Res* 2016;474(12):2714-2721.

14. Finch DJ, Pellegrini VD Jr, Franklin PD, Magder LS, Pelt CE, Martin BI: The effects of bundled payment programs for hip and knee arthroplasty on patient-reported outcomes. *J Arthroplasty* 2020;35(4):918-925.e7.

15. Agarwal R, Liao JM, Gupta A, Navathe AS: The impact of bundled payment on health care spending, utilization, and quality: A systematic review. *Health Aff (Millwood)* 2020;39(1):50-57.

16. Navathe AS, Emanuel EJ, Venkataramani AS, et al: Spending and quality after three years of medicare's voluntary bundled payment for joint replacement surgery. *Health Aff (Millwood)* 2020;39(1):58-66.

17. Dummit LA, Kahvecioglu D, Marrufo G, et al: Association between hospital participation in a medicare bundled payment initiative and payments and quality outcomes for lower extremity joint replacement episodes. *J Am Med Assoc* 2016;316(12):1267-1278.

18. Barnett ML, Wilcock A, McWilliams JM, et al: Two-year evaluation of mandatory bundled payments for joint replacement. *N Engl J Med* 2019;380(3):252-262.

19. Iorio R, Clair AJ, Inneh IA, Slover JD, Bosco JA, Zuckerman JD: Early results of Medicare's bundled payment initiative for a 90-day total joint arthroplasty episode of care. *J Arthroplasty* 2016;31(2):343-350.

20. Dundon JM, Bosco J, Slover J, Yu S, Sayeed Y, Iorio R: Improvement in total joint replacement quality metrics: Year one versus year three of the bundled payments for care improvement initiative. *J Bone Joint Surg Am* 2016;98(23):1949-1953.

21. Medicare Program: Comprehensive Care for Joint Replacement Model Three-Year Extension and Changes to Episode Definition and Pricing. Available at: https://www.federalregister.gov/documents/2020/02/24/2020-03434/medicare-program-comprehensive-care-for-joint-replacement-model-three-year-extension-and-changes-to. Accessed October 15, 2020.

22. Rozell JC, Courtney PM, Dattilo JR, Wu CH, Lee GC: Should all patients be included in alternative payment models for primary total hip arthroplasty and total knee arthroplasty? *J Arthroplasty* 2016;31(9 suppl):45-49.

23. Phillips JLH, Rondon AJ, Vannello C, Fillingham YA, Austin MS, Courtney PM: How much does a readmission cost the bundle following primary hip and knee arthroplasty? *J Arthroplasty* 2019;34(5):819-823.

24. Urish KL, Qin Y, Li BY, et al: Predictors and cost of readmission in total knee arthroplasty. *J Arthroplasty* 2018;33(9):2759-2763.

25. Clair AJ, Evangelista PJ, Lajam CM, Slover JD, Bosco JA, Iorio R: Cost analysis of total joint arthroplasty readmissions in a bundled payment care improvement initiative. *J Arthroplasty* 2016;31(9):1862-1865.

26. Bernstein JA, Yeroushalmi D, Slover JD, Bosco JA 3rd: The cost of an episode of care in a total knee arthroplasty patient is more than a total hip arthroplasty patient within an alternative payment model. *J Arthroplasty* 2020;35(8):1964-1967.

27. Courtney PM, Edmiston T, Batko B, Levine BR: Can bundled payments be successful in the Medicaid population for primary joint arthroplasty? *J Arthroplasty* 2017;32(11):3263-3267.

28. Courtney PM, Huddleston JI, Iorio R, Markel DC: Socioeconomic risk adjustment models for reimbursement are necessary in primary total joint arthroplasty. *J Arthroplasty* 2017;32(1):1-5.

29. Karas V, Kildow BJ, Baumgartner BT, et al: Preoperative patient profile in total hip and knee arthroplasty: Predictive of increased Medicare payments in a bundled payment model. *J Arthroplasty* 2018;33(9):2728-2733.e3.

30. Humbyrd CJ: The ethics of bundled payments in total joint replacement: "Cherry picking" and "lemon dropping". *J Clin Ethics* 2018;29(1):62-68.

31. Cairns MA, Moskal PT, Eskildsen SM, Ostrum RF, Clement RC: Are Medicare's "Comprehensive Care for Joint Replacement" bundled payments stratifying risk adequately? *J Arthroplasty* 2018;33(9):2722-2727.

32. Ryan SP, Plate JF, Black CS, et al: Value-based care has not resulted in biased patient selection: Analysis of a single center's experience in the care for joint replacement bundle. *J Arthroplasty* 2019;34(9):1872-1875.

33. Plate JF, Ryan SP, Black CS, et al: No changes in patient selection and value-based metrics for total hip arthroplasty after comprehensive care for joint replacement bundle implementation at a single center. *J Arthroplasty* 2019;34(8):1581-1584.

34. Haas DA, Kaplan RS: Variation in the cost of care for primary total knee arthroplasties. *Arthroplast Today* 2016;3(1):33-37.

35. Boylan MR, Chadda A, Slover JD, Zuckerman JD, Iorio R, Bosco JA: Preferred single-vendor program for total joint arthroplasty implants: Surgeon adoption, outcomes, and cost savings. *J Bone Joint Surg Am* 2019;101(15):1381-1387.

36. Collins KD, Chen KK, Ziegler JD, Schwarzkopf R, Bosco JA, Iorio R: Revision total hip arthroplasty: Reducing hospital cost through fixed implant pricing. *J Arthroplasty* 2017;32(9 suppl):S141–S143.

37. Gurnea TP, Frye WP, Althausen PL: Operating room supply costs in orthopaedic trauma: Cost containment opportunities. *J Orthop Trauma* 2016;30(suppl 5):S21–S26.

38. Siegel GW, Patel NN, Milshteyn MA, Buzas D, Lombardo DJ, Morawa LG: Cost analysis and surgical site infection rates in total knee arthroplasty comparing traditional vs. single-use instrumentation. *J Arthroplasty* 2015;30(12):2271-2274.

39. Capra R, Bini SA, Bowden DE, et al: Implementing a perioperative efficiency initiative for orthopedic surgery instrumentation at an academic center: A comparative before-and-after study. *Medicine (Baltimore)* 2019;98(7):e14338.

40. EXPAREL is a cost-effective option for postsurgical pain management in the hospital and ambulatory (outpatient) settings. Available at: https://www.exparel.com/hcp/value/total-hip-arthroplasty. Accessed October 8, 2020.

41. Danoff JR, Goel R, Henderson RA, Fraser J, Sharkey PF: Periarticular ropivacaine cocktail is equivalent to liposomal bupivacaine cocktail in bilateral total knee arthroplasty. *J Arthroplasty* 2018;33(8):2455-2459.

42. Ellis TA 2nd, Hammoud H, Dela Merced P, et al: Multimodal clinical pathway with adductor canal block decreases hospital length of stay, improves pain control, and reduces opioid consumption in total knee arthroplasty patients: A retrospective review. *J Arthroplasty* 2018;33(8):2440-2448.

43. Memtsoudis SG, Poeran J, Zubizarreta N, et al: Association of multimodal pain management strategies with perioperative outcomes and resource utilization: A population-based study. *Anesthesiology* 2018;128(5):891-902.

44. Auyong DB, Allen CJ, Pahang JA, Clabeaux JJ, MacDonald KM, Hanson NA: Reduced length of hospitalization in primary total knee arthroplasty patients using an updated enhanced recovery after orthopedic surgery (ERAS) pathway. *J Arthroplasty* 2015;30(10):1705-1709.

45. Stambough JB, Nunley RM, Curry MC, Steger-May K, Clohisy JC: Rapid recovery protocols for primary total hip arthroplasty can safely reduce length of stay without increasing readmissions. *J Arthroplasty* 2015;30(4):521-526.

46. Slover JD, Mullaly KA, Payne A, Iorio R, Bosco J: What is the best strategy to minimize after-care costs for total joint arthroplasty in a bundled payment environment? *J Arthroplasty* 2016;31(12):2710-2713.

47. Glaser D, Lotke P: Cost-effectiveness of immediate postoperative radiographs after uncomplicated total knee arthroplasty: A retrospective and prospective study of 750 patients. *J Arthroplasty* 2000;15(4):475-478.

48. Campbell ML, Gregory AM, Mauerhan DR: Collection of surgical specimens in total joint arthroplasty: Is routine pathology cost effective? *J Arthroplasty* 1997;12(1):60-63.

49. Tuttle JR, Ritterman SA, Cassidy DB, Anazonwu WA, Froehlich JA, Rubin LE: Cost benefit analysis of topical tranexamic acid in primary total hip and knee arthroplasty. *J Arthroplasty* 2014;29(8):1512-1515.

50. Evangelista PJ, Aversano MW, Koli E, et al: Effect of tranexamic acid on transfusion rates following total joint arthroplasty: A cost and comparative effectiveness analysis. *Orthop Clin North Am* 2017;48(2):109-115.

51. Gillette BP, Maradit Kremers H, Duncan CM, et al: Economic impact of tranexamic acid in healthy patients undergoing primary total hip and knee arthroplasty. *J Arthroplasty* 2013;28(8 suppl):137-139.

52. Slover J, Bosco J: Cost analysis of use of tranexamic acid to prevent major bleeding complications in hip and knee arthroplasty surgery. *Am J Orthop (Belle Mead NJ)* 2014;43(10):E217-E220.

53. Agaba P, Kildow BJ, Dhotar H, Seyler TM, Bolognesi M: Comparison of postoperative complications after total hip arthroplasty among patients receiving aspirin, enoxaparin, warfarin, and factor Xa inhibitors. *J Orthop* 2017;14(4):537-543.

54. Springer BD, Odum SM, Fehring TK: What is the benefit of tranexamic acid vs reinfusion drains in total joint arthroplasty? *J Arthroplasty* 2016;31(1):76-80.

55. Sousa RJG, Abreu MA, Wouthuyzen-Bakker M, Soriano AV: Is routine urinary screening indicated prior to elective total joint arthroplasty? A systematic review and meta-analysis. *J Arthroplasty* 2019;34(7):1523-1530.

56. Parvizi J, Koo KH: Should a urinary tract infection be treated before a total joint arthroplasty? *Hip Pelvis* 2019;31(1):1-3.

57. Scotting OJ, North WT, Chen C, Charters MA: Indwelling urinary catheter for total joint arthroplasty using epidural anesthesia. *J Arthroplasty* 2019;34(10):2324-2328.

58. Garbarino LJ, Gold PA, Anis HK, et al: Does intermittent catheterization compared to indwelling catheterization decrease the risk of periprosthetic joint infection following total knee arthroplasty? *J Arthroplasty* 2020;35(6 suppl):S308–S312.

59. Elbuluk AM, O'Neill OR: Private bundles: The nuances of contracting and managing total joint arthroplasty episodes. *J Arthroplasty* 2017;32(6):1720-1722.

60. Jubelt LE, Goldfeld KS, Blecker SB, et al: Early lessons on bundled payment at an academic medical center. *J Am Acad Orthop Surg* 2017;25(9):654-663.

61. Joynt Maddox KE, Orav EJ, Zheng J, Epstein AM: Evaluation of Medicare's bundled payments initiative for medical conditions. *N Engl J Med* 2018;379(3):260-269.

Condition-Based Payment

Erik Y. Tye, MD • John P. Andrawis, MD, MBA
Richard C. Mather III, MD, MBA
Prakash Jayakumar, MD, PhD

INTRODUCTION

The United States spends more per capita on health care than any other country, yet fails to achieve a commensurate improvement in many population health outcomes.[1] Most payment systems continue to incentivize volume and procedural performance rather than value, defined as the health outcomes benefiting patients relative to cost. Centering care around a patient's preferences, values, and needs related to their condition[2] is one of the key components of higher value care. Thus, there has been a gradual shift among stakeholders in the public and private sector toward redefining incentives and developing value-based alternatives to payment and practice. Alternative payment models (APMs) were created to improve health care value by transitioning from traditional fee-for-service (FFS) medicine and shifting financial risk and reward for both health care costs and quality onto medical providers. Pioneered by Medicare in 1982 with the adoption of the diagnosis-related group system for hospital inpatient services, bundled payments served as a type of APM to tackle the inefficiencies brought about by FFS models. By encouraging providers to work collaboratively with payers and adopt innovative approaches to care delivery, these APMs aimed to focus care on improving value across the entirety of a condition.

In a bundled payment system, clinicians assume accountability for the quality and cost of care where those who keep costs below a risk-adjusted price share a portion of the resulting savings, and those who exceed the target price incur financial penalties.[3] Bundled payments encourage physicians to collaborate and improve efficiency, coordinate care, and limit low-value services in a more cost-effective matter. Bosco et al,[4] in their review of bundled arrangements, described seven principles that are critical to the success of the bundled payment: (1) preoperative identification and modification of patient risk factors, (2) adoption of evidence-based clinical pathways, (3) collection and dissemination of robust data, (4) identifying variations in outcomes and costs, (5) handling postdischarge costs, (6) maximizing quality, and (7) configuring gainsharing arrangements. Over the past 5 years, the Affordable Care Act allowed the Center for Medicare & Medicaid Innovation to create different payment reforms and an opportunity to expand bundled payments. APMs in musculoskeletal care have included the voluntary Bundled Payment for Care Improvement Initiative and the mandatory Comprehensive Care for Joint Replacement model (CJR).[5] These procedure-based payment models involve a payment bundle for all services delivered by provider groups managing an entire surgical episode of care, for example, index hospitalization until 90 days after total joint replacement (TJR) for patients with degenerative joint disease (DJD) of the hip or knee.[6] Implemented in 2013, the Bundled Payment for Care Improvement Initiative program has since shown cost reductions through reduced use of postacute care facilities such as inpatient rehabilitation facilities and skilled nursing facilities without negatively affecting clinical outcomes.[7,8] The Comprehensive Care for Joint Replacement model, since its introduction in 2016, has shown reductions in total spending through a similar approach with lower utilization of postacute care while refining and increasing the efficiency of operational practices.[9]

LIMITATIONS OF CURRENT PROCEDURE-BASED BUNDLES

Episodic bundled payments for procedures such as total joint replacement have demonstrated improved operational efficiency and reduced total costs among participating hospitals without having a detrimental effect on clinical outcomes. However, the overall magnitude of cost reductions is modest with limited improvement in clinical outcomes, especially considering the investment of time and resources within these programs.[8,10,11] Further, procedure-based bundled episode payments address a limited part of the care continuum and fall short in engaging patients further upstream, prior to the phase of preoperative optimization. Critical opportunities exist around utilizing a range of evidence-based nonsurgical strategies, enhancing appropriate surgical selection through shared decision making, and integrating both surgical and nonsurgical strategies into consensus-based standards and more comprehensive practice guidelines for managing persistently painful musculoskeletal conditions.

Current nonsurgical management of common musculoskeletal conditions, such as DJD, frequently involves the overutilization of low-value services such as MRI and hyaluronic acid injections. Further, substantial underutilization of evidence-based, clinical guideline supported, nonsurgical modalities exists, including arthritis education, structure exercise programs, and dietary and weight management.[12,13] Populations with chronic musculoskeletal conditions also exhibit high levels of psychological distress.[14,15] Such stressors have shown to negatively affect functional outcomes and patient experience.[16-18]

Procedure-based bundles also fundamentally do little to address the issue of surgical appropriateness.[19] Current procedure-based APMs lack incentive structures that reward specialists around appropriate treatment selection, thereby tackling the issue of overuse, or mitigate negative side effects such as preferential patient selection ("cherry picking") to maximize gains.[20] Notably, the number of total knee replacement (TKR) cases performed in the United States and worldwide has continued to rise. Data suggest up to 30% of TKRs performed in the United States may not be appropriately indicated based on standardized criteria, leaving a proportion of patients dissatisfied with their surgery[21,22] (**Figure 1**). This problem is further compounded by the lack of implementation of the aforementioned nonsurgical care strategies.

Payment and care models that center around the procedure not only limit exposure of the range of potentially beneficial services available to patients, but also the prospect of surgeons and patients to engage in shared decision-making—a concept where the latest knowledge (nature of the condition and details of all potential treatment options including their risks and benefits) are discussed using expert communication and surgeon-patient interaction before arriving at an informed decision aligned with the patient's preferences, values, and needs. Shifting toward a model configured to provide a comprehensive and longitudinal condition-based approach, including optimal nonsurgical strategies and appropriate surgery, promises to enhance the experience and outcomes for patients (**Figure 2**).

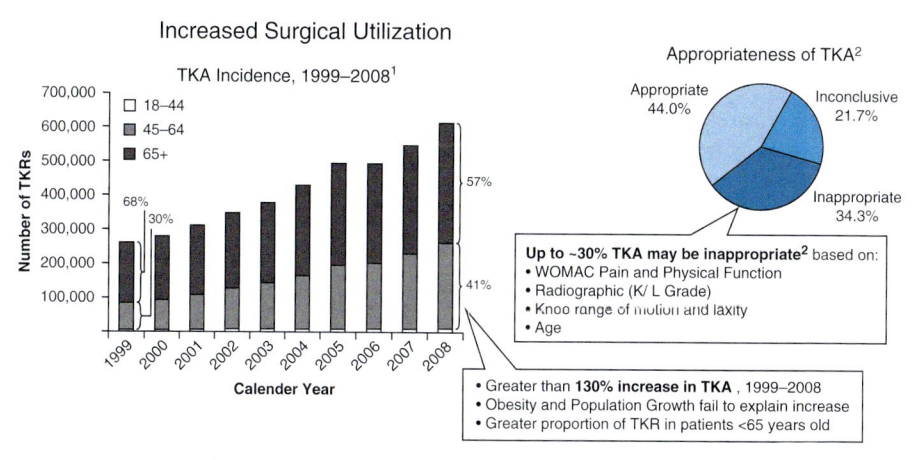

FIGURE 1 Bar graph and pie chart indicate the growing number of total knee replacements performed in the last 2 decades with 34.3% of cases inappropriately indicated. K/L = Kellgren-Lawrence, TKA = total knee arthroplasty, TKR = total knee replacement, WOMAC = Western Ontario and McMaster Universities Arthritis Index. (Bar graph reproduced with permission from Losina E, Thornhill TS, Rome BN, Wright J, Katz JN: The dramatic increase in total knee replacement utilization rates in the United States cannot be fully explained by growth in population size and the obesity epidemic. *J Bone Joint Surg Am* 2012;94[3]:201-207. Pie chart data from Riddle DL, Jiranek WA, Hayes CW: Use of a validated algorithm to judge the appropriateness of total knee arthroplasty in the United States: A multicenter longitudinal cohort study. *Arthritis Rheumatol* 2014;66[8]:2134-2143.)

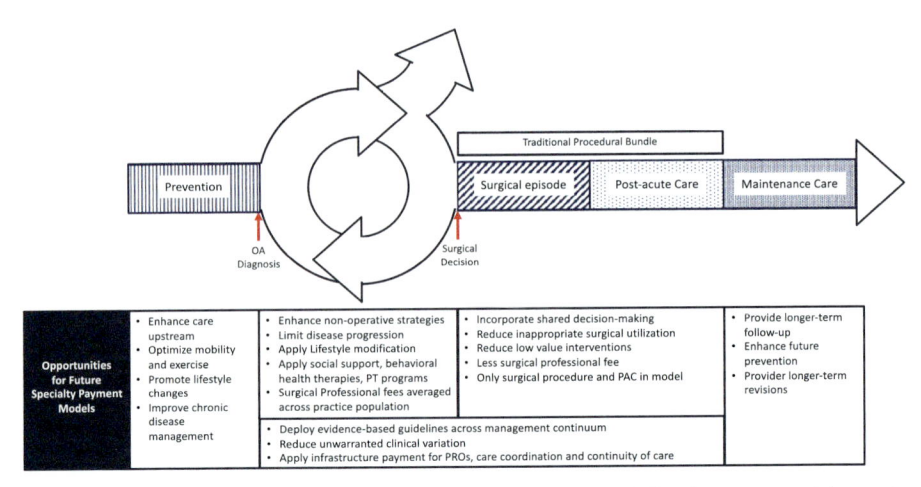

FIGURE 2 Illustration shows opportunities to improve specialized care not addressed through current payment models. PROs = patient-reported outcomes. (Reproduced with permission from Jayakumar P, O'Donnell J, Manickas-Hill O, et al: Critical considerations for condition-based alternative payment models: A multi-stakeholder perspective. *Health Affairs Blog* 2020. Available at: https://www.healthaffairs.org/do/10.1377/hblog20200714.732842/full/. Accessed July 12, 2023.)

Transitioning bundled episode payment models toward an outcomes-driven, patient-centered, and condition-focused approach, from one oriented around the procedure, signals opportunities to overcome perpetual cost containment strategies and limitations in access to evidence-based low-cost interventions, while also promising significant cost savings. Failure to do so, either through bundled episode payments in specialty care or via models involving primary care or accountable care organization arrangements with specialty care, is ultimately unlikely to result in the change that is needed. Condition-based bundled episode payments (CBEPs) are an emerging payment and practice framework that hope to address the shortcomings of procedure-based bundled payment systems. CBEPs expand the scope of care through incentivizing appropriate utilization of procedures, evidence-based treatment selection based on a patient's holistic needs, care coordination involving a range of services, and reimbursement based on health-related outcomes achieved, thereby reducing inappropriate procedures, variation in care, and total costs of care (**Figure 3**).

CBEP AND PRACTICE MODELS

The concept of CBEPs is gaining traction across US health care with a critical need for evidence to garner payer-provider engagement and commitment from stakeholders to invest in change. Few healthcare systems have successfully oriented themselves toward CBEPs. This section highlights both national and international exemplars at various stages of the transition toward a condition-based approach to the management of musculoskeletal conditions.

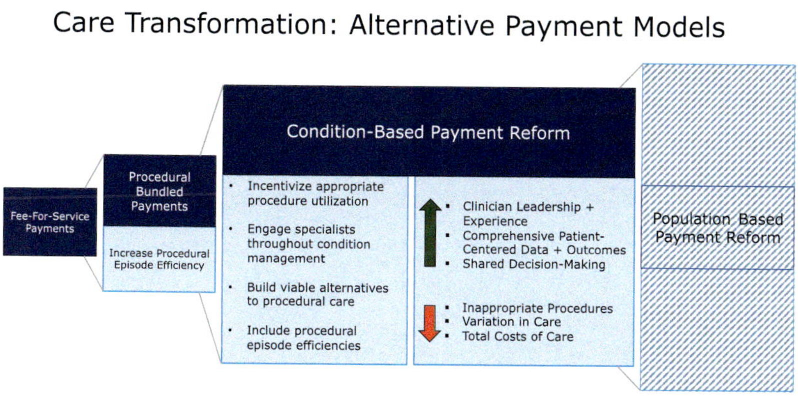

Care Transformation: Alternative Payment Models

FIGURE 3 Chart showing the chapter authors' analysis of condition-based payment reform widens the scope of care.

CONDITION-FOCUSED CARE MODELS

Case Study A: The Musculoskeletal Institute at The University of Texas Health Austin, Dell Medical School—A True Condition-Based Bundled Episode Payment and Practice Model

The Musculoskeletal Institute at the University of Texas Health at Austin, Dell Medical School is composed of multiple integrated practice units (IPUs) providing condition-based care for patients with a broad range of musculoskeletal conditions. Leaders of the institution established a partnership with their county health district and local taxpayers, serving a vested interest by multiple stakeholders in using resources more effectively for patients with joint pain of the lower extremity, upper extremity, back, and neck, alongside sports injuries (**Figure 4**).

Each IPU has a dedicated group of professionals including an orthopaedic surgeon and associate clinician (or advanced practitioner, chiropractor, or nurse practitioner) alongside physical therapists, a dietician, a behavioral health-trained social worker, and medical assistants serving multiple roles including care navigation and coordination. Other medical specialists such as psychiatrists, pharmacists, and anesthesiologists are also available to assist with the patient's care. The IPU team works in a co-located common workspace within a single facility and enables patients to seek counsel from a multidisciplinary team "on-demand" from the outset and throughout their full cycle of care. The multidisciplinary team is accountable for outcomes and costs associated with the condition-based episode of care. The bundle is initially priced based on evaluations of historical specialist claims data (incorporating diagnostic and procedural codes) for patients referred to a specialist managing hip or knee arthritis. As the bundle evolves, more accurate micro-cost accounting approaches, such as time-driven, activity-based costing, can be utilized to ascertain the true total costs of care based on patient-focused events and resources used for patient care along their entire care journey.

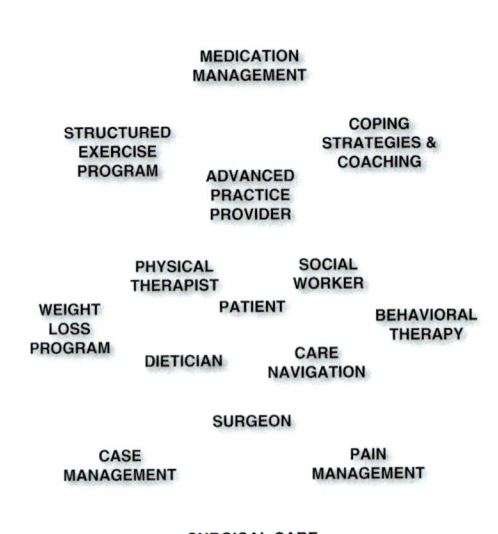

FIGURE 4 Word cloud depicting the Musculoskeletal Institute Integrated Practice Unit at the University of Texas at Austin, Dell Medical School Care Delivery Model. (Data from Keswani A, Koenig KM, Bozic KJ: Value-based healthcare: Part 1 – Designing and implementing integrated practice units for the management of musculoskeletal disease. *Clin Orthop Relat Res* 2016;474[10]:2100-2103.)

The episode price of the CBEP is based on 12 months commencing with the initial referral and includes a range of nonsurgical strategies from physical therapy, structured exercise programs and patient education, imaging, physician-administered medications including injections, to social support with case management and behavioral therapy, and lifestyle modification (including nutritional guidance, weight loss counseling, and smoking and alcohol cessation), outcomes tracking, shared decision-making using a technology-enabled patient decision aid, in-office procedures including image-guided injections, alongside surgical professional fees. The IPU aims to meet needs such as lifestyle management, nutrition, behavioral health, social wellbeing that are shown to dominantly influence health outcomes. Based on this holistic approach, the IPU model takes on the full risk based on the premise that patient outcomes will be improved when patients are treated appropriately with such a wide selection of services.

This configuration incentivizes clinicians to deliver treatments geared toward optimizing patient outcomes and tailoring treatment choice to the patient's physical, emotional, and social needs rather than focusing on driving procedural volume. If a full range of evidence-based nonsurgical strategies have been exhausted at any point during the episode of care (ie, 1 year in the case of the musculoskeletal IPU), the patient's biopsychosocial needs are met, and they are deemed appropriate for surgical intervention following a shared decision-making consultation, the patient can undergo surgery as part of a new surgical bundle. The surgical bundle encompasses costs of the surgical workup, procedure including implant, and intra-operative and postoperative care (up to 90 days) minus the surgeon's professional fees. Surgical care includes a standardized clinical pathway for perioperative management including the Preoperative Assessment and Global Optimization program.[22] This program is a surgical home managed by the team's anesthesiologists that covers the entire episode of care and includes design features to guide not only patients, but also family members through the perioperative care process. The entire care model mandates the longitudinal capture of patient-reported outcome measures (PROMs) as a requisite for the condition-based bundled episode payment from baseline through the entire episode of care.

Analysis was conducted on 2,364 new patients who presented to the IPU during an analysis period between October 2017 to October 2020. Of a subset of patients with DJD of the hip (n = 259), 220 (85%) completed Hip dysfunction and Osteoarthritis Outcome Score for Joint Replacement (HOOS JR) surveys at baseline and 6-month follow-up, and 214 (83%) completed baseline and 1 year. HOOS JR scores increased from baseline to 6 months ($\Delta = 19.1 + 2.1$, $P = 0.065$) and baseline to 1 year ($\Delta = 35.8 + 2.9$, $P < 0.001$) (**Figure 5**). At 1 year, 72.7% (IPU-based non-surgical care only or IPU only) and 88% (IPU-based nonsurgical care plus THA or IPU-based THA) of patients achieved minimal clinically important difference (MCID), and 62.3% (IPU only) and 88% (IPU-based THR) achieved substantial clinical benefit (SCB) (**Figures 6** and **7**). At each interval, HOOS JR ($P < 0.05$) were significantly higher for those receiving IPU care alone as well as those receiving IPU-based THA. Multivariable regression demonstrated baseline HOOS JR scores, undergoing surgery, and greater symptoms of generalized anxiety explained most of the variance in achieving MCID and SCB at 1 year.

Of a subset of patients with DJD of the knee (n = 429), 392 (91%) completed Knee injury and Osteoarthritis Outcome Score for Joint Replacement (KOOS JR) surveys at baseline and 6 months, and 371 (86%) at baseline and 1-year. KOOS JR scores increased from baseline to 6 months ($\Delta = 13.8 + 2.4$, $P < 0.001$) and baseline to 1 year ($\Delta = 33.1 + 2.3$, $P < 0.001$) (**Figure 5**). At 1 year, 81.2% (IPU only) and 92.9% (IPU-based TKR) achieved MCID ($P - 0.006$), and 79% (IPU care only) and 83.6% (IPU-based TKR) achieved SCB ($P = 0.024$) (**Figures 6** and **7**). In multivariable regression, age, baseline KOOS JR, undergoing surgery, and greater symptoms of generalized anxiety and depression explained most of the variance in achieving MCID and SCB at 1 year. Lower baseline anxiety (Generalized Anxiety Disorder-7 [GAD-7]) and depression (Patient Health Questionnaire [PHQ-2/-9]) resulted in greater likelihood of achieving MCID and SCB.

Thus, significant improvements in functional outcomes were attained via a comprehensive, team-based approach focused on nonsurgical strategies, regardless of whether TJR was performed during the episode of care.

Assessment of utilization and unit costs demonstrated reductions in optimal use of treatment modalities compared to traditional care (**Table 1**), cost savings (**Figure 8**), and overall reductions in total cost of care (**Figure 9**).

Key drivers of patient savings include the expansion of virtual touchpoints to reduce low-value in-person visits, appropriate utilization of surgery as an effective treatment option, and elimination of costly, unnecessary treatments and diagnostics (eg, judicious use of joint injections, MRI).

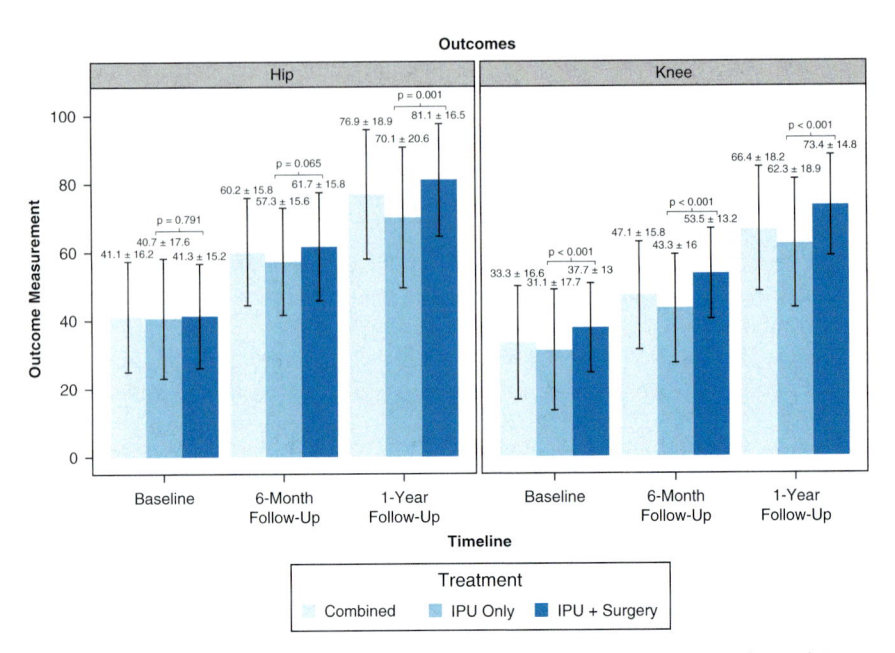

FIGURE 5 Bar graft showing functional outcomes at baseline, 6-month, and 1-year follow-up with integrated practice unit (IPU) only, IPU-based total joint replacement surgery, and all patients combined. (Data from the University of Texas at Austin, Dell Medical School, Orthopaedic Integrated Practice Unit.)

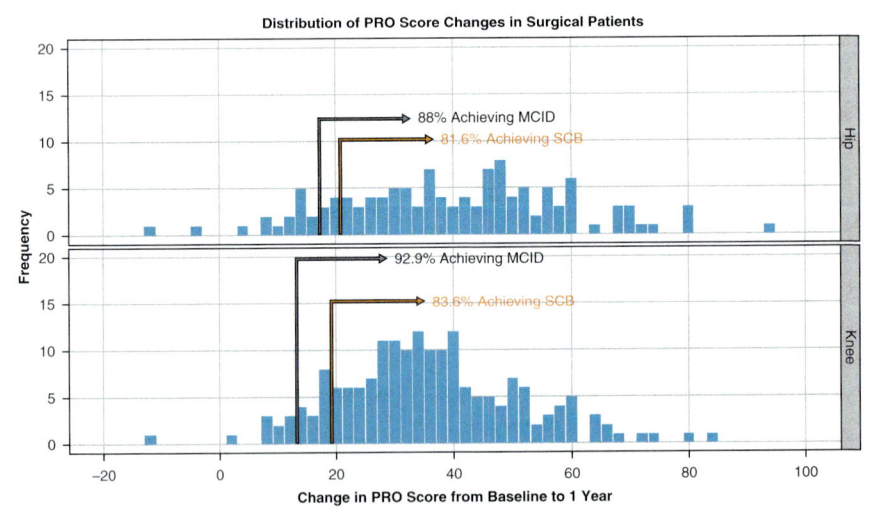

FIGURE 6 Bar graph showing proportion of patients achieving minimal clinically important difference (MCID) and substantial clinical benefit (SCB) among patients with degenerative joint disease of the hip or knee undergoing total joint replacement surgery. PRO = patient-reported outcome. (Data from the University of Texas at Austin, Dell Medical School, Orthopaedic Integrated Practice Unit.)

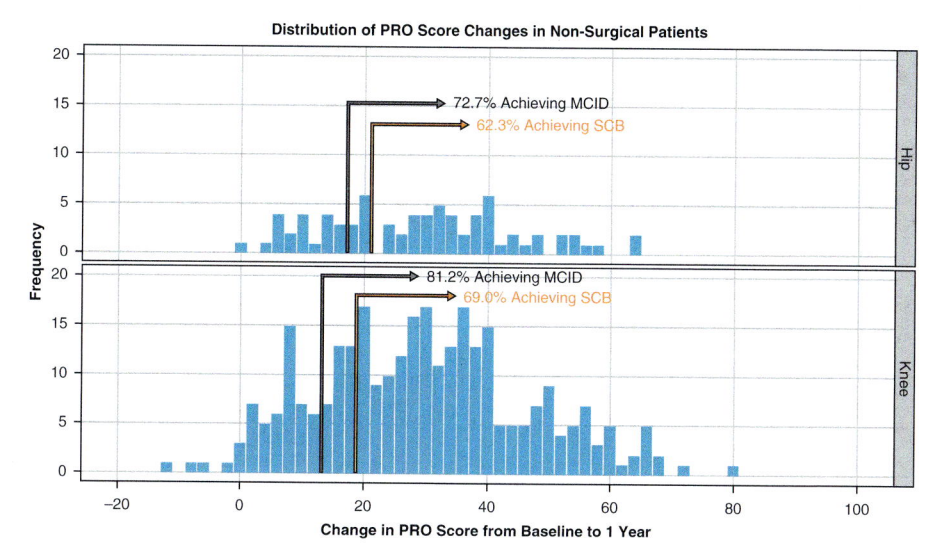

FIGURE 7 Proportion of patients achieving minimal clinically important difference (MCID) and substantial clinical benefit (SCB) among patients with degenerative joint disease of the hip or knee receiving integrated practice unit-based nonsurgical care only. PRO = patient-reported outcome. (Data from the University of Texas at Austin, Dell Medical School, Orthopaedic Integrated Practice Unit.)

TABLE 1 Level of Utilization Comparing the Musculoskeletal Integrated Practice Unit Model With Traditional Care

Musculoskeletal Treatment Utilization

Treatment Modalities	Traditional Care Model		UTHA MSKI Care Model	
	% of Patients	# per Patient	% of Patients	# per Patient
Office visits/telehealth	100	4.8	100	2.8
Integrated behavioral health	Zero	0	21	1.8
Physical therapy	18	8.7	67	4.8
Simple imaging	67	1.6	50	1.3
Advanced imaging	8	1	2	1
Injections	75	1.2	18	1.5
Laboratory	18	1.9	15	1.4
Durable medical equipment	29	1.8	6	1.0
Inpatient/outpatient surgery	18	1.0	15	1.0

Based on historical Austin/Central Texas commercial utilization and internal University of Texas Health Austin (UTHA) utilization data. MSKI = musculoskeletal infection

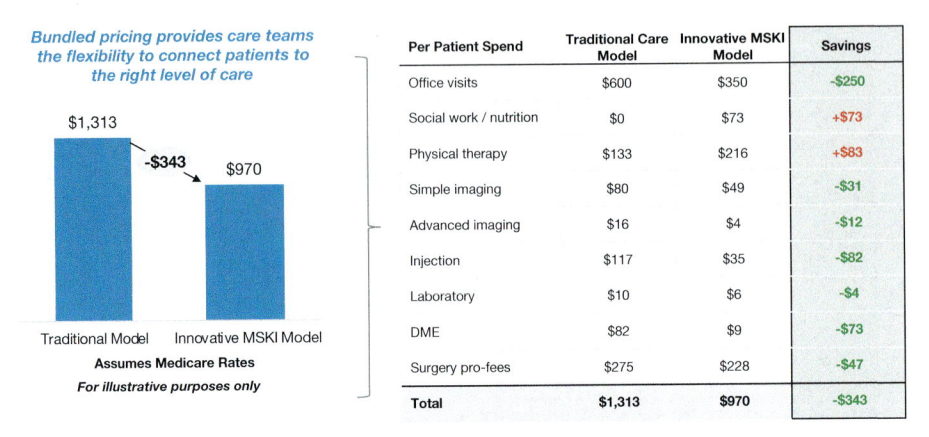

Bundled pricing provides care teams the flexibility to connect patients to the right level of care

Per Patient Spend	Traditional Care Model	Innovative MSKI Model	Savings
Office visits	$600	$350	-$250
Social work / nutrition	$0	$73	+$73
Physical therapy	$133	$216	+$83
Simple imaging	$80	$49	-$31
Advanced imaging	$16	$4	-$12
Injection	$117	$35	-$82
Laboratory	$10	$6	-$4
DME	$82	$9	-$73
Surgery pro-fees	$275	$228	-$47
Total	**$1,313**	**$970**	**-$343**

FIGURE 8 Chart showing level of cost savings comparing the musculoskeletal (MSK) integrated practice unit model with traditional care. DME = durable medical equipment. (Data from the University of Texas at Austin, Dell Medical School, Orthopaedic Integrated Practice Unit.)

Case Study B: Duke University School of Medicine Joint Health Program

At the Duke University Health System, researchers developed a comprehensive Joint Health Program (JHP) designed to identify and treat musculoskeletal, physiological, and psychosocial problems related to patients with musculoskeletal conditions causing hip and knee pain, such as DJD. The program was designed to offer longitudinal, coordinated, comprehensive evidence-based nonsurgical treatments (**Figure**

Annual Per Patient MSK Spend Categories

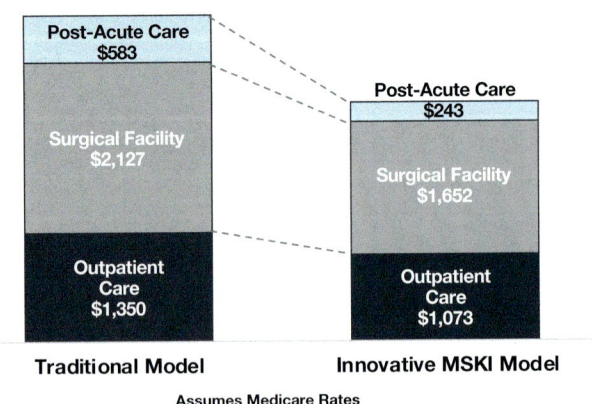

FIGURE 9 Chart showing total costs of care based on annual per patient spend comparing the musculoskeletal (MSK) integrated practice unit model with traditional care. (Data from the University of Texas at Austin, Dell Medical School, Orthopaedic Integrated Practice Unit.)

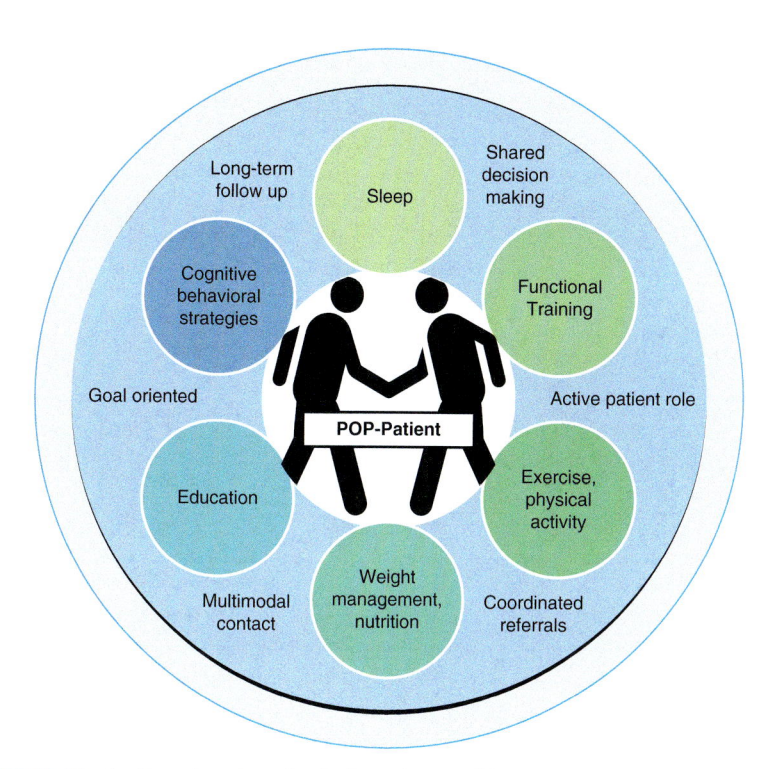

FIGURE 10 Illustration showing the Duke Joint Health Program Model of Care. (Reproduced with permission from Malay MR, Lentz TA, O'Donnell J, Coles T, Mather Iii RC, Jiranek WA: Development of a comprehensive, nonsurgical joint health program for people with osteoarthritis: A case report. *Phys Ther* 2020;100[1]:127-135.)

10). The program centers on the development of a multidisciplinary clinician, rather than a multidisciplinary clinic. The multidisciplinary clinician, or primary osteoarthritis clinician, is a physical therapist who receives comprehensive training on well-established evidence-based guidelines for nonsurgical management of DJD: pain education, physical activity and prescriptive exercise, sleep health, nutrition and weight management, and cognitive behavioral therapy-based strategies for managing pain associated with psychological distress as it relates to DJD.[23] The model was inspired by a Duke psychologist who developed and tested in a randomized controlled trial a formal training model to teach cognitive behavioral therapy to physical therapists.[24] A standardized set of PROMs as well as experience measures are collected through each patient's episode of care. A total of 2,065 patients were enrolled in the program within the first 2 years of its inception. Preliminary results demonstrate that a substantial percentage of patients with DJD of the hip and knee were satisfied with this type of care and a high number of patients achieved clinical improvement following this more comprehensive management program prior to, or in certain cases, in lieu of, surgical intervention (**Figures 11** and **12**). Their program also highlighted a substantial incidence of psychosocial comorbidities in their DJD

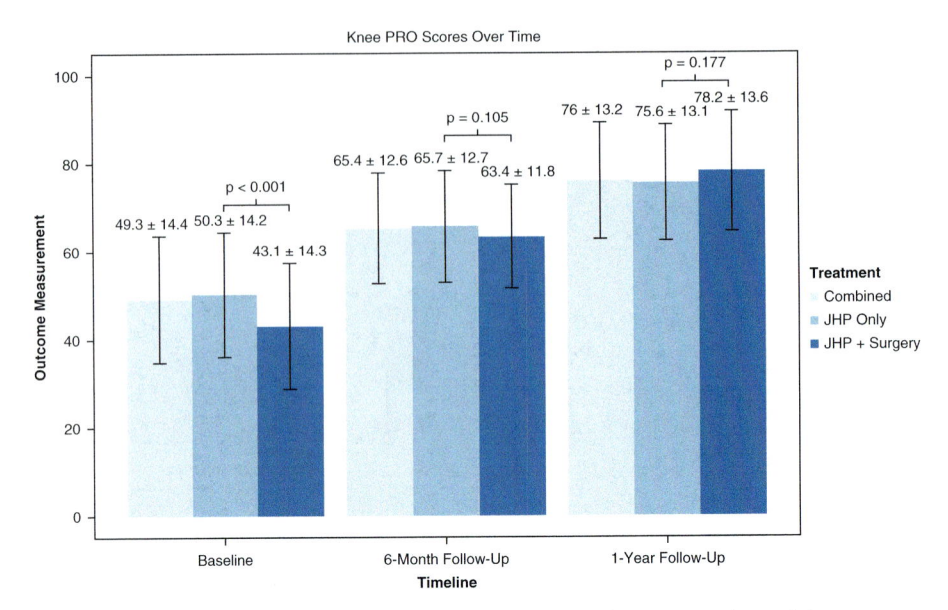

FIGURE 11 Chart showing functional outcomes at baseline, 6-month, and 1-year follow-up with the Duke Joint Health Program (JHP) only, JHP-based total joint replacement surgery, and all patients combined. PRO = patient-reported outcome.

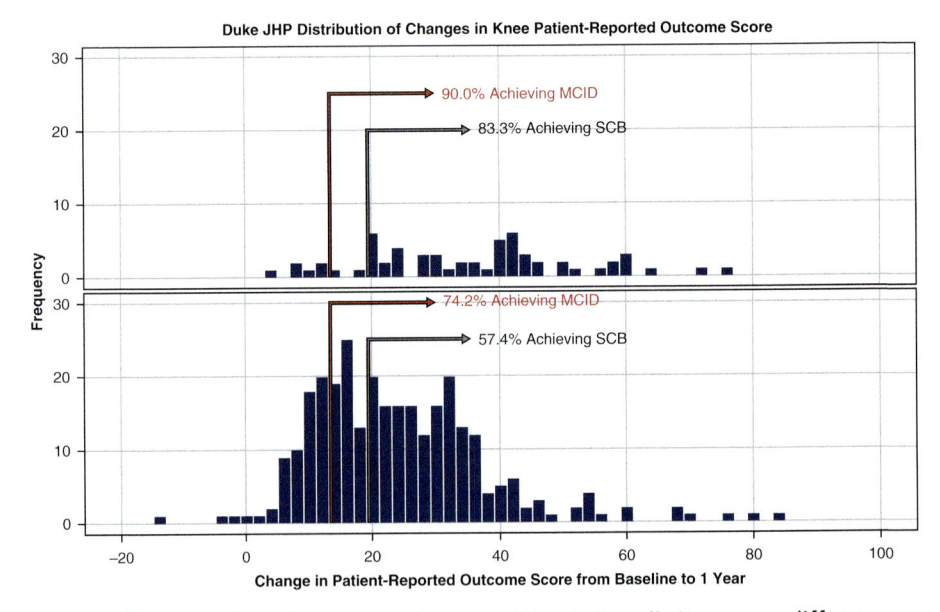

FIGURE 12 Proportion of patients achieving minimal clinically important difference (MCID) and substantial clinical benefit (SCB) among patients with degenerative joint disease of the hip or knee within the Duke Joint Health Program (JHP).

patient population.[25] As mentioned previously, these psychosocial conditions have been implicated with worse outcomes after TJR and highlight the role of addressing these comorbidities in condition-based care models.

Case Study C: Lessons From Abroad

Australia

In Australia, the osteoarthritis chronic care program was created through a grant by the Ministry of Health and provides approximately 1 year of comprehensive services (eg, exercise, weight loss, disease management, psychological management) managed by a musculoskeletal coordinator for patients with hip or knee DJD drawn from a surgical waitlist. The aim is to provide a system-level, best-practice management framework for DJD that is informed and approaches DJD care on a continuum from early to advanced disease management. The model recognizes that consumers will require different components of care at different times and focuses on integrating services to optimize care and to make best use of health resources. The program demonstrated an 11% reduction in total knee replacement surgeries and 4% reduction in hip replacements and was associated with lower rates of obesity and hypertension with slight reductions in patient-reported pain, mobility, and function after 1 year.[26]

Denmark

Denmark launched the Good Life with osteoArthritis in Denmark initiative in 2013 with the aim of standardizing clinical care guidelines for the treatment of patients with DJD of the hip and knee nationwide. Their protocol consisted of three mandatory elements: 2-day course for physiotherapists to receive rigorous training in all elements regarding musculoskeletal care of patients with DJD; 8 weeks of education and supervised neuromuscular exercises for patients with knee and hip DJD symptoms provided by a trained physiotherapist; and the use of quality-of-life outcome scores starting from each patient's initial visit. Their results over a nationwide sample demonstrated that conservative nonsurgical care resulted in an improvement in pain, physical function, physical activity, and quality of life for patients and reduced patient use of opioids and work disability.[27]

VALUE-ORIENTED MODELS OF HEALTH CARE

Although certain programs both in the United States and abroad have begun to develop comprehensive, conservative DJD care models with promising results, others have noticed a real benefit behind these care models and have gradually shifted focus on value-based health care by incorporating critical elements of CBEP within a procedure-based model utilizing PROMs, virtual care, and multidisciplinary care coordination.

Dartmouth-Hitchcock GreenCare: PROMs Help Decision Making

Leaders at Dartmouth-Hitchcock Medical Center implemented a coordinated clinical care pathway for primary TJR in 2011 in an effort to appropriately address evolving reimbursement policies. The program created standardized care delivery models that address health care from initial surgeon referral through 1 year after surgery, with attention placed on appropriately aligning providers, measuring compliance with clinical evidence for each patient, incorporating PROMs into clinical decisions, using formal shared decision making, and addressing per appointment and per case cost reductions.[28,29] Their use of PROMs into clinical decision making to help shared decision making was revolutionary at the time. Since then, the use of PROMs has expanded and formal shared decision making now has the ability to use artificial intelligence to aid decision making about DJD.[30]

Geisinger Medical Center: Create a Surgical Home

Geisinger Medical Center was designated a Center of Excellence (COE) for TJR in the Employers Center of Excellence Network by Health Design Plus, which is a national leader in the creation and management of employer-sponsored health plan offerings. As part of the Employers Center of Excellence Network joint replacement program, patients visit a multidisciplinary team including surgeons, primary care providers, and physical and occupational therapists. Geisenger tag-lined their approach the ProvenCare model. This was one of the first models that created a surgical home where services are bundled around the consumer/patient and their family. A registered nurse coordinator serves as a resource for the patient and coordinates the care of all medical specialists for the patient. Hospital providers utilize bundled rates, and the hospital and surgeons are measured on quality and outcomes data with a focus on clinical outcomes, patient experience, and shared decision making.[31]

Walmart COE: Virtual Care

Walmart's COE program pays for employees to travel and receive care at designated facilities and was expanded in 2014 to include hip and knee replacements. Leaders of the program have begun integrating and expanding telehealth capabilities to push the continuity and coordination of multifaceted care, which are basic principles in APMs. Members eligible for the COE program are now offered digital physical therapy in which patients are able to do physical therapy online with credentialed providers; this offers a form of care delivery that can be more cost-effective than many in-person office visits and provides convenience for patients.[32]

FRAMEWORK FOR CONDITION-BASED BUNDLES

The Basics

Building CBEP models clearly requires substantial engagement among key stakeholders and some important facilitators at interpersonal, structural, functional, and technological levels. Strong payer-clinician engagement around a shared vision and mission driven by actionable guidance and evidence is crucial to achieving a CBEP model from the outset. National coalitions driven by groups, such as the Consortium for Next Generation Alternative Payment models,[33] underline the importance of a playbook for navigating this engagement, spanning discovery of the nature, scale and opportunity for a CBEP model, understanding competing priorities, appreciating the challenges of specifying the program, and defining who is going to participate (payers, clinicians, vendors) and how (contracting arrangements). Further, there is a need for an analytical approach encompassing the primary and secondary condition scope, using diagnostic coding, procedural codes for defining the scope of services, and performance evaluation. These analytical outputs set the stage for defining and communicating savings assumptions, before developing model specifications (**Table 2**). Model specifications include the definition of episode triggers, episode timing, population and risk adjustment, service configuration, accountability and accountable entities and the flow of finance and payment alongside program pricing, type and level of risk, and performance and quality measurement.

Design Features for a Condition-Based Model—DJD

The design features of a condition-based model first requires an analytical approach and subsequent analytical outputs to generate initial evidence of current performance measures, which can help to drive the configuration of a program for full implementation and scaling. Such a framework applied to degenerative joint disease includes key considerations such as condition scope, diagnostic coding, service scope, performance evaluation, and timeframe. Utilizing DJD as the primary condition scope, diagnostic coding through either region-specific codes (International Classification of Diseases, Tenth Revision [ICD-10]) or global musculoskeletal codes are selected along with the types of services provided relevant to the treatment of DJD. Types of services may include some or all types of interventions (low and high value) provided at a designated range of service locations (inpatient, outpatient, office, surgery centers, etc.) Performance evaluation is then conducted over a designated time period wherein APM eligibility, attribution, and accountability are adjudicated. An analytics team of the health plan is then designated to generate quantitative outcomes based on the analytical approach put forth by the participating service providers. The interested parties can then utilize the data to specify what modalities provide opportunity, how those opportunities are used in their service delivery configuration, and the projected outcomes related to quality, finances, and/or experience.

Comprehensive model specifications are then generating using the prior insights and savings assumptions taken from the analytical output from the initial design stages. First, an episode definition must be clearly delineated, which in the example of DJD would be defined as management of hip or knee DJD from first diagnosis (**Table 3**). The episode definition or "trigger" will most likely depend on the member's diagnosis or provision of a service type. Second, designating a duration of the episode of care is critical and can be negotiated with interested parties. Episode timing may cover a given calendar year, 90 days since initial eligible claim, etc. Different options for the episode timing may include fixed time (days/months/years), fixed event (issue resolution, objective clinical improvement, patient completion of certain activity), and patient choice/election. Third, defining the eligible patient population along with the range of services included and the inclusion/exclusion criteria regarding complication and comorbidities should be clearly outlined (**Table 4**). Fourth, service configuration of what patients receive, how they are seen, and what insurance entities are covered will need to be clearly delineated. Enhancing patient experience by adapting current care models with more developed and targeted services to reflect patient needs will be paramount, whether that be onsite or virtual

TABLE 2 **Analytical Approach to Generate Scope of Services, Performance Evaluation, and Ultimately Savings Assumptions Prior to Large-Scale Condition Based-Model Development**

1. Primary Condition Scope

Musculoskeletal degenerative joint disease and derangement

2. Secondary Condition Scope

Minor inflammation and sprains
Osteoporosis
Malignancy (primary or metastatic)
Major injury (eg, MVAs, trauma)
Autoimmune arthroses (eg, RA, lupus) or other major inflammation

Illustration
Include:
- MSK degeneration and derangement
- Osteoporosis
- Minor inflammation and sprains

Exclude
- Minor inflammation and sprains
- Malignancy (primary or metastatic)
- Major injury (motor vehicle accidents, trauma)
- Autoimmune arthrosis (eg, RA, lupus) or other inflammation

3. Diagnostic Coding

Option 1: Anatomic region-specific codes (ICD-10) – the partnership intent by payer and provider is to initially focus solely on a specific anatomic region (eg, lower extremity, upper extremity) at the exclusion of other anatomic regions. This scope may be preferred if payer and/or provider seeks a narrower, focused scope.

Option 2: Global MSK codes (ICD-10) – the partnership intent is to effectively capture all relevant MSK diagnoses together (eg, hip and neck and back and knee and shoulder and other). (See Appendix G)

4. Service Scope

Type of service (some or all)
1. All CPT codes
2. Specific CPT codes (eg, surgery, physical therapy, anesthesia)
3. Low value interventions (eg, utilization MRI, hyaluronic acid, arthroscopy)

Geographic
1. Zip code/county level
2. State level
3. MSA level
4. Other strategic level

TABLE 2 **Analytical Approach to Generate Scope of Services, Performance Evaluation, and Ultimately Savings Assumptions Prior to Large-Scale Condition Based-Model Development** **(Continued)**

Place of service (some or all)
1. Inpatient
2. Outpatient
3. Office
4. Ambulatory Surgical Center (ASC)
5. Emergency department

Illustration
Include all CPT codes that evidence an eligible diagnosis (defined earlier by scope considerations) within a prespecified claim level (eg, first four positions), at any place of service, in as wide a geography as feasible. More is better to create critical mass for clinicians, patients, and finances (practice revenue potential, medical expense savings potential; spread out fixed costs for everyone for this transformation).

5. Performance Evaluation

Performance Start-Stop
1. Performance year – predefined 12-month period wherein APM eligibility, attribution, and accountability are adjudicated. Most obvious is calendar year (January 1 – December 31).
2. Episode basis – member-specific starting date when initial eligible diagnosis/trigger starts. Unique for each member (eg, one member on March 13, another on April 3, etc.)

Duration of Performance
1. 90 days
2. 6 months
3. 12 months

Illustration
12-month performance year on a calendar year basis with 90-day and 6-month evaluations

physical therapy, imaging, professional fees, physician administered medications, and behavioral health interventions including smoking cessation, weight loss, or pain management. Finally, elements of the supporting infrastructure include the need for a robust health information technology platform spanning an electronic medical record system capable of supporting the multidisciplinary model of care, telehealth platform to enable remote connection and continuity of care, coding and cost accounting platform fit for integrated models of care delivery, and perhaps most importantly a patient-reported outcome measurement solution either built into the electronic medical record or delivered via a third party (**Table 5**).

The accountable entity can be based on voluntary participation and include surgeons, primary care providers, or a single accountable entity in which payments are

TABLE 3	Episode Definition for a Selected Population Including Timing of Services and Accountable Entities	
Payment Model Design		
Episode Definition: Management of hip or knee osteoarthritis from first diagnosis, including nonsurgical and surgical services		
Target Patient Population	**Timing & Duration**	**Accountable Entity**
Patients with diagnosed hip or knee osteoarthritis (OA), excluding co-existing rheumatoid arthritis	Inclusion Criteria: • First instance of hip or knee OA diagnosis • Equation visit	Voluntary participation Orthopaedic surgeon
Patients already affiliated with accountable provider OR patients who meet clinical criteria and voluntarily associate with accountable provider	One-year episode renewed for subsequent years at appropriate rate	Single accountable entity (payments may be divided internally among coordinating care team)

divided internally among the coordinating care team. The CBEP must balance incentives to perform procedures by distributing professional fees across all patients evenly, build infrastructure and alternative care pathways to attract providers and payers to implement the payment model, and shift revenue from facilities to decision makers in the form of shared savings with more appropriate utilization of intensive procedures. More importantly, however, the most effective approach is a dyad between a savvy administrator and clinical champion with a focus on leading a multidisciplinary team that is measured on a single platform of success while achieving appropriate patient reported clinical outcomes. It is very important to allow the team to be led from within and to elevate the best performers into leadership roles within their professional discipline. Rather than a top-down approach, a true multidisciplinary team will allow those on the front lines to help suggest and implement solutions to challenges. Most interactions with central services such as information technology, electronic medical records management, billing, and compliance offices is managed through the leadership dyad, but selection of the appropriate subject matter experts from within the team allows everyone to feel engaged and present their best selves for the group. Overall, functioning as a single team on behalf of the patients rather than a group of individuals is critical to the success of implementing this type of payment reform.

With regard to finance and payment flow, a baseline benchmark is negotiated between the payer and provider/hospital system. This will include all of the evidence-based services that may be used in the treatment of the condition, whether provided by the team or subcontracted to others when needed. Prospective periodic (monthly or quarterly) payments are assigned based on historical per patient annual spend on relevant services (according to the program specifications regarding included ICD-10 codes, Current Procedural Technology codes, sites, types, provider, geographies, lines of businesses, etc.) The payments are for nonsurgical management,

TABLE 4 Examples of Services Included Within the Musculoskeletal Case Illustration Involving Degenerative Joint Disease of the Hip and Knee

Surgery	Medical	Radiology	Pathology and Laboratory	Evaluation and Management
Arthroplasty	Behavioral Services	Radiography	Complete blood	Ampuatory
Total	Durable medical	MRI	count	Hospital
Partial	equipment	CT	Comprehensive	Inpatent
Revision	Physician-Adm Meds	Ultrasono-	metabolic panel	Observation
Removal	Hyaluronic acid	graphy	Surgical	Critical care
Nonarthroplasty	Corticosteroids		pathology	Emergency
Arthroscopy	Patelets		C-reactive	Skilled nursing
Osteotomy	Nutrition services		protein	facility
Arthodesis	Procedures		Erythrocyte sedi-	Other
Arthrotomy	Arthrocentesis		mentation rate	Rest home
Acetabuloplasty	Stimulaton		Infectious agent	Case manage-
	Rehab		detection	ment
	Physical therapist/			Remote care
	occupational			Home health
	therapist			
	Chiropractor			
	Physical medicine			
	and rehabilitation			
	Other			
	Orthosis			
	Complementary			
	medical services			

infrastructure support, surgical episodes including surgical professional fees averaged across attributed practice population and surgical episodes (ie, a population-based payment promoting greater efficiencies). It is important to note that although the condition-based bundle is designed to provide a range of nonsurgical and surgical treatments tailored to the physical, emotional, and social needs of the patient, sometimes early surgery is the highest value approach. If a patient comes into the office with end-stage arthritis and quality of life is severely diminished, then a discussion about surgery is appropriate and timely and there is no reason to force failure of nonsurgical treatment in preparation for surgery. The pricing is set up to accommodate the surgical bundle whenever it is triggered. Discount rates are offered to attract providers and hospitals to adopt and buy in to the payment model. Similar to the principles that allow for original bundled payments to succeed, condition-based bundling would use evidence-based care pathways, standardized treatment processes, and shared decision-making tools to train staff members to work at the top of their license.

TABLE 5 Elements of a Supportive Infrastructure

A. Episode Definition (Trigger)

Key Q. How does an eligible patient "trigger" this initiative?

Key Q. Under what conditions is an eligible member excluded before triggering, or during the initiative?

Key Points. This trigger will most likely depend on the member's diagnosis or provision of a service type, potentially at a certain location and by a certain provider or set of providers.

MSK Illustration. Referral for treatment of hip or knee osteoarthritis

B. Episode Timing (Anchor)

Key Q. Over what time is the program?

Key Q. Are we tending toward a defined episode of care with a patient-specific start/stop – Or are we looking a population health model?

Key Q. Once in the initiative, how long does a patient remain in the initiative?

Key Q. Under what conditions does the member exit the initiative?

Key Points. Episode timing may cover a given calendar year, 90-days since initial eligible claim, etc. In any event, the answer to the timing question also depends on eligibility and the line drawn between who is and who isn't eligible among the population served. Different options for the anchor may include fixed time (days/months/years), fixed event (issue resolution, objective clinical improvement, patient completion of certain activity), and patient choice/election. There is also a need to define renewal terms and who, how, and at what price to renew for subsequent years, if applicable.

MSK Illustration. On the same date of the specialist visit (eg, orthopaedic surgeon); and diagnosis of hip or knee osteoarthritis with duration being one-year, renewable.

C. Patient Population and Risk Adjustment

Key Q. Who is eligible?

Key Q. How will everyone affected know that a patient could be impacted by this new initiative?

Key Q. Where does the patient live?

Key Points. This can be centered on patient diagnosis/condition via ICD-10, lab or other data and clinical characteristics. There may also be geographical considerations with patients from certain counties, certain states, certain regions (eg, ACA), certain lines of business (fully insured, ASO) in the configuration. Exclusion should also be defined, such as for death, co-morbidities, insurance status change, assignment to another strategic program or initiative that may better serve the member.

MSK Illustration. Diagnosed hip or knee osteoarthritis but exclude patients with concomitant rheumatoid arthritis.

D. Service Configuration

Key Q. What does the patient get/who do they see/how are they engaged?

Key Q. How is the patient covered by insurance?

Key Q. What is the location of service(s)?

TABLE 5 Elements of a Supportive Infrastructure (Continued)

Key Points. Based on service utilization (by CPT, HCPCS, other codes) — as all (total costs of care) or certain service codes (provided any which way/only for specific diagnoses, by specific providers (practice entity, specialty type), at specific locations. Servicing provider may be only a certain service provider type, such as medical oncologist; or anyone who touches the patient. The type or place of service may include all types of service; all locations, only an office setting (versus facility), or only a professional claim (versus facility), etc.

The health plan line of business can be focused on an individual market (U65), fully insured (small group, large group, national employer accounts), administrative services only, Medicare, Medicaid, special clients (eg, state health plan, federal employee plan, student groups). Each line of business may be run as a distinct profit-and-loss center, with its own leadership, funding, membership, regulations, business dynamics, and more. They can have widely different considerations depending on the patient population.

Critical to incorporate the engagement of patients and teams using longitudinal measurement of patient reported outcomes, advanced patient experience measures, shared decision-making.

MSK Illustration. All services appropriate and necessary for the treatment of hip or knee osteoarthritis (derived from clinical consensus, evidence-based practice guidelines, claims data analysis).

E. Accountability and Accountable Entity

Key Q. To whom is the patient's care attributed and what is the attribution model?
Key Q. How might you develop models for overlapping accountability involving specialty care in conjunction with different primary care payment and delivery arrangements/integrated care delivery reforms?
Key Q. How will everyone affected know that a patient is impacted by this new initiative?
Key Q. How will accountability be configured and reconciled and is this sustainable?
Key Q. How do you deal with healthcare practice changes?

Key Points. Attribution entails taking nontrivial accountability for the financial, quality, and/or experience. This needs a definition of the providers receiving attribution, and an understanding why these providers and not others. This component also requires an examination of what accountable care programs already exist for the provider and/or health plan for which a patient eligible for this initiative may also be eligible for another program (eg, primary care-based accountable care organization (ACO), integrated delivery network (IDN). There is a need to configure financial or quality "credit" for efficiency/care improvements and defining how it will be trickled down, charged back and whether double payment (ie, equal credit for everyone) will be accepted (whether only in a temporary fashion or permanent). A strategy should be in place for changes in health practices in relation to new drugs or devices, innovations or technology, advances in evidence-based care delivery, professional/clinical practice guidelines, and changing regulations.

Overlapping accountability might take different forms eg, (i) within traditional FFS arrangement (condition-based bundled) (ii) advanced primary care ACOs and specialty model (primary care provider incentivized to work with specialists in this model but leaning toward taking on more risk/savings and services); (iii) integrated/consolidated health system (whole health system may move toward risk-adjusted capitated payment with the aim to improve MSK models within ecosystem).

(Continued)

TABLE 5 Elements of a Supportive Infrastructure (Continued)

Specialty partnerships being considered might irk or excite existing accountable partners (eg, primary care ACOs) by adding the specialty model leveraging their existing benefits toward even greater and more considerable gains (ie, widening the net on opportunities for cost savings). Generally, any subsequent model that removes (1) membership or (2) money from an existing model is resisted. So how can the model be setup to be a win-win-win for the health plan – specialty model – primary care model? Careful consideration and some enterprise architectural changes, including harmonization of the current ACO configurations, are needed with balance reached in contractual specifications around partnership relationships, financial accounting, "fairness"/platonic ideas, and administrative complexity. Technical modifications are also needed ie, – what does the health plan need to incrementally do to identify and record a member's attribution to two or more models? Notably, depending on the specificity of current ACO accountability, specialty model expense may be ineligible to be included. For example, if the ACO contract only permits "medical claims" to be counted in accountability, the health plan may not be able to charge back specialty model shared savings/incentives payments to the ACO.

Finally, it's also important to set appropriate targets over time eg, advanced ACO may focus in the first few years on (a) transformation of primary care through increased access and team-based care; (b) bolstering practice-based case management; (c) reducing utilization of specialty care services eg, avoidance ED reattendance; (d) developing new roles and value-enhancing activities

MSK Illustration. Simply the orthopaedic practice could be the accountable entity but also different designs based on clinician/clinician teams by institutional design for independent practices, health systems, employed physicians, and other risk-bearing entities (including vendors).

F. Finance and Payment Flow

Key Q. What are the key considerations around finance and payment?

Key Points. In an overlapping model situation, options include double-payment (to each the primary and specialty accountable entities) – not ideal, but easiest solution. If affected population is small, but with massive savings opportunity, then it may be sustainable (eg, through adjusting prospective trends). Enables value for the clinical partners, but this dilutes value reaped by health plan; Charge back – create a hierarchy of specialty-then-primary-care medical expense and savings/losses reconciliation, such that specialty experience is charged back to the primary care ACO. Carve out – remove from primary care ACO the affected specialty population. Generally undesirable, but there may be effective use cases. Adjust future primary care ACO trend based on specialty model expense – for the first few years, health plan may be double-paying savings to ACO and specialty model; but over time as savings become more predictable from the specialty model, the primary care ACO trend rate could be adjusted to incorporate the specialty model impact, thus eliminating double-payment by the health plan. 3-way gain share – health plan, specialty model accountable entity, and affected primary care ACO together workout specific gainsharing (eg, 33/33/33 or something similar). This may be fair but adds significant administrative complexity.

Ideally no specialty model would exist that significantly hampers the primary care ACO financially – ie, a specialty program should add fuel to the fire to lower medical expense further and improve quality more broadly.

TABLE 5 Elements of a Supportive Infrastructure (Continued)

MSK Illustration. Prospective periodic (monthly or quarterly) payments based on (a) historical medical expense for eligible population and (b) market trend. The payments are for (1) non-surgical management, (2) infrastructure support, (3) surgical episodes including surgical professional fees averaged across attributed practice population and (4) surgical episodes (ie, a population-based payment promoting greater efficiencies in terms of providers, site of service (eg, ASCs versus outpatient versus. inpatient surgery), and judicious use of surgery

G. Program Pricing

Key Q. What should the episode price be inclusive of and what are withholding criteria?

Key Points. The price is inclusive of:
- Historical per-patient annual spend on relevant services (according to the program specifications regarding included ICD-10s, CPTs, sites, types, provider, geographies, lines of business, etc.)

MSK Illustration

Include surgical professional fee distributed across all patients as fraction of utilization rate (eg, $1,000 fee, 15% utilization rate = $150 added to each per-member per-period payment
- For the related-but-separate surgical bundle, there will exist a separate target price (less the surgical professional fee)

Apply withholds for (1) episode completion/attribution and (2) quality measurement
Balance provider-specific and multi-provider/regional utilization history
Also need to include correction for under-utilization of relevant services (eg, nutrition, mental health)

"Traditional" procedural bundle (eg, facility, PAC) could exist as a separate payment construct, but tied to this one via risk.

H. Type and Level of Risk

Key Q. What are the key considerations around type and level of risk?

Key Points. Likely begin with initial upside for 1 to 2 years, introduce downside years 2 to 3 and beyond, moving eventually toward risk-adjusted capitated payment. Scope of risk to be defined by program parameters (diagnosis, service, site, type, provider, geography, etc.).

I. Performance and Quality Measurement, Evaluation, and Impact

Key Q. How will we measure quality and integrate patient generated health data? Outcomes versus process versus patient self-report

Key Q. What are the types of data required for evaluation and impact assessment?

Key Points.
Process measures and/or outcomes measures
- HEDIS/MIPS measures
- Patient-reported outcomes/experience/engagement/decision-making
- Utilization rates
- Relative utilization intensity (eg, site of service, substitutable utilization)
- Diversity/equity

(Continued)

TABLE 5 Elements of a Supportive Infrastructure (Continued)

Data type ie, how to collect/identify/transmit.
- Utilization/claims
- Patient-reported outcomes measures and instruments
- Provider submitted
  - I (preferred)
  - Self-report (not preferred)

If there are new measures/instruments/measurement approaches being considered for the provider/health plan then it is important to consider whether existing tools can be repurposed, whether one or more existing measures are "good enough", and for new/modified measures to better understand the level of effort/cost required to develop (usually by health plan) and the timeline for doing so.

MSK Illustration. Achieve minimum patient-reported outcome improvement for minimum percentage of practice's patients in key domains: Pain, anatomic site-specific disability (eg, for knee, for shoulder distinctly), general health/quality of life, mental health. Relevant measures include: KOOSJR, HOOSJR, PROMIS physical function, PROMIS Global-10, NPRS, SF 12v12, HKSS. Require race/ethnicity reporting. Consider performance guarantees for per-capita utilization around opioids, advanced imaging, global surgical utilization, etc. Relevant HEDIS measures include: Advanced care planning, care for older adults, appropriate use of imaging studies for low back pain, among others.

J. Quality Reporting, Impact and Socialization

Key Q. How will quality impact the program?
Key Q. Will there be performance guarantees?
Key Q. What is the reporting structure?
Key Q. How will the program be socialized?

Key Points.
Assessing the impact of quality on the program requires setting benchmarks (based on data type and time); setting accountability (considering that until benchmarks are reliably established, how is accountable entity responsible for quality; and once benchmarks established, how the accountable entity will be responsible – eg, beat absolute threshold, maintain rates, beat target rate or improvement (eg, 5% improvement). Also considering for a given performance against a benchmark, what the reward or penalty will be and whether there will be a bonus pool. Existing shared savings/losses arrangement impact will also require consideration, such that post-quality-reconciliation earned sharing rate is increased/maintained/decreased. Will need to define how much of the sharing rate is impacted? 5%, 50%, 100%?

In terms of performance guarantees, need to consider process-related service level agreements such as data exchange, member engagement, member program completion.

TABLE 5 Elements of a Supportive Infrastructure (Continued)
In terms of program reporting need to consider how the health plan reports to the accountable entity; how the accountable entity reports to the health plan; what the health plan/accountability will report to the member; what the health plan/accountability entity will report to the health plan customer (eg, employers). This can build on reporting system that currently exists but also factor in reporting elements that will be net new and the level of effort, cadence, and specification of contemporary reporting approach.
In terms of program socialization, key considerations will include how the program will be socialized to the provider community in relation to ACOs, independent practices, health systems and who will socialize and to what extent. Plus, how the program will be socialized to the health plan customers and to members.

Some Key Considerations

Risk Adjustment

First, in designing a condition-based bundle, recognizing the potential risks inherent of a heterogenous population that could affect resource utilization becomes critical. In a procedure-based bundle, the risk stems from patients with complex medical issues that could potentially extend length of stay, influence higher intensity after discharge disposition, and potentially result in higher readmission. These risks are still present in a condition-based bundle. However, with a Condition Bundled Payment intended to move upstream from a patient's condition, there is now risk that centers around determining the likelihood of needing surgery among these patients enrolled in the payment model. Moreover, patients may have varying pain severities attributed by their DJD and consequently use disproportionate amounts of nonsurgical care. This issue is mitigated somewhat by having a broader population included in the bundle. Nevertheless, the factors that influence the likelihood of utilizing nonsurgical care versus surgical care remain unknown and need further study to inform effective risk adjustment.

Population Identification

Second, to create a sustainable APM, the condition-based bundle will need to attract interested and willing payers, purchasers, clinicians, and patients all with varying practice types, market shares, and financial situations. Designing payment model pricing and flow options for CBEPs will require use of empirical claims analysis to help identify and characterize high-prevalence, high-cost chronic conditions that could benefit from improved efficiency, outcomes, and potential savings. Additionally, identifying the right patient population that would ideally benefit from the model will be critical to the success of the CBP model. This can be centered on patient diagnosis/condition via ICD-10, laboratory, or other data and clinical characteristics. Exclusion should also be defined, such as for death, comorbidities, insurance status change, assignment to another strategic program or initiative that may better serve the member.

Attribution

A third challenge will be how model developers define return on investment and how to distribute cost savings within the program. Any case for CBEP should include how providers can attribute patients, how the structure improves on fee-for-service, the pathways available once patients are attributed, and example opportunities for achieving savings. Determining how these models will function in different organizations will be challenging, but critical. Integrated hospital systems and independent practices have inherent differences with regards to infrastructure and resource-utilization. Distinguishing how to design a model suitable for a clinician-entity's needs will be a challenge for parties interested in adopting this type of payment reform. Considerations for solvency and acknowledging that higher payment may be required to help equip smaller, independent practices will be an important consideration in promoting the adoption of CBEPs. Furthermore, an emphasis on PROMs will be critical as they offer one of the most effective tools to measure meaningful outcomes, which drives patient satisfaction. To date, however, many organizations have yet to make significant progress collecting and reporting PROMs. The lack of standardization and creating universally precise, efficient PROMs to track longitudinal outcomes will limit the progress of condition-based reform. Moreover, it will be important to streamline existing reporting processes to make PROMs easier to generate, report and analyze for improving payer transmission.

Breaking Away From Old Models

Fourth, fighting certain stigmas with regard to novel payment reform will be a challenge in the years to come. Proponents of CBEPs have found that many payers are not prepared to adapt to the nontraditional type of billing and payment attributed with CBEPs. Bundles should be built with a strong payer-clinician partnership with an aligned vision and mission. These particular bundled programs are set up to help health care specialists to behave more rationally in the best interests of their patients instead of having uphill battles to deliver the care that patients need. It gives them more stake in the game so that they can pay more attention to appropriate resource management while continuing to require accountability on the side of patient outcomes. Ultimately, those who are not interested will take longer to adopt these reformed payment models. However, the obvious benefits of these strategies will slowly force them into the market as well. Continuing down a fee-for-service path will perpetuate payment for a multitude of unnecessary services without any data on the true outcomes of patients, which is not a sustainable strategy in the current stream of payment reform.

FUTURE OF CONDITION-BASED PAYMENTS

The implementation of condition-based bundling has been slow to develop, but early results show that it provides a promising alternative to FFS and procedure-based bundling to improve outcomes and focus on true cost-saving value-based care. Key drivers for success require the presence of a strong, motivated leadership of clinicians and ancillary staff to establish well-defined goals with a clear emphasis on patient engagement and the desire to push for access to valid, reliable data on costs and outcomes in real time.

The framework of condition-based payment is intended to provide financial support for the necessary care delivery models and generate the incentives to deliver condition-based rather than procedure-based care. It offers a viable and exciting path forward for specialist-driven, value-based health care but efforts are still in the early stages. In its current form, CBEPs in orthopaedics have been limited to mostly managing hip and knee arthritis as standardized care pathways exist and are defined. However, there are standardized care pathways for other chronic diseases in orthopaedics and these CBEPs will need to be defined, adopted, and studied. Payers are beginning to take steps to make value-based contracting for patients with specialized chronic disease more routine. The Center for Medicare and Medicaid Innovation is developing models for direct provider contractor, which is one promising avenue to build a specialized condition-based platform. Additionally, refining the use of PROMs through predictive analytics solution using artificial intelligence are already underway to enhance the informed decision-making process by generating personalized benefit-risk and complication for patients.

SUMMARY

As efforts ramp up, enabling clinician, practice, and payer champions will be essential for informing practice-based business decisions and organization-specific care redesign. Ongoing efforts are underway to push the goals of condition-based bundling, which is to improve preventative/conservative care delivery, tackle appropriateness of surgery/procedure, and ultimately improve outcomes regardless of whether patients pursue nonsurgical or surgical care pathways.

REFERENCES

1. Papanicolas I, Woskie LR, Jha AK: Health care spending in the United States and other high-income countries. *J Am Med Assoc* 2018;319(10):1024-1039.

2. Porter ME: What is value in health care? *N Engl J Med* 2010;363(26):2477-2481.

3. Agarwal R, Liao JM, Gupta A, Navathe AS: The impact of bundled payment on health care spending, utilization and quality: A systematic review. *Health Aff (Millwood)* 2020;39(1):50-57.

4. Bosco JA, Harty JH, Iorio R: Bundled payment arrangements: Keys to success. *J Am Acad Orthop Surg* 2018;26(23):817-822.

5. Press MJ, Rajkumar R, Conway PH: Medicare's new bundled payments: Design, strategy, and evolution. *J Am Med Assoc* 2016;315(2):131-132.

6. CMS.gov: Comprehensive care for joint replacement model [Internet]. Available at: https://innovation.cms.gov. Accessed April 25, 2023.

7. Navathe AS, Song Z, Emanuel EJ: The next generation of episode-based payments. *J Am Med Assoc* 2017;317(23):2371-2372.

8. Dummit LA, Kahvecioglu D, Marrufo G, et al: Association between hospital participation in a Medicare bundled payment initiative and payments and quality outcomes for lower extremity joint replacement episodes. *J Am Med Assoc* 2016;316(12):1267-1278.

9. Barnett ML, Wilcock A, McWilliams JM, et al: Two-year evaluation of mandatory bundled payments for joint replacement. *N Engl J Med* 2019;380(3):252-262.

10. Kivlahan C, Orlowski JM, Pearce J, Walradt J, Baker M, Kirch DG: Taking risk: Early results from teaching hospitals' participation in the center for Medicare and Medicaid innovation bundled payments for care improvement initiative. *Acad Med* 2016;91(7):936-942.

11. Bannuru RR, Osani MC, Vaysbrot EE, et al: OARSI guidelines for the non-surgical management of knee, hip, and polyarticular osteoarthritis. *Osteoarthritis Cartilage* 2019;27(11):1578-1589.

12. Skou ST, Roos EM: Physical therapy for patients with knee and hip osteoarthritis: Supervised, active treatment is current best practice. *Clin Exp Rheumatol* 2019;37(5 suppl 120):112-117.

13. Rathbun AM, Shardell MD, Ryan AS, et al: Association between disease progression and depression onset in persons with radiographic knee osteoarthritis. *Rheumatology (Oxford)* 2020;59(11):3390-3399.

14. Hawker GA: Osteoarthritis is a serious disease. *Clin Exp Rheumatol* 2019;37(5 suppl 120):3-6.

15. Straub LE, Cisternas MG: Psychological well-being among US adults with arthritis and the unmet need for mental health care. *Open Access Rheumatol* 2017;9:101-110.

16. Jaiswal P, Railton P, Khong H, Smith C, Powell J: Impact of preoperative mental health status on functional outcome 1 year after total hip arthroplasty. *Can J Surg* 2019;62(5):300-304.

17. Perneger TV, Hannouche D, Miozzari HH, Lübbeke A: Symptoms of osteoarthritis influence mental and physical health differently before and after joint replacement surgery: A prospective study. *PLoS One* 2019;14(6):e0217912.

18. Inacio MCS, Paxton EW, Graves SE, Namba RS, Nemes S: Projected increase in total knee arthroplasty in the United States – An alternative projection model. *Osteoarthritis Cartilage* 2017;25(11):1797-1803.

19. Riddle DL, Jiranek WA, Hayes CW: Use of a validated algorithm to judge the appropriateness of total knee arthroplasty in the United States: A multicenter longitudinal cohort study. *Arthritis Rheumatol* 2014;66(8):2134-2143.

20. Ghomrawi HMK, Mushlin AI, Kang R, et al: Examining timeliness of total knee replacement among patients with knee osteoarthritis in the US: Results from the OAI and MOST longitudinal cohorts. *J Bone Joint Surg Am* 2020;102(6):468-476.

21. Jayakumar P, Uhler L, Galea V, Hoff M, Koenig K: *Improving Value in Musculoskeletal Health Care.* The University of Texas at Austin, Dell Medical School Musculoskeletal Institute Experience. White Paper, 2020.

22. Vetter TR, Uhler LM, Bozic KJ: Value-based healthcare: Preoperative assessment and global optimization (PASS-GO) – Improving value in total joint replacement care. *Clin Orthop Relat Res* 2017;475(8):1958-1962.

23. Malay MR, Lentz TA, O'Donnell J, Coles T, Mather Iii RC, Jiranek WA: Development of a comprehensive, nonsurgical joint health program for people with osteoarthritis: A case report. *Phys Ther* 2020;100(1):127-135.

24. Bennell KL, Ahamed Y, Jull G, et al: Physical therapist-delivered pain coping skills training and exercise for knee osteoarthritis: Randomized controlled trial. *Arthritis Care Res (Hoboken)* 2016;68(5):590-602.

25. Lentz TA, George SZ, Manickas-Hill O, et al: What general and pain-associated psychological distress phenotypes exist among patients with hip and knee osteoarthritis? *Clin Orthop Relat Res* 2020;478(12):2768-2783.

26. Victorian Osteoarthritis Model of Care. Available at: https://msk.org.au/wp-content/uploads/2018/07/MoC_Final-report.pdf. Accessed March 09, 2021.

27. Skou ST, Roos EM: Good Life with osteoarthritis in Denmark (GLA:D™): Evidence-based education and supervised neuromuscular exercise delivered by certified physiotherapists nationwide. *BMC Musculoskelet Disord* 2017;18(1):72.

28. Van Citters AD, Fahlman C, Goldmann DA, et al: Developing a pathway for high-value, patient-centered total joint arthroplasty. *Clin Orthop Relat Res* 2014;472(5):1619-1635.

29. Dartmouth-Hitchcock Medical Center: Dartmouth-Hitchcock "Green Care." Available at: https://www.dartmouth-hitchcock.org/about. Accessed March 09, 2021.

30. Jayakumar P, Moore MG, Furlough KA, et al: Comparison of an artificial intelligence-enabled patient decision aid vs educational material on decision quality, shared decision-making, patient experience, and functional outcomes in adults with knee osteoarthritis: A randomized clinical trial. *JAMA Netw Open* 2021;4(2):e2037107.

31. Geisinger Medical Center chosen as hip and knee replacement Center of Excellence. Available at: https://www.geisinger.org/about-geisinger/news-and-media/news-releases/2020/07/21/19/36/geisinger-medical-center-chosen-as-hip-and-knee-replacement-center-of-excellence. Accessed March 09, 2021.

32. Stewart A: Walmart's centers of excellence program cut joint replacement costs by 15% – 5 things to know. *Becker Spine Review*. March 18, 2019. Available at: https://www.beckersspine.com/beckers-orthopedic-and-spine-review/45089-walmart-s-centers-of-excellence-program-cut-joint-replacement-costs-by-15-5-things-to-know.html. Accessed April 25, 2023.

33. Jayakumar P, O'Donnell J, Manickas-Hill O, et al: Critical considerations for condition based alternative payment models: A multistakeholder perspective. Available at: https://www.healthaffairs.org/do/10.1377/hblog20200714.732842/full/. Accessed April 25, 2023.

CHAPTER 10

Global Capitation and the US Healthcare Landscape

Eugenia Lin, MD • Prakash Jayakumar, MD, PhD

INTRODUCTION

The escalation of health care costs in the US and the exacerbation by economic and public health crises has placed value-based reimbursement at the forefront of the health care policy and practice agenda. This chapter provides a brief history and evolution of global capitation in US health care, compares and contrasts this model with value-based bundled payment, assesses the pros and cons of global capitation, and explores key considerations for implementing capitated models in current orthopaedic practice.

BACKGROUND

Global capitation is a type of payment model designed for integrated health care delivery. Capitated payment models (also termed global payments or global budgets) are usually structured as a single, fixed prospective payment made by payers to provider organizations to cover the costs of a predefined set of services delivered to patients periodically, usually as a per-member per-month arrangement.[1,2] Provider organizations include integrated care organizations, physicians, or large physician groups that aim to deliver all the necessary services to meet a patient's health care needs (eg, diagnostics, home health, and inpatient and outpatient services) over a designated period of time. The total payment does not vary based on the services provided, and provider organizations are themselves simultaneously assessed for quality and outcomes of care delivered. Common features of global capitation models include the administration and oversight of cost and performance by clinicians, financial infrastructures configured around a baseline global budget, and broad stakeholder engagement between payers, clinicians, and policymakers.

In the broader context of US health care, the rapid escalation in health care spending (approximately 17% of gross domestic product in 2018) has failed to achieve a commensurate improvement in many population health outcomes[3] (**Figure 1**). This vulnerability has stimulated a need to rethink health care payment and practice, which remains embedded in an unsustainable but

Neither of the following authors nor any immediate family member has received anything of value from or has stock or stock options held in a commercial company or institution related directly or indirectly to the subject of this chapter: Dr. Lin and Dr. Jayakumar.

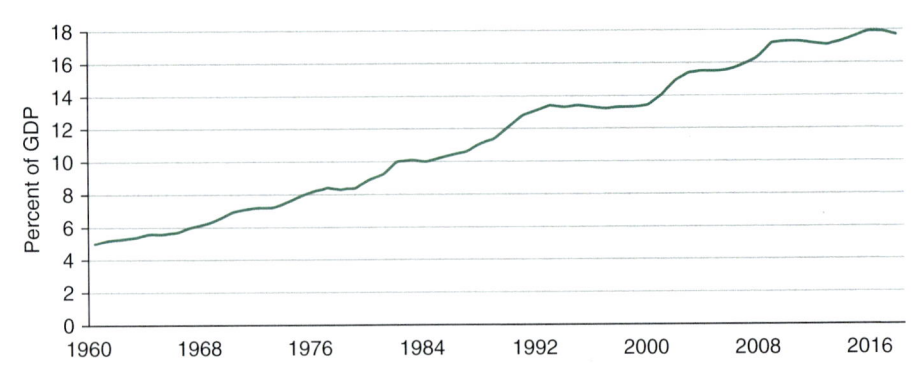

FIGURE 1 US health care expenditure as a share of gross domestic product (GDP), 1960 to 2018. (Reproduced with permission from Nunn R, Parsons J, Shambaugh J: A dozen facts about the economics of the US health-care system. Brookings. Available at: https://www.brookings.edu/research/a-dozen-facts-about-the-economics-of-the-u-s-health-care-system/. Accessed February 3, 2021.)

dominant fee-for-service (FFS) infrastructure.[3] Global capitation offers one type of value-based reimbursement strategy for containing costs without sacrificing quality and striving to achieve outcome-based reimbursement benefiting both patients and clinicians (**Table 1**). Compared with FFS, global capitation aims to reduce the use of expensive or duplicative resources and low-value

TABLE 1 Types of Value-Based Models

Bundles	Shared Savings	Shared Risk	Global Capitation
Health care provider receives a fixed amount for services per episode of care (ie, irrespective of number of clinicians or services) Bundles encourage collaboration and delivery of a range of services to meet patient needs, reduce low-value interventions (eg, redundant, non–evidence-based tests and treatments), and reduce costs for patients and clinicians	Payers reimburse clinicians or provider organizations based on performance (quality and spending targets) Also known as upside risk, clinicians share in net savings that accrue to payer when actual spending for defined population is less than target amount. If clinicians spend above the target, they do not incur penalties from payers	Payers reimburse clinicians or provider organizations based on performance (quality and spending targets) Also known as downside risk, clinicians gain greater financial rewards when actual spending is less than target amount, but also take on greater risk and losses (covering all or part of excessive costs) if spending above target	Clinicians paid a single, fixed amount per patient covering all services Clinician takes on 100% risk but keeps all savings

interventions, issues that are prevalent in current orthopaedic practice. Capitation also provides an opportunity for sustainable value-based payment, capable of remaining buoyant amid various crises in health care from economic recessions to pandemics; these disruptions can affect volumes of inpatient and outpatient care, especially in the wide variety of preference-sensitive conditions, such as osteoarthritis.

A BRIEF HISTORY OF GLOBAL CAPITATION IN THE UNITED STATES

In 1965, the US government enacted Medicare, government-funded health insurance programs, and the use of retrospective FFS payments. An exponential increase in use and costs of care in subsequent years resulted in the government and private payers seeking alternative reimbursement models that could curb this medical inflation. In the early 1970s, the Nixon presidential administration enabled the development of health maintenance organizations (HMOs) and some competitive medical plans.[4,5] HMOs used capitated payment and aimed to reduce waste in the medical system while also increasing market competition. Competitive medical plans, although less commonly used, are a type of managed care organization that offers a prepaid capitated delivery similar to HMOs; however, they are not federally certified and therefore face less regulation compared with HMOs.

Following the HMO Assistance Act of 1973, HMOs became more common from the mid to late 1970s, garnering federal backing with additional supportive legislation and financial public assistance. In subsequent decades, HMOs saw substantial growth, influenced in part by the conversion of HMOs from nonprofit organizations to for-profit, private sector entities that experienced high volumes of enrollment. HMOs were primarily owned by insurance companies with employers paying the HMOs for services on a capitated basis, most commonly via per-member per-month payment arrangements. HMOs, in turn, continued to pay care delivery groups by using FFS, and in some cases, passed along a portion of the capitated insurance payment directly onto clinician groups, sharing some of the financial risk. Different strategies to limit health care consumption have been employed by HMOs, including mandates set for primary care providers to act as gatekeepers on the front lines, and some HMO plans formed stringent criteria for specialist-to-specialist referrals.

HMOs waned after reaching peak utilization around 1996 to 1998 (approximately 16% of all payment method types) before leveling off to approximately 7% in 2007 and 5.3% by 2013.[6,7] Although HMOs were successful in mitigating the increase in national health care expenditures, critics flagged delays to treatment, rationing of care, and potential undertreatment as reasons to shift from these arrangements toward alternative payment models (APMs) focused on providing appropriate interventions in line with the patient's needs. A growing number of patients and physicians expressed dissatisfaction with the quality of care with a sense that profits were driving the model, rather than care configured around the patient's condition.[8] HMOs decreased in utilization because of inadequate risk adjustments, resulting in ineffective accounting of the disease burden, and inaccurate budgeting and side effects such as physician groups taking on more risk than they could manage. Ultimately, HMO use declined as FFS, preferred provider organizations (PPOs), and other open-access models continued to grow and increase market competition in the United States.[7]

CAPITATION MODELS AND THE TRANSFORMATION TOWARD VALUE

Value in health care is defined as the health outcomes benefiting patients relative to cost.[9] Passage of the Patient Protection and Affordable Care Act (colloquially known as Obamacare) enacted by the 111th US Congress and signed into law in 2010, allowed the creation of accountable care organizations (ACOs): groups of doctors, hospitals, and other medical specialists that are voluntarily committed to providing coordinated high-value care to Medicare patients.[10] ACOs now have different forms based on the local health care environment and existing level of competition among clinicians. These include those piloted through the Centers for Medicare & Medicaid Services (CMS) and the Center for Medicare and Medicaid Innovation, such as the Medicare Shared Savings Program, as well as those developed by private payers. The goals of commercial ACOs mirror those of CMS ACOs. ACOs can use FFS billing approaches with productivity-based compensation, incentive-based compensation, or straight salaries, or structure payment through global capitation.[10] Variable integration of bonus payments for achieving quality benchmarks can also be instituted.

Additional legislation supporting the transition from volume-based reimbursement toward that which is value-based includes the 2015 enactment of the Medicare Access and Children's Health Insurance Program Reauthorization Act (MACRA). MACRA replaces Medicare's reimbursement system originally implemented in 1992 and revised in 1997 as the Sustainable Growth Rate Formula.[11-13] Termed the permanent "doc fix," this legislation authorized the implementation of an incentive payment program known as the Quality Payment Program (QPP).[14,15] The QPP has two value-based payment tracks known as the Merit-Based Incentive Payment System (MIPS) and the advanced APM.[15]

The MACRA legislation is a pay-for-performance program but allows opportunities for capitation-based models. The aim of MACRA and the QPP is to transform payment for care based on quality, cost, promoting interoperability, care coordination, and improvement activities. The two tracks of the QPP allow the opportunity to blend different model configurations to mitigate unwarranted errors from processing different payment structures.[14-17] Other programs such as CMS's Medicare-Medicaid Financial Alignment Initiative, which began in 2015, implement capitated-payment reimbursement models in different states.[18,19] This model enables CMS, a state, and a health plan to jointly enter a three-way contract to provide coordinated care. CMS and the state pay for the health plan and prospective capitated payment. This capitated model by CMS involves a blended capitated rate for Medicare-Medicaid enrollees (or dual-eligible individuals), whereas the health plans oversee coordinated care across the spectrum of Medicare and Medicaid services.[19]

Similar to previous capitated models such as HMOs, the current CMS Capitated Models aim for overall cost savings through improved management, decreased use of high-cost services, and increased administrative and clinical efficiency. In contrast to HMOs, these newer models implement and use measures of quality improvement. To incentivize providers to meet quality thresholds, CMS and the state utilize withholding of a portion of the capitated payment to the participating health plan.[20] More recently, an option that aligns with both payment tracks includes the Direct Contracting model that commenced in 2021, a 5-year Medicare ACO that explores partially and fully capitated payment models.[21] The next generation of ACOs and newer care delivery models developed by government and commercial payers oriented toward improving outcomes relative to cost may participate in capitated payment mechanisms such as the All-Inclusive Population-Based Payment (AIPBP).

GLOBAL CAPITATION VERSUS VALUE-BASED BUNDLED PAYMENT

Global capitation covers a range of services that can be used to manage the health care needs of a specific patient population (**Figure 2**). The financial risk largely falls on providers: although they benefit from the total savings for costs of care that remain less than a single, fixed prospective payment set for services required by the population served, they also experience a financial loss if costs exceed this target payment. The amount of payment is based on historical data or prospective actuarial assessment. In contrast, bundled episode payment, a single payment

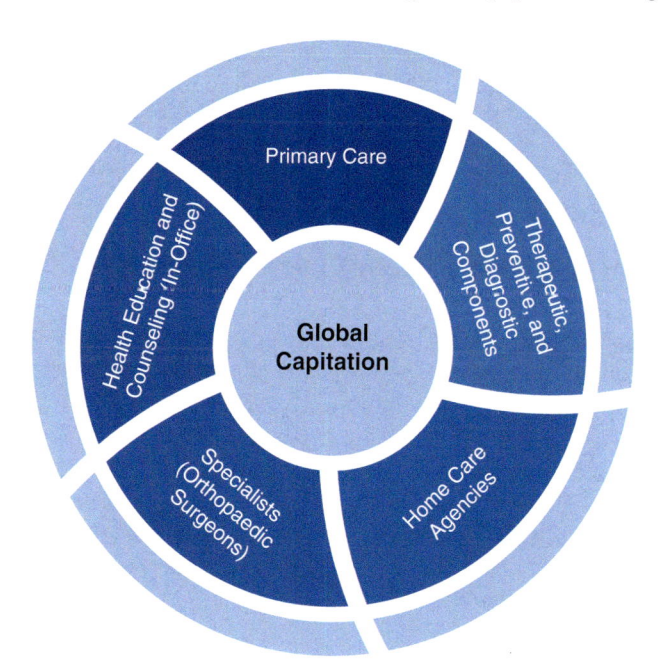

FIGURE 2 Global capitation services. An example of services that global capitation payment models may cover including primary care services, health education and counselling (in-office), specialist care (such as orthopaedics), home care agencies, and therapeutic, preventive, and diagnostic components.

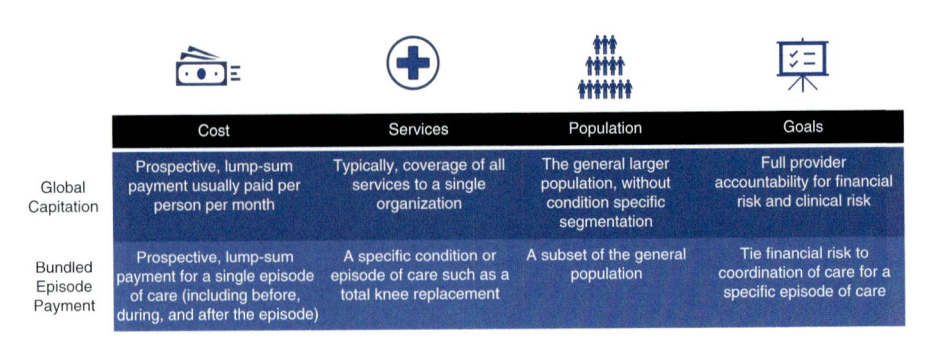

FIGURE 3 Global capitation versus bundled episode payment models. A comparison of two value-based care models, global capitation and bundled episode payments by cost, services, population, and overall goals of the two models.

made to cover the cost of services delivered by multiple providers over a defined time period for an episode of care (eg, total knee arthroplasty), offers an alternative model for value-based reimbursement. Although bundled episode payments have traditionally been targeted toward high-volume, high-cost procedures such as those piloted nationally in joint arthroplasty, they can also be configured around conditions, such as persistent joint pain secondary to osteoarthritis. Both approaches involve prospective lump-sum payments to cover the cost of care delivered, but they can differ in terms of population, scope of services, and duration of coverage (**Figure 3**). The debate continues around the optimal choice for a given health system in achieving value between global capitation and bundled episode payments.[22] This chapter focuses on the strengths and weakness of global capitation and these are reflected against aspects of bundled episode payment.

STRENGTHS AND WEAKNESSES OF GLOBAL CAPITATION

Payment, Incentives, and Costs of Care

Global capitation represents a fundamental shift away from FFS, in which providers are held accountable for providing necessary services and achieving an expected level of quality improvement for a designated population at a fixed cost. The prospective payment in capitated models offers some tolerance against socioeconomic crises. This contrasts with FFS structures, which depend on volume and become heavily affected by reductions or suspensions of interventions during such crises. Effectively, the prepayment in capitated models affords a steady flow of cash, enabling systems to continue business, in the short-term at least, allowing both providers and patients to budget for health care expenses in a more predictable manner.[2,23]

In global capitation, providers are incentivized to avoid unnecessary tests and low-value interventions (which contain costs rather than generating profit) via a system of prepayment that covers a range of medical services. For instance, if medical imaging such as MRI is appropriate for assessment of a given condition, patients do not need to consider the costs of this test, which will be included in the suite of services provided. However, if evidence is lacking for the benefit of performing MRI, providers are less inclined to order it. Patients may also appreciate that the costs of their care are more effectively aligned with their clinical needs rather than secondary financial gains for the provider.

As a counterpoint, some experts underline the potential for abuse of global capitation by the underutilization of services to contain costs, and the risk of providers being less intent on treating more complex patients. The effects of "rationing" and "cherry picking" in capitated models were evident in the HMO era.[24] Because clinicians are prompted to lower health care expenditures by selecting only appropriate care, there is a potential for restricting services, regardless of appropriateness. In the case of HMOs, the rationing of care tended to occur by the insurance plans and not providers themselves.[25] More recent models of capitation shift responsibility and insurance risk onto providers, along with aspects such as prior authorizations and denials.[2] Although some models assert that greater financial responsibility can incentivize providers to minimize waste and optimize efficiency, other models contend that this increased pressure can trickle down to negatively affect patient-provider relationships.[26]

As an alternative, bundled episode payments allow both clinicians (who better understand clinical risk and provide optimal care for patients) and payers (who better understand financial risk and provide actuarial assessment) to perform their roles and play to their strengths. Proponents think that bundled episode payments also offer a more effective purchasing mechanism for consumers, giving them a stake in the process of engaging with value-based purchasing by providing the opportunity to calculate the portion of the bundled price upfront. However, these models may also run the risk of overuse and a tendency to seek further episode-based payments, which may risk slipping into a volume-based approach to care. Although the barriers to entry may be considered lower for bundled episode payments compared with capitated models incorporating large health systems, both models have the potential to amass market power.

Both global capitation and bundled episode payments support a fundamental shift toward quality improvement and an outcomes-driven approach to care delivery and payment that extends beyond increasing efficiency and cost-containment alone. This effort requires a more comprehensive patient-centered approach that engages patients in education, self-management, and prevention as much as managing their condition with a range of evidence-based interventions. Effective countermeasures will also be beneficial in limiting underuse or overuse of resources, plus additional controls against amassing market power to drive up prices while promoting drivers for appropriate treatment selection, and instilling trust between clinicians and payers to set the right price at the outset. Strategies to achieve the right balance may include adjustment of payment amounts for volume increases, price ceilings or regulatory oversight over price increases, prior authorizations for particular procedures, and the institution of stop loss coverage and risk corridors. Stop loss, also known as excess insurance, is coverage for catastrophic or unpredictable claims. Particularly in capitation, stop-loss coverage refers to protection against financial loss incurred based on a capitation agreement between the plan and the clinician.[27] Risk corridors are a provision in risk-sharing agreements whereby a clinician's financial losses or profits are limited to a specified percentage above and below their break-even point, to prevent them from experiencing excessive profits or catastrophic losses (especially relevant in the case of smaller clinician groups from taking on too much financial risk).[27]

Clinical Care Delivery

Capitated models provide care that is integrated and coordinated around the patient's needs. Care delivery is organized at various levels, from a hospital or healthcare system to clinician groups. For example, a multidisciplinary group of clinicians across different service lines could comprise a care delivery network whereby patients receive care across treatment settings by using a designated set of resources.[28] The structural and functional integration within capitated models also offers a degree of versatility and the capability to include novel approaches, therapies, and treatments of proven efficacy that may otherwise be challenging to integrate into other payment and practice settings. One example is the introduction of telemedicine for video consultations to improve continuity of care and convenience, while also saving cost and time without incurring the billing challenges that could arise in more traditional FFS models. Another example involves more effective interactions among specialty care, primary care, community-based organizations, which may be crucial for assessment and taking action around social determinants of health, preventive care, and effective care coordination between primary and secondary care. One example in the inpatient setting is the program implementation for comprehensive care of geriatric hip fractures at the University of Colorado, in which geriatric patients historically were treated by different service lines during their inpatient stay.[29] Historically, the lack of care coordination resulted in surgical delay and discharge, difficulties with complications and recovery, and poor coordination following discharge. Length of stay was the primary outcome and was significantly improved, with hospitalist comanagement and redesign of workflow for optimal care coordination. Notably, patient follow-up with primary care providers for osteoporosis also increased significantly.

Considering bundled episode payments, procedure-focused bundles may more effectively bring the clinical team and hospital together to develop specific service lines around the intervention. Over time, these services are performed with greater efficiency without sacrificing quality, as observed in models such as the CMS CJR bundle. However, experts have expressed caution around the potential for these models to proliferate into focused factories fueling a so-called medical arms race with competition over the newest technologies and this stimulating overuse rather than controlling spending. In contrast, bundled episode payments focused on the condition rather than procedure and driven by patient outcomes promise to achieve better value for patients.

Proponents of global capitation recognize the complexities around bundled payments when it comes to handling overlapping or concurrent episodes, and how these conditions evolve over time could be complicated to manage operationally. New clinical issues arising over time (termed the woodwork effect) may add to this complexity. This naturally requires a comprehensive definition of the episodes, episode trigger, and how multiple concurrent conditions (and potential episodes and movement between these episodes) are controlled and shared. Although supporters of global capitation suggest that the provider network may offer a more pragmatic approach to treating a broader mix of patients with a spectrum from single discrete conditions to multiple comorbidities, proponents of bundled episodes think that careful configuration including allowances (eg, for high-complexity patients and complications) will prevent the system from becoming overwhelmed. Bundles may also enable closer control over the provision of certain services without burdening the clinicians with insurance risks. Both global capitation and bundled episode payments require effective risk-adjustment strategies.

From the population perspective, it is also important to recognize the potential for different value-based reimbursement arrangements for commercial versus Medicare patients who have distinct clinical and insurance characteristics (eg, the effect of increasing co-pays and deductibles). Further, considerations for these arrangements include the integration of social factors (unmet needs and social determinants of health) alongside considerations around health equity and access for vulnerable populations.

Data Systems and Administration

Implementing the organizational infrastructure for value-based reimbursement that delivers an optimal set of services and enables performance measurement aligned with value (standardized outcome measurement sets and quality metrics) naturally requires a level of upfront investment. Global capitation aims to decrease the administrative burden by providing an initial payment that serves as a simple prospective transaction covering the patient's care pathway. However, the model still depends on substantial actuarial planning and adjustments for risk that can be developed based on information learned from earlier versions of these models.[2]

Risk adjustment is a process of adjusting payments to clinicians to reflect patient characteristics, especially health status, age, sex, and other demographic characteristics. Although existing risk adjustment techniques have their limitations, the capture of a wide range of measures quantifying physical, psychological, and social determinants of health should be incorporated to improve this function.[30,31] Standardized sets of measures for social determinants and/or indexed social risk data could be used in this instance.[32] Calculations using traditional risk adjustment models can be challenging when also trying to incorporate uncontrollable and unforeseen risks. An effective system should be configured to ensure payers retain insurance risk (ie, the risk of whether patients have serious health problems) and that providers accept performance risk (ie, the risk of whether care for a particular health problem is delivered effectively).

A critical component in enabling value-based reimbursement models is a system (or more specifically, a suite of tools) that provides actionable data that monitors and manages utilization, outcomes and costs. Both bundles and capitated models depend on a departure from legacy transaction systems managing FFS billing toward solutions capable of managing alternative performance-based forms of payment. In global capitation, although the responsibility of care delivery and payment risk still remains with the provider or provider group, the tools to enact this model can be facilitated by external support from the payer and some third-party companies. With the backdrop of clement regulations due to the coronavirus disease 2019 (COVID-19) pandemic and broad overhaul of anti-Stark laws to enable reform to make room for value-based care, data analytic companies have begun to develop tools to mitigate the administrative complexity of value-based contracting and payment arrangements.

More robust data analysis will also guide further definition of the payment model, which may involve the development of a fully capitated model or transitions toward hybrid configurations (eg, partial capitation, in which clinicians are paid a single monthly payment to cover certain services for patients on a capitated basis). Capitated services may include laboratory testing, preventive care by contracting with groups of clinicians delivering all enrollees outpatient care, whereas other services are covered on a FFS basis, such as reimbursement of hospitals in their network for inpatient care. Other combinations include part capitated, part ACO-style shared-savings arrangements.

KEY CONSIDERATIONS FOR IMPLEMENTING CAPITATION IN CURRENT ORTHOPAEDIC PRACTICE

Implementing capitation-based models in current orthopaedic practices should consider perspectives at the policy, payer, and patient-clinician level.

Policy Level

The federal commitment for states to implement innovative capitated models is ongoing with legislation including MACRA, the institution of MIPS, advanced APMs, and CMS's Financial Alignment Initiative. Years of federal legislation have also called for the use of capitated payments in the form of block grants for states to limit Medicaid expenditure.[13,14] The stimulus for policymakers to move toward capitated models of payment and value-based reimbursement has been further emphasized by the fragility of the FFS system exposed by the COVID-19 pandemic.[23,33]

Orthopaedic practices considering a move toward fully or partially capitated models require a degree of overhaul of existing infrastructures, greater regulatory guidance from policymakers, and upfront investment. The 2015 MACRA legislation provides federal policy guidance to address various payment-related and practice-related aspects toward value-based delivery. First, the legislation itself superseded the previous Medicare SFG formula for reimbursement, which was unpopular with both providers and legislators.[12] Second, the MIPS and Advanced APMs provide options for providers to align with capitated delivery models.[14,33]

Policymakers need to gauge whether current legislation such as MACRA are sufficient enough for guiding practices toward capitated payment. Some experts think that capitated payment options through MIPS and Advanced APMs are too few and may be too slow to implement.[13,34] Most capitation-based models to date have occurred in primary care, whereas specialty services have focused more on using bundled payment arrangements.[21] There is mixed evidence for global capitation achieving effective coordination of appropriate care delivery in primary care as well as other clinical settings.[35-37] Capitated models may be aligned with the current state of orthopaedic practices in the United States. Orthopaedic surgeons are treating an increasing Medicare population in the midst of an escalation in surgical procedures, while gaining an increasing awareness of the multifaceted, biopsychosocial nature of musculoskeletal problems. The delivery of effective global capitation in orthopaedic practice will require transparency and clear and appropriate rewards for quality and accountability tailored to musculoskeletal conditions at the policy level.[38]

Payer Level

A shift toward capitated models of care by payers requires a substantial change in the business model (cost structures, market competition, and profit margins) compared with well-established FFS systems. Traditionally, under an FFS model, payers are insurance companies, HMOs, managed care organizations, or any entity that pays or arranges payment for medical services. However, in a global capitated model, payers are required to transition from being insurers offering coverage of services toward delegating insurance risk to clinicians (**Figure 4**). Thus, orthopaedic practices working under global payments should appreciate the need for strong collaborative relationships with payers in configuring the payment model, risk arrangement, bonus opportunities, gainsharing thresholds, and service lines.[34,37] Practices should also recognize that the transition of cost accounting

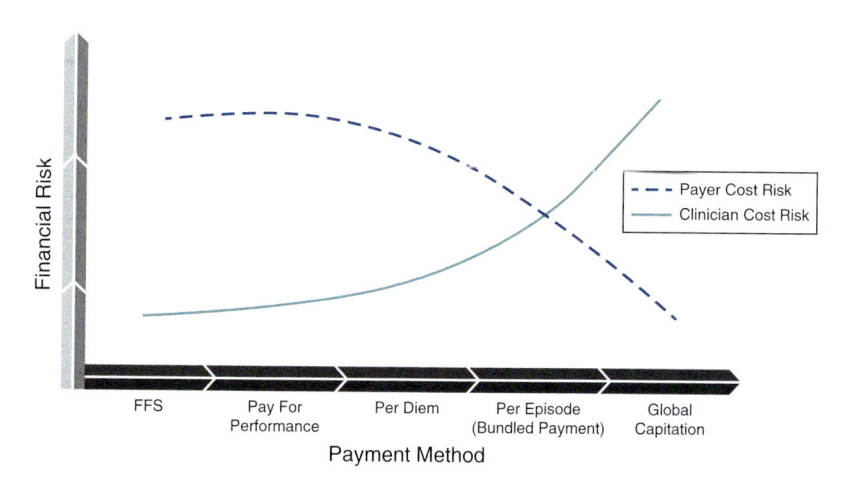

FIGURE 4 Clinician and payer financial risk sharing by payment method. From left to right, payment method starts from fee-for-service (FFS) to global capitation, representing the two extremes for clinician and payer cost risk. The blue dashed lines represent payer cost risk, The green solid line represents clinician cost risk. For global capitation, payers have the least financial risk and clinicians have the most financial risk.

under capitation is based on actuarial accounting and a prospective risk-adjusted payment through financial forecasts centered around utilization and quality standards rather than income alone where payments are received through retrospective claims.

Another consideration for orthopaedic practices at the payer level relates to risk adjustment. For high-cost users or for circumstances in which unpredictable costs are incurred, risk modeling may grossly undercalculate the cost needed to treat a patient. In these instances, there are a few methods to limit financial loss. Reinsurance has been used to cover care costs for patients who may exceed certain amounts and breach a specific amount in costs to clinicians.[27] Clinicians should be aware of strategies such as including risk corridors and stop loss described earlier in optimizing their practices as well as the continued actuarial adjustments of payment rate that go into future payment arrangements.

Depending on the structure of the capitated payment, orthopaedic practices have the option to contract with other clinician groups. For example, partial capitation or subcapitation can be used as a hybrid model in which certain encounters are covered under the monthly lump sum, and other services could be paid by bundled payments or even FFS. In an orthopaedic setting, patients could be covered for standard radiographs, preoperative appointments, surgery, and follow-up appointments in a specified window, and covered using FFS for medical imaging modalities such as MRI or medications not related to the orthopaedic condition or procedure. Capitated models also allow different approaches to compensate clinicians, from salary-based payment, productivity and relative value units, toward forms of subcapitation depending on specialty or size of clinician groups and organizations. Incentive payments for meeting quality measures can also be incorporated and should be recognized by practices. Hybrid options for capitated payment include partnering with managed service organizations, practice management companies, or health information technology companies.

Capitated models also allow some flexibility around the choice of services delivered, which remains at the discretion of clinicians and health service organizations. This should assist orthopaedic practices in configuring the optimal set of evidence-based treatments for various musculoskeletal conditions alongside tools and technologies to optimize pathways. Telemedicine and telehealth are being launched in the mainstream and provide opportunities to connect clinicians to patients during new patient visits as well as follow-up consultations, something that has been difficult to bill for under a traditional FFS environment.

Commercial payers are able to innovate rapidly and have greater ability to include or exclude clinicians who do not meet performance standards. Notably, the CMS framework allows private payers to construct their own frameworks similar to QPP track goals. One of the greatest challenges of the orthopaedic specialty regarding MACRA and QPP frameworks was the content of quality reporting measures. Initially, orthopaedic practitioners were required to report quality based on nine measures, where only four or five of these measures applied directly to orthopaedics.[39] The 2019 metrics readjusted this reporting standard, with orthopaedic practices required to submit data for six measures or a complete specialty measure set.[40]

In the commercial payer space, the potentiality to allow for fast-paced innovation and dynamic adjustments affords the orthopaedic practices to use more relevant performance measures. For instance, Humana's global capitation model for primary care physicians instituted a quality initiative called "Star Recognition," by adding bonuses for meeting quality and outcome benchmarks. This model also supports the creation of medical homes to generate further shared-savings before potentially transitioning to value-based models of care where clinicians assume full accountability for a patient's outcomes and total cost of care.[41]

Orthopaedic practices should have systems with a clear focus on outcomes and payments, especially in capitated models where the responsibility of financial risk is predominantly on the provider. For example, orthopaedic surgeons can proactively manage the costs of patients with severe osteoarthritis undergoing total knee arthroplasty if they are empowered with comparative information on both performance and episode costs, including the variable inpatient facility costs, proportion of costs from readmissions or errors, and so on. These data will help consolidate payment for evidence-based services that result in a healthier population while rejecting services that are less efficacious.

Patient and Clinician Level

Global capitation aims to foster more transparent and supportive relationships among patients and clinicians.[38] These models also serve to enhance the engagement between clinician groups and other clinical entities (eg, clinically integrated networks, ACOs) and payers (integrated delivery networks, government, health plans). Capitated models are most effective when they are fully integrated and provide enhanced access to interdisciplinary care delivered by clinical teams. Networks and payer relationships change as administrative and financial risk falls under the clinician who takes on much of the administrative burden.[42]

Effective orthopaedic practices under global capitation incorporate comprehensive performance measurements, including mandatory reporting of quality metrics and patient experience. Practices should be rewarded for achieving optimal outcomes, appropriate treatment selection, controls over underutilization and rationing, and include incentives for providers exceeding quality thresholds.[34,38,43] These measurement frameworks should also account for high-risk, high-cost patients.[34,38] Orthopaedic physician groups should consider tools and techniques enabling risk stratification of their patient populations while using outcome measures and other clinical data. Preoperative assessment using a range of patient and clinical factors at baseline can allow surgeons to appropriately identify patients that have increased needs and thus work to optimize patients prior to surgery, potentially reducing costly health expenditures postoperatively.

Clinician management of medical needs under global capitation aims to focus on care coordination, multidisciplinary treatment of disease, and decision making aligned with performance measurement.[42] Ideally, preventive care should be reinforced alongside a reduction in use of low-value interventions and strategies to avoid unwarranted use of expensive services such as emergency room readmissions. It is important for such strategies to maintain the focus on the needs of the population served instead of cherry-picking healthier patients to meet the bottom line. Notably, it is important to recognize the concerns of orthopaedic surgeons around reimbursement, demand, reductions in referrals, and potential loss of autonomy in managed care settings.[44,45] This may be the case in any reimbursement model that shifts away from unsustainable FFS care delivery.

Positive effects for patients depend on effective care integration, coordination, and individualization of care. Failure to achieve these can result in redundant services and administrative processes, poor patient experience, and potential error and disruption in patient safety. Global capitation can also provide opportunities for orthopaedic practices to benefit individuals in relation to patient-facing payments, such as deductibles or copayments. Lowering costs of copayments and deductibles may increase access to care and also prioritize opportunities for patient consumers to receive a range of services including preventive therapies and treatments. Effective capitated models rely on consumer involvement in the development and implementation of these models.

In a 2020 analysis of more than 5 million enrollees within United Healthcare's Medicare Advantage program, primary care physicians paid under a capitation-based model were found to influence provider behavior by prioritizing preventive services while avoiding unnecessary interventions and lowering use of inpatient services.[46] As the right incentives are optimized, private payers may have more flexibility to incorporate specialty services within capitated payment models to provide services outside the typical FFS payment structure. This may be especially useful in practicing high-value, whole person care for preference-sensitive orthopaedic conditions such as osteoarthritis where there is more than one viable evidence-based treatment option.

Case Study: Kaiser Permanente, Irvine Orthopaedic Surgery

Kaiser Permanente is an exemplar of a vertically integrated care delivery system in the United States that has brought together a range of clinicians under one roof, on a salary basis, setting internal incentives around production. The organization has been a major proponent for the use of capitation models since the introduction of HMOs. In 2013, the Kaiser Permanente Irvine orthopaedic surgery group included 21 orthopaedic surgeons performing 900 total joint replacements annually at a 250-bed general acute care hospital. The orthopaedic surgeons are contracted and paid as salaried employees of the Permanente Medical Group, with payment on a capitated basis for professional services. Bonus payment opportunities based on achieving quality criteria are also available. The capitated payment covers all professional services per member, per month but excludes medical devices, such as orthopedic implants, which are paid for from other hospital budgets. The physicians have no stake in the ownership of their local hospital system and no financial gainsharing or financial consulting opportunities based on their contract. Payment in Kaiser Permanente's system provides consistent, prepaid cash flow that is designed to avoid complex, convoluted billing administration.

Rapid growth was observed on inception of the program with long wait times for procedures. In 2011, after contracting with DePuy, the group restructured surgery scheduling to improve efficiency and mitigate capacity constraints. They streamlined operating room procedures and postoperative processes with designated personnel to improve consistency, maximized postoperative efficiency through discharge planning prior to admission, and optimized postsurgical care by breaking down postoperative stays into hourly segments and contracting with subacute, rehabilitation, and skilled nursing facilities. The Kaiser Permanente orthopaedic surgeons also invested resources to optimize patients. The Osteoarthritis Care Pathway designated patients into different categories based on disease severity, functional limitations, surgical preference, and behavior (eg, willingness to lose weight). This approach allowed the integration of surgical and nonsurgical care strategies such as steroid injections, nutrition counseling, and physical therapy.[47] The capitated model at Kaiser Permanent Irvine Orthopaedics is aligned with the broader focus by Kaiser Permanente on outcomes and quality of care which aims to track patients using multiple orthopaedic registries (eg, registries for anterior cruciate ligament reconstruction, shoulder arthroplasty, spine surgery, and total joint replacement).[48] Despite concerns about patients lacking choice and the perceived barriers of signing up to a closed network model, the organization continues to deliver high-value services and positive outcomes.

SUMMARY

Global capitation is a model aligned with the principles of value-based health care in forming payment arrangements and benefits designs for patients to have easily accessible and affordable evidence-based services. Capitated models can demonstrate some resilience during times of stress in orthopaedic practices and health care in general, such as that demonstrated by the COVID-19 pandemic.

In historical context, HMOs were the last widespread versions of capitated models used as a chief delivery strategy, with its peak in the late 1990s and early 2000s. Based on concerns over care rationing, gatekeeping restrictions by primary care providers, and complaints about insurance companies putting profit over patient health, preferred provider organizations, and FFS payments eventually usurped the market share held by HMOs.

Moving forward from the HMO era, both commercial and public payers are once again exploring the use of capitation delivery models. Capitated models represent the largest shift and transformation away from volume-based payments and towards value-based payments. The strengths of capitation models include the potential for substantial cost savings by minimizing inappropriate, low-cost care, lowering cost and increasing higher quality care, conferring greater controls for providers with less third-party involvement by payers in clinical decision-making, and financial security with prospective payments.

There are several key considerations for orthopaedic practices considering global capitation as a payment model. Orthopaedic practices should consider collaborative, upstream approaches that include regular interactions with primary, community, and preventive care, alongside better integration of social factors and social determinants of health to mitigate risk. Orthopaedic practices should aim to reduce redundancy, and low-value or inappropriate interventions. The US health care agenda continues to support a move away from FFS toward value-based care models, including global capitation. The debate continues around the optimal value-based reimbursement model. Whether orthopaedic practices use bundled payment episodes or if there will be a general transition in the wider healthcare system toward global capitation remains to be seen.

REFERENCES

1. Berenson RA, Rich EC: US approaches to physician payment: The deconstruction of primary care. *J Gen Intern Med* 2010;25(6):613-618.

2. Berenson RA, Upadhyay D, Delbanco SF, Murray R: *Global Capitation to an Organization.* Urban Institute, 2016.

3. Papanicolas I, Woskie LR, Jha AK: Health care spending in the United States and other high-income countries. *J Am Med Assoc* 2018;319(10):1024-1039.

4. Gruber LR, Shadle M, Polich CL: From movement to industry: The growth of HMOs. *Health Aff (Millwood)* 1988;7(3):197-208.

5. Langwell KM, Hadley JP: Capitation and the Medicare program: History, issues, and evidence. *Health Care Financ Rev* 1986;1986(Spec No):9-20.

6. Zuvekas SH, Cohen JW: Paying physicians by capitation: Is the past now prologue? *Health Aff (Millwood)* 2010;29(9):1661-1666.

7. Zuvekas SH, Cohen JW: Fee-for-service, while much maligned, remains the dominant payment method for physician visits. *Health Aff (Millwood)* 2016;35(3):411-414.

8. Wilensky GR, Rossiter LF: Coordinated care and public programs. *Health Aff (Millwood)* 1991;10(4):62-77.

9. Porter ME, Teisberg EO. *Redefining Health Care: Creating Value-Based Competition on Results,* ed 1. Harvard Business Review Press, 2006, p 528.

10. Chernew ME, Conway PH, Frakt AB: Transforming Medicare's payment systems: Progress shaped by the ACA. *Health Aff (Millwood)* 2020;39(3):413-420.

11. Casalino LP: The Medicare access and CHIP Reauthorization Act and the corporate transformation of American medicine. *Health Aff (Millwood)* 2017;36(5):865-869.

12. Findlay S: Implementing MACRA. Health Affairs, 2017.

13. O'Shea J: Salvaging MACRA implementation through Medicare advantage: Health Affairs Blog. Health Affairs. Available at: https://www.healthaffairs.org/do/10.1377/hblog20171017.462746/full/. Accessed November 20, 2020.

14. Centers for Medicare & Medicaid Services: Quality payment program. Available at: https://www.cms.gov/Medicare/Quality-Payment-Program/Quality-Payment-Program. Accessed November 20, 2020.

15. U.S. Centers for Medicare and Medicaid Services: MIPS Alternative Payment Models (APMs). Available at: https://qpp.cms.gov/apms/mips-apms. Accessed November 20, 2020.

16. Hobson CE, Bihorac A, Hadian M, et al: The impact of changes in Medicare's physician payment system on critical care. *Crit Connect* 2017;15:18-19.

17. Association of American Medical Colleges: MACRA frequently asked questions. Available at: https://www.aamc.org/what-we-do/mission-areas/health-care/macra/faq. Accessed November 20, 2020.

18. The Innovation Center: Financial alignment initiative for Medicare-Medicaid enrollees. Available at: https://innovation.cms.gov/innovation-models/financial-alignment. Accessed November 20, 2020.

19. Mann C, Bella M: Financial models to support state efforts to integrate care for Medicare-Medicaid enrollees SMDL# 11-008 ACA #18. U.S. Centers for Medicaid, CHIP, and Survey and Certification Medicare-Medicaid Coordination Office. Available at: https://www.cms.gov/Medicare-Medicaid-Coordination/Medicare-and-Medicaid-Coordination/Medicare-Medicaid-Coordination-Office/Downloads/Financial_Models_Supporting_Integrated_Care_SMD.pdf. Accessed February 24, 2023.

20. U.S. Centers for Medicare and Medicaid Services Medicare-Medicaid Coordination Office: Joint rate-setting process for the capitated financial alignment model. Available at: https://www.cms.gov/files/document/capitatedmodelratesetting process03192019.pdf. Accessed February 24, 2023.

21. Costello AM, Smith B: Value-based care opportunities in Medicaid SMD #20-004. U.S. Centers for Medicare and Medicaid Services. Available at: https://www.medicaid.gov/Federal-Policy-Guidance/Downloads/smd20004.pdf. Accessed February 24, 2023.

22. Berenson RA, de Brantes F, Burton RA: Payment reform: Bundled episodes vs. global payments. The Urban Institute. Available at: https://www.urban.org/research/publication/payment-reform-bundled-episodes-vs-global-payments. Accessed February 3, 2021.

23. Houston R, Brykman K: Addressing provider viability: The case for prospective payments during COVID-19. Center for Health Care Strategies. Available at: https://www.chcs.org/addressing-provider-viability-the-case-for-prospective-payments-during-covid-19/. Accessed December 2, 2020.

24. Schrijvers G: Competition supports integrated care. *Int J Integr Care* 2007;7(1):e49.

25. Frakt AB, Mayes R: Beyond capitation: How new payment experiments seek to find the 'sweet spot' in amount of risk providers and payers bear. *Health Aff (Millwood)* 2012;31(9):1951-1958.

26. Spector JM, Studebaker B, Menges EJ. Provider payment arrangements, provider risk, and their relationship with the cost of health care. The Society of Actuaries. Available at: https://www.soa.org/globalassets/assets/Files/Research/Projects/research-2015-10-provider-payment-report.pdf. Accessed November 20, 2020.

27. Goodson JD, Bierman AS, Fein O, Rask K, Rich EC, Selker HP: The future of capitation: The physician role in managing change in practice. *J Gen Intern Med* 2001;16(4):250-256.

28. Shortell SM, Gillies RR, Anderson DA: The new world of managed care: Creating organized delivery systems. *Health Aff (Millwood)* 1994;13(5):46-64.

29. Anderson ME, McDevitt K, Cumbler E, et al: Geriatric hip fracture care: Fixing a fragmented system. *Perm J* 2017;21:16-104.

30. Committee on Accounting for Socioeconomic Status in Medicare Payment Programs, Board on Population Health and Public Health Practice, Board on Health Care Services, Institute of Medicine, National Academies of Sciences, Engineering, and Medicine: Accounting for Social Risk Factors in Medicare Payment: Identifying Social Risk Factors. National Academies Press, 2016.

31. Rice N, Smith PC: Capitation and risk adjustment in health care financing: An international progress report. *Milbank Q* 2001;79(1):81-113.

32. Jones J, Miller S: Social determinants of health and Medicaid payments. Deloitte Insights. Available at: https://www2.deloitte.com/us/en/insights/industry/public-sector/medicaid-social-determinants-of-health.html. Accessed February 3, 2021.

33. Hinton E, Rudowitz R, Stolyar L, Singer N: 10 things to know about Medicaid managed care. KFF. Available at: https://www.kff.org/medicaid/issue-brief/10-things-to-know-about-medicaid-managed-care/. Accessed November 18, 2020.

34. Arora VS, Jain SH: What US medicine needs to do to finally embrace capitation: Health Affairs Blog. Health Affairs. Available at: https://www.healthaffairs.org/do/10.1377/hblog20201029.440795/full/. Accessed December 2, 2020.

35. Roberts ET, McWilliams JM, Hatfield LA, et al: Changes in health care use associated with the introduction of hospital global budgets in Maryland. *JAMA Intern Med* 2018;178(2):260-268.

36. Duff-Brown B: Exploring the capitation reimbursement model for primary care. Scope. Available at: https://scopeblog.stanford.edu/2017/09/12/exploring-the-capitation-reimbursement-model-for-primary-care/. Accessed December 2, 2020.

37. Paul DP III, Brunoni J, Dolinger T, Walker I, Wood D, Coustasse A: How effective is capitation at reducing health care costs? 41st Annual Meeting of the Northeast Business and Economics Association. Available at: https://mds.marshall.edu/cgi/viewcontent.cgi?article=1123&context=mgmt_faculty. Accessed December 2, 2020.

38. Baveja L, Bazell C, Counihan A: Six challenges to successful adoption of value-based care in the Middle East. Milliman. Available at: https://www.milliman.com/en/insight/six-challenges-to-successful-adoption-of-value-based-care-in-the-middle-east. Accessed December 2, 2020.

39. Small orthopedic practices aim to succeed with implementation of MACRA. Available at: https://www.healio.com/news/orthopedics/20161006/small-orthopedic-practices-aim-to-succeed-with-implementation-of-macra. Accessed February 3, 2021.

40. Quality payment program. Available at: https://www.aaos.org/advocacy/federal-advocacy-issues/quality-payment-program/. Accessed February 3, 2021.

41. Humana: Value-based care payment models. https://www.humana.com/provider/news/value-based-care/payment-models#:~:text=The%20Humana%20Star%20Recognition%20program,achievements%20for%20specific%20quality%20measures. Accessed November 20, 2020.

42. Friedberg MW, Chen PG, White C, et al: Effects of health care payment models on physician practice in the United States. *Rand Health Q* 2015;5(1):8.

43. Novikov D, Cizmic Z, Feng JE, Iorio R, Meftah M: The historical development of value-based care: How we got here. *J Bone Joint Surg Am* 2018;100(22):e144.

44. Leslie BM, Blau ML: Survival strategies in a changing practice environment. *J Hand Surg Am* 2014;39(5):1012-1016.

45. Jacofsky DJ, Haas DA: A Payment Model that Prevents Unnecessary Medical Treatment. *Harvard Business Review*. Available at: https://hbr.org/2016/12/a-payment-model-that-prevents-unnecessary-medical-treatment. Accessed December 2, 2020.

46. UnitedHealth Group: Physicians provide higher quality care under set monthly payments instead of being paid per service, UnitedHealth Group Study shows. Available at: https://www.unitedhealthgroup.com/newsroom/2020/uhg-study-shows-higher-quality-care-under-set-monthly-payments-403552.html. Accessed November 20, 2020.

47. Robinson JC: Case studies of orthopedic surgery in California: The virtues of care coordination versus specialization. *Health Aff (Millwood)* 2013;32(5):921-928.

48. Paxton L, Funahashi T: Kaiser Permanente National Implant Registries 2019 Report. Kaiser Permanente National Implant Registries. Available at: https://deviceassessment.kaiserpermanente.org/wp-content/uploads/2023/07/2019_ImplantRegistry_AnnualReport-1.pdf. Accessed November 23, 2020.

Accountable Care Organizations

David N. Bernstein, MD, MBA, MEI
Mary Lynch Witkowski, MD, MBA

INTRODUCTION

In 2018, health care expenditures in the United States continued to increase at an alarming rate (4.6%), now accounting for almost 18% of gross domestic product (GDP).[1] Perhaps even more concerning is the current projected annual growth rate of health spending, estimated to be 5.4% each year through 2028.[1] The unfortunate reality is that this concerning level and growth in health care spending has been noted for many years and outpaces the growth of GDP and wages both in the United States and globally.[2] This means that for every dollar earned, individuals and governments are dedicating an increasingly larger share to health care spending every year. In addition, not only has concern focused on the growth of health care spending but also on the inconsistent quality of care provided. Research demonstrates that despite the money spent on health care, the United States has among the highest number of hospitalizations from preventable causes and avoidable deaths, as well as a shorter life expectancy.[3] Over the years, these concerning findings have led policymakers and other health care stakeholders to take action to attempt to tackle "fixing" health care through a variety of initiatives and programs.

The need for meaningful and sustainable health care reform is not new. However, to successfully achieve desired changes, health care delivery systems must alter how they pay for health care, including orthopaedic care. Currently, the incentives are drastically misaligned, rewarding high-cost surgeons who deliver more services regardless of quality or appropriateness. Significant transformation is needed to address these health care delivery challenges and volume-driven incentives. By making the shift toward a system based on value, progress in health equity can be made as well, which is critical given the large health disparities in medicine, including within orthopaedic surgery. Ultimately, the goal of high-value care for patients, defined as health outcomes achieved per dollar spent across the full cycle of care, has been adopted by many clinicians across the globe.[4] For example, there has been progress made in bundled payment initiatives within orthopaedic surgery to reduce spending while ensuring quality,[5-8] as well as other value-based health care intervention.

Dr. Bernstein or an immediate family member serves as a paid consultant to or is an employee of CAPADEV, Institute For Strategy And Competitiveness at Harvard Business School, National Academy of Medicine, and The Heritage Foundation and serves as a board member, owner, officer, or committee member of J. Robert Gladden Society. Neither Dr. Witkowski nor any immediate family member has received anything of value from or has stock or stock options held in a commercial company or institution related directly or indirectly to the subject of this chapter.

One of the key structural programs introduced in the ongoing shift from rewarding volume toward rewarding health care value is Accountable Care Organizations, or ACOs. The United States Centers for Medicare & Medicaid Services (CMS) defines an ACO as, "…groups of doctors, hospitals, and other health care providers, who come together voluntarily to give coordinated high-quality care to their Medicare patients."[9] These health services networks share medical and financial responsibility for a large group of patients, receiving a capitated payment to keep a patient population healthy.

This chapter delves into the history of ACOs, focusing on a brief background on and robust definition of this payment model; illustrates the role of orthopaedic surgery care in ACOs and how this may vary across different ACOs and patient populations; and provides insight into more recent developments and future directions, including how ACOs and other forms of value-based payment models, such as bundled payments, have overlapped and been integrated.

HISTORY OF ACOs
ACO Precursors

Numerous attempts to reform health care payment models over recent years have focused on the transition away from the traditional fee-for-service (FFS) health care reimbursement model, which financially rewards the quantity of services provided instead of quality, toward incremental layering of process and quality metrics on top of a FFS system. The results of policy interventions have been mixed, without lasting financial and clinical outcomes improvement identified. Current alternative payment structures, including ACOs, may have a long-term positive effect as they are optimized over time. However, understanding the path to ACOs is vital to moving forward.

With the desire to control health care costs and improve clinical outcomes, the origins of ACOs arguably began with health maintenance organizations, or HMOs, in the late 1980s and early 1990s. HMOs took a managed care approach, whereby patients would have lower premiums in exchange for only having insurance coverage when they sought care with physicians or other health care professionals who contracted with that specific HMO. Thus, clinical care was only covered if it was provided by health care professionals who were in network.[10] HMOs also focused on preventive services and wellness as a means of reducing overall cost of care for a given patient population. Many managed care organizations struggled early in their evolution for a variety of reasons. First, many had poor financial management, with revenues far underperforming outlays.[11] These financial issues caused notable strain, ultimately resulting in many HMOs falling behind on payments to physicians, among other problems. These effects cascaded, as physicians and other health care professionals severed ties with HMOs as reimbursements faltered. Second, in many cases, patients suddenly became severely limited in their choice of doctor,[12] causing severe backlash and discontent. Many health care consumers who previously had much greater freedom of choice now found themselves in narrow-network HMOs. Third, the

goal of HMOs to manage patient populations in their respective networks efficiently and effectively demonstrated the need for robust health-related information technology that simply was not available.[13] Fourth, HMOs were not tied to
clinical outcomes, limiting any incentive for physicians or health care providers
to truly drive "better health."

Based in part on some of the challenges faced by HMOs in the 1990s, a key
step toward an ACO-type model was the Medicare Physician Group Practice
(PGP) Demonstration, the first physician pay-for-performance initiative introduced by CMS.[14] Beginning in 2005, the 5-year program included 10 physician
groups. This initiative was the first of its kind to begin to shift risk to health
professionals by offering financial bonus incentives if preestablished cost reduction and/or 32 quality measures were achieved. Although a step in the right
direction toward value-based health care, it is important to note that 7 of these
quality metrics were claims-based and 25 were medical record–based; therefore,
they did not accurately measure the outcomes most important to patients. For
example, patients are more likely to care about their ability to resume activities of daily life or have decreased daily pain, and less likely to be concerned
with whether antibiotics were given on time or whether certain safety protocols and regulatory requirements were met.[15] Although all outcomes measures
(eg, claims-based, medical record–based, or patient-reported) can be of value,
it is crucial to remember that the patient should be the focus of health care so
outcomes most important to the individual should be measured. However, the
requirement of measuring any metrics was a pivotal innovation and continued
the transition toward a value-based health care system. As part of this transformation, it also provided the framework for transition to the ACO model of care.

The Rise of ACOs

The term ACO was first coined by Elliott Fisher, MD, MPH during a Medicare
Payment Advisory Committee (MedPAC) public meeting in 2006 and further
described in an early 2007 *Health Affairs* article.[13,16] Ultimately, the idea was to ensure
that the accountability of patient care be shared across all health care professionals involved. The goal with the ACO approach was to accomplish the "triple aim"
proposed by Donald M. Berwick, MD, MPP - "improving the experience of care,
improving the health of populations, and reducing per capita costs of health care."[17]

In 2009, MedPAC moved beyond discussion and recognized ACOs as an alternative approach to traditional Medicare reimbursement structure. MedPAC recommended a reimbursement structure that utilized FFS but also created financial
incentives to try to drive decreased cost and improved quality of care.[18] The desire
to drive higher-value health care in the United States paired with favorable scoring of key ACO components by the Congressional Budget Office led to the ACO
model of care being included in the Medicare program in the Patient Protection
and Affordable Care Act (ACA) of 2010 (colloquially known as Obamacare).
Specifically, ACOs were included in Title XVIII of the Social Security Act (42 USC
§1,395 et seq.).

A more recent CMS program also created through the ACA is the Medicare Shared Savings Program (MSSP), which enables and encourages the creation of ACOs. Since its inception in 2012, the program has resulted in notable growth of 220 ACOs covering 3.2 million assigned beneficiaries to 517 ACOs covering 11.2 million beneficiaries.[19] In addition, CMS has continued to innovate further in the ACO space with the introduction of the Next Generation ACO Model in 2016,[20] which was designed for experienced ACOs seeking the potential for higher financial reward than that which was available under the MSSP. A key feature of this model is that it allowed its member ACOs to improve care for and better engage with patients by waiving certain Medicare services rules, allowing for telehealth and home visits following discharge, for example. However, the Next Generation ACO Model also requires participating ACOs to assume higher levels of financial risk through their payment mechanisms and cost benchmarking. Currently, 41 ACOs participate in the Next Generation ACO Model.

Overall, the use of ACOs across the United States continues to increase. When examining hospitals currently engaged in ACOs, 59% (1,625 of 2,749) of non-federal general hospitals across the United States are active in an ACO, either as a lead or a participant.[21] This varies from no reported participation in Alaska to 100% participation of non-federal, general hospitals in Vermont and Rhode Island.[21] Indeed, these data demonstrate the growth and widespread use of ACOs as a care delivery model in the United States; therefore, it is important for orthopaedic surgeons to understand them and how they may affect musculoskeletal care delivery and reimbursement.

Defining an ACO

After establishing an understanding of how ACOs became part of the health care fabric of the United States, an ACO can be clearly defined. From a more practical standpoint, ACOs are financial entities that provide all health care for a cohort of patients over a period of time in exchange for a capitated payment. The ACO is held to a fixed per capita payment and therefore holds the risk for the utilization of resources while also holding the ACO accountable for quality, and in some cases, clinical outcomes. When designed in a true value-based health care fashion, ACOs can allow physicians, including orthopaedic surgeons, the capability to be rewarded financially when clinical outcomes are optimized in an efficient manner but also be held accountable for the financial cost of inefficient care and/or poor clinical outcomes. However, not all ACOs are built the same, and the key design differences have significant effects on the underlying incentives of the ACO.

Although the core components of the CMS definition of ACOs are, of course, accurate, there are nuances and vagueness in this definition that should be acknowledged. First, the ACO model is not limited only to Medicare. It can be implemented as part of a private payor's strategy to move toward value-based payment for health care services. Second, ACOs can be led by different groups, such as hospitals or physicians. The structural differences in how ACOs are built have a significant effect on the underlying incentives behind these models. Hospital-led ACOs are often built around the historical footprint of the facility and service line mix of the existing enterprise; thus, they often have greater incentives to maintain the viability of the system as a whole. Physician-led ACOs often focused on certain patient segments that are treated by those physicians, who have incentives that are more closely aligned with the needs of those particular patients.

Success of ACOs have, in fact, differed based on whether they are physician-led or hospital-led, with the latest analyses demonstrating that physician-led ACOs produce a Medicare savings almost sevenfold greater than that of hospital-led ACOs ($180.41 versus $26.76 saved per beneficiary).[22] Third, the size and services provided within an ACO (eg, the number of physicians or specialties included) can vary widely. Generally, the ACO structure can more easily adapt to a value-based approach if it is focused on a patient segment and not only the financial needs of a large, diversified health system. Fourth, although the goal of an ACO is to increase risk-sharing with health care professionals and incentivize higher quality care at a decreased cost, the current level of risk-sharing, and therefore the pressure of incentives, varies greatly. The current CMS MSSP program offers four possible ACO options (Track 1, Track 1+, Track 2, Track 3), ranging from Track 1, in which participants do not assume downside financial risk, to Track 3, in which participants share a great deal of risk but have the highest possible financial upside if cost saving and quality metrics are achieved.[19] Currently, the most popular ACO option is Track 1, with 82% of participants falling into this category.[23] Overall, although the overarching general components of what constitutes an ACO are clearly laid out by CMS, orthopaedic surgeons should also consider the continually shifting and variable elements previously noted as they engage with and deliver care through ACOs during the ongoing shift toward value-based health care.

OVERLAP AND INTEGRATION OF ACOs WITH OTHER VALUE-BASED HEALTH CARE CONCEPTS: CURRENT PRACTICE AND FUTURE DIRECTIONS

The skyrocketing health care spending in the United States and globally without robust and transparent measurement of consistent outcomes important to patients will not be fixed solely by the innovative ACO models and initiatives currently in use and under development. "The Value Agenda," as coined by Professor Michael E. Porter and Dr. Thomas H. Lee, includes organizing into integrated practice units, measuring outcomes and costs for every patient, bundling payments for care cycles and patient segments, integrating care delivery across separate facilities, expanding high-value services across geography, and building an enabling information technology platform.[24] Although ACOs begin to move toward accomplishing some of the goals established in "The Value Agenda," such as the use of enabling information technology platforms and expanding services across sites and geographies, more work is required.

Bundled payments within ACO agreements are already being used in orthopaedic surgery. Bundled payments refer to lump monetary sums designed to cover the full cycle of care around a specific medical condition.[25] However, bundled payments (similar to ACOs) differ in how they are currently defined in practice. Currently, several initiatives exist that incorporate bundled payments into routine health care delivery, including by CMS and private payors. The push to increase the use of bundled payments and ACOs has led to an overlap of both in certain instances.

Utilizing bundled payments as the reimbursement mechanism for orthopaedic surgeons participating in an ACO is likely the "sweet spot" as health care systems transition away from a focus on quantity toward value for patients. In such a setting, orthopaedic surgeons will have the opportunity to earn the financial benefit associated with delivering exceptional, high-value musculoskeletal care. Thus, orthopaedic surgeons will be more highly rewarded based on what they can control and/or are involved in from a patient care standpoint, instead of being penalized or rewarded for global, hospital-level outcomes not associated with orthopaedic care (eg, rates of hospital-acquired pneumonia). Importantly, in this situation, the potential financial risk faced by orthopaedic surgeons would be much more appropriately based on clinical outcomes and resource utilization directly associated with the care of musculoskeletal conditions. Aligning incentives based on the role and responsibilities of orthopaedic surgeons is crucial, and the approach of integrating bundled payments within ACOs has remarkable potential to accomplish this objective.

As the integration of different value-based payment models progresses, they must work for all patients, not just a select few. However, early research shows that beneficiaries in both ACOs and part of a CMS bundled payment program were less likely to be older than 85 years, African American, of low socioeconomic status, and burdened with clinical complications.[26] In addition, hospitals with greater overlap of ACO and CMS bundled payment program participation were more likely to be nonprofit and less likely to be a safety net provider.[26] This raises notable concern about how these alternative value-based payment models, as currently designed and implemented, may result in adverse patient selection and increased health disparities and inequities, at least on a minimal scale.[27] These initial findings demonstrate that more work needs to be done in better defining, designing, and implementing value-based payments to ensure that they benefit all patients.

There remains a high probability that many of the principles of value-based health care will continue to be implemented within different programs and initiatives across health systems in the United States and globally. Thus, it is unlikely that care delivery and payment mechanisms, such as ACOs and bundled payments, will revert completely to traditional FFS. Indeed, it is more likely that a greater number of value-based health care programs will be developed and implemented. To ensure orthopaedic surgeons are able to continue to deliver high-quality musculoskeletal care and remain fairly compensated, they must be active in guiding adjustments to these care delivery and payment model innovations. Specifically, it is imperative to ensure that orthopaedic surgeons assist in developing appropriate risk-adjustments for orthopaedic patients. This important work will help ensure that the implementation of such reimbursement models do not worsen, but rather improve, health care disparities.

ORTHOPAEDIC CARE AND ACOs

The primary objective of an ACO to increase clinical care quality while reducing cost through better coordinated care has the potential to create substantial value for patients. However, as with many health policy endeavors, numerous challenges exist in appropriately designing, fully implementing, and reaping the potential benefits in practice. One of the major challenges is determining how subspecialty services, such as orthopaedic surgery, best fit into and engage with primary care physicians and hospitals as part of the ACO structure. This is especially vital for orthopaedic surgeons given the importance of musculoskeletal medicine in the United States, where more than one of every two persons older than 18 years are affected and almost three of every four persons older than 65 years are affected.[28] A more robust understanding by orthopaedic surgeons of how they fit into the ACO puzzle will not only allow them to continue to deliver excellent clinical care but be rewarded financially in a manner that is consistent with the value they deliver.

The Role of Orthopaedic Surgeons in an ACO

ACOs seek to provide patients with primary and specialty care, including orthopaedic surgical evaluation and treatment. However, ACOs are not required to include orthopaedic surgeons within the ACO itself. Nonetheless, ACOs must still manage the cost and quality of specialty care being provided for each patient it covers.

Orthopaedic surgeons can deliver care to patients in different ways as part of an ACO, which depends partially on the surgeon's practice. In some cases, orthopaedic surgeons will not experience much, if any, change to their daily clinical practice. However, in other instances, involvement in an ACO may have a notable effect. It is crucial for orthopaedic surgeons to plan ahead and be aware of how they can be involved with ACOs. Although there are certainly nuances and variations in how involved an orthopaedic surgeon can be with ACOs, the following four examples provide a brief illustration of the possibilities.

1. **ACO With Employed Orthopaedic Surgeons**
   Many large medical centers and health systems have created ACOs whereby all physicians employed by the institution are part of the ACO. In such cases, the effect of ACO implementation may not necessarily be felt at the individual orthopaedic surgeon level as much. This is because internal referral patterns and systemwide contracts are unlikely to change drastically, at least in the short term. In addition, orthopaedic surgeons may continue to be paid using relative value unit–driven payment methods. Thus, orthopaedic surgeons participating in an ACO in this way may not even realize they are part of an ACO, let alone appreciate whether or not the ACO, as a whole, saved money over time through risk-sharing contracts.

2. **ACO Contracted With Orthopaedic Surgeons in Private Practice or Physician Groups**
   Orthopaedic surgeons can also contract directly with an ACO to deliver care through agreements between ACOs and their private specialty group

or individual practice. Orthopaedic practices or individual surgeons may have relationships with one or many ACOs. When truly a part of an ACO, orthopaedic surgeons may have the opportunity to be financially rewarded when the ACO as a whole saves money. However, the opposite is true as well when the ACO loses money. In such two-sided risk arrangements, orthopaedic surgeons may be effectively accountable for the management of musculoskeletal conditions for those patients covered in the ACO. The terms of these arrangements may differ, and the financial upside (or downside), for participating in an ACO should be determined a priori.

3. **ACO With FFS Contracts With Orthopaedic Surgeons**
   In another approach to contracting with ACOs, orthopaedic surgeons can continue with FFS payments. When this occurs, prices for orthopaedic care are noted as part of the contract when it is first agreed on. This guarantees a set price for each encounter, procedure, or intervention. However, orthopaedic surgeons cannot share in savings created by the ACO through their care pathways or other means.

4. **ACO With Bundled Payment Contracts With Orthopaedic Surgeons**
   As the use of bundled payments in health care continues to expand, they have also become one avenue for subspecialists (eg, orthopaedic surgeons) to take on higher levels of risk for potentially higher reward in ACOs. For example, instead of agreeing to FFS contracts, orthopaedic surgeons can contract with ACOs and set a bundled payment price. In such agreements, orthopaedic surgeons are provided a lump sum by the ACO in exchange for guaranteeing the set of services required to care for a patient's condition (eg, knee osteoarthritis), as bundled payments were originally described, or procedure and its respective perioperative timeframe. In this approach, if the orthopaedic surgeon and their team can deliver care more efficiently and ensure high-quality outcomes, they would reap the financial benefits.

Potential Benefits of Delivering Orthopaedic Care in an ACO

Especially for musculoskeletal care, sustainable and meaningful health care delivery reform to optimize the time and energy of orthopaedic surgeons is not possible without true payment reform. This is especially important to accomplish because researchers predict a growing shortage of orthopaedic surgeons as the United States' population continues to age.[29] Delivering orthopaedic care as part of an ACO, either directly as a member physician or through a contract arrangement, may help achieve this goal.

When delivering musculoskeletal care to a patient who is covered by an ACO, orthopaedic surgeons will likely benefit from the enhanced communication among care team members in conjunction with the payment structure. Orthopaedic care is expensive and unnecessary evaluation and treatment should be avoided whenever possible. Because ACOs incentivize cost-effective, high-quality care, there may be increased focus on ensuring that patients are referred to specialists such as orthopaedic surgeons only when warranted. Orthopaedic surgeons and primary care physicians, as well as advanced practice providers, can mutually benefit from enhanced collaboration and focus on ensuring all nonsurgical management approaches have been attempted by the primary care physician or advanced practice provider before an official referral has been placed. For example, in a physician-led primary care ACO model (capitated in a manner similar to Medicare Advantage for primary care), ACO delivery organizations focus on meeting the primary care needs of their patients, often with innovative and efficient approaches. When their patient's condition (eg, knee osteoarthritis) is severe enough that it warrants specialty care, they should be referred to high-value specialists in the area and the physician is responsible for the bundled payment amount within their capitated framework. This frees up the primary care ACO to focus its own efforts on effective primary care and on the integration of condition-based care through collaboration with these high-value, specialty-focused providers. In addition, increased communication will reduce the likelihood of duplicate imaging studies, for example, because they will be available to the entire care team; this will streamline the evaluation and treatment process and save money. This is possible outside of an ACO with better integrated information technology; however, the team-based focus on patient outcomes while ensuring appropriate use of funds makes this even more likely in an ACO-type payment structure. Ultimately, these savings can then be shared appropriately among all health care professionals involved.

As ACOs become ever more commonplace, the number of patients covered through an ACO will increase. Orthopaedic surgeons who join one or more ACOs or who routinely engage with ACOs may benefit from frequent patient referrals from them.

Orthopaedic surgeons who are active members of or participants in an ACO or multiple ACOs also play a crucial role in charting the future of alternative value-based payment models. It is likely that ACOs and other value-based payment initiatives, such as bundled payments, will be part of the fabric of United States health care payment strategy and policy moving forward. Orthopaedic surgeons who have experienced both the benefits and limitations of ACOs as they have previously been or are currently structured will be highly incentivized to drive greater positive change moving forward. Advocacy cannot be underestimated, and active participation on a policy level will help shape the future of musculoskeletal care in these evolving health care delivery and reimbursement models.[30] This will not only act to support the profession but continue to ensure that patients have access to high-quality musculoskeletal care.

Potential Challenges and Possible Pitfalls for Orthopaedic Surgeons in an ACO

Although current and future benefits exist for participating in or engaging with ACOs, there are also a number of possible pitfalls and areas of concern that orthopaedic surgeons should keep in mind. Importantly, these are likely to change over time as new ACO models are introduced by CMS and private payers. However, the core principles of these challenges and possible pitfalls are likely to remain relevant for some time.

A major challenge faced by orthopaedic surgeons in ACOs is demonstrating their value through the quality metrics outlined by CMS that are considered as part of reimbursement. This is mainly driven by the fact that many ACOs are often built around broad patient populations with a wide range of conditions and health care service needs. This leads to the use of many general hospital-wide metrics (eg, urinary tract infection rate) in many instances, which may not have much meaning to the quality of care provided by orthopaedic surgeons. Indeed, most of the almost three dozen quality measures that are provided by the government do not truly fall within the purview of orthopaedic surgeons. Nonetheless, the care that is being provided by an orthopaedic surgeon is likely of high cost even when it is cost-effective, as well as beneficial to patient health and well-being. It can also play a vital role in patient satisfaction. As ACO models continue to develop, it is possible that outcome measures that matter most to patients undergoing orthopaedic procedures, such as functional status and pain level, will be incorporated into payment models. Additionally, objective metrics such as radiographic measurements and range of motion may also be included. In the meantime, orthopaedic surgeons should strive to demonstrate their value to the overall care of a patient by highlighting the improved well-being patients experience following musculoskeletal care, whether surgical or nonsurgical.

Another major obstacle in engaging with ACOs as an orthopaedic surgeon is grounded in the current structure of many of the ACOs. There is an incentive to keep care inside the ACO to have a greater amount of control, allow for the flexibility to have internal payment rates when desired (including to specialists such as orthopaedic surgeons), and ensure a level of patient volume that will cover overhead costs. Such incentives lead to ACOs attempting to minimize "leakage" of patients to health professionals outside the ACO. This is not always in the best interest of the patient, an independent, high-value orthopaedic surgeon, or small surgical practice in the marketplace looking to contract with ACOs in the community. In such a situation, investing in creating a world-class orthopaedic surgical team may not result in increased business given the lack of incentives to send patients outside of the ACO. In addition, if the incentives are not in place to reward high-value orthopaedic surgeons, but rather to keep care internal to the ACO irrespective of care quality, those outside of the ACO will unfairly be in a weaker negotiating position to become part of a different ACO. This means they may care for more patients. Ultimately, such a situation may result in independent orthopaedic surgeons and surgeon practices accepting less favorable contract terms.

Orthopaedic surgeons should also seek to measure and provide data about their outcomes and resource utilization, including readmissions and cases that require a return to the operating room. These are important metrics in the setting of an ACO because of the set amount of funds used to cover each patient's health care services over a given timeframe (eg, 1 calendar year). In addition, as ACOs become more common, it is likely that greater risk may fall on health systems and physicians. Thus, complication rates and instances of returning to the operating room, as well as other potentially costly elements of musculoskeletal care delivery, will likely become even more crucial measures to evaluate frequently. Part of this work will entail routinely measuring and assessing patient-reported outcome measures, which can be used to measure pain, functional status, and quality of life, among other outcomes most important to patients. These instruments provide a patient-centric perspective on health outcomes and have been shown to improve the patient experience.[31] It may become necessary in the future to provide such information to demonstrate added value to participate in a given ACO. Orthopaedic surgeons should be transparent and upfront with ACOs regarding their expectations when considering joining one or contracting with one. Specifically, there are going to be patients at high risk for needing access to increased levels of health care resources, including those with complications and those with the possibility of requiring multiple surgeries. Orthopaedic surgeons should not be penalized financially for providing the necessary care for these patients. Agreements regarding risk adjustment must be made a priori to ensure that patients continue to receive the care they need. Additionally, orthopaedic surgeons should not be overburdened or placed at higher financial risk by treating patients whose treatment may potentially be more costly.

Conducting the necessary homework and forming appropriate agreements prior to delivering orthopaedic care as part of an ACO can be both time consuming and frustrating to orthopaedic surgeons, who likely entered medicine to deliver care and not to figure out the best way to adjust to a changing reimbursement landscape. However, both goals are likely critical for continued financial stability, which will ultimately allow for continued high-quality patient care. First, orthopaedic surgeons should be direct in negotiating their rates. As part of this endeavor, they should ensure that if they are involved in risk-sharing, the other members of the care team are appropriately involved as well. This is likely to be a larger issue as ACO programs from CMS and other payors continue to develop and increase risk-sharing in their models. Second, individual orthopaedic surgeons may find it more challenging to join ACOs, as their negotiating power will likely be much less than large practice or academic health system departments. However, if more and more patients end up being covered by ACOs, it will be imperative for individual orthopaedic surgeons to join or contract with such organizations. This can be done via collaboration among fellow local orthopaedic surgeons to truly create a larger clinical entity with greater negotiating power or through being transparent in quality metrics to demonstrate to ACOs the added value provided. Transparency with quality metrics may drive others, including larger orthopaedic practices, to also measure and report quality metrics so they can compete. Further, individual orthopaedic surgeons or smaller group practices can collaborate with other specialists to create a multispecialty group that works together to deliver much of the subspecialty care required by patients in ACOs.

Overall, there are potential benefits of ACOs for orthopaedic surgeons, but it requires them to also understand areas that may pose challenges and cause pitfalls. However, by considering the elements noted in this chapter, orthopaedic surgeons can be well positioned to thrive in an era of ACOs, even as they adapt. Ultimately, ensuring high-value care to patients by delivering high-quality musculoskeletal care at the best possible cost is the goal of orthopaedic surgeons. Therefore, they deserve to be appropriately and fairly compensated, including in the setting of ACOs.

SUMMARY

ACOs are an innovative health care payment model that aim to promote the collaboration of health care professionals for coordinated, high-value health care. They became a core transformational component of healthcare systems following the passage of the ACA in 2010. Currently, many patients across the United States are part of an ACO in an effort to better contain costs while ensuring high-quality care.

Given the large number of musculoskeletal concerns in the general population, orthopaedic care is a crucial component of general health care in the United States. Orthopaedic surgeons may actively participate as part of ACOs or by contracting with ACOs. Referral patterns and region-specific conditions may lead an individual orthopaedic surgeon or orthopaedic surgery practice to select one route over the other. It is crucial for orthopaedic surgeons to be well versed in terminology around ACOs and what they can mean for their practice, while avoiding pitfalls such as not negotiating terms at the beginning.

ACOs have a few key benefits for orthopaedic surgeons. First, collaboration among physicians and health care professionals in an ACO can help ensure that only appropriate patients (those who most likely need surgery) see an orthopaedic surgeon. Second, redundancy may be reduced with increased communication inherent to an integrated ACO model. Third, by being active in ACOs, orthopaedic surgeons can play a crucial and vocal role in the continued innovation needed around alternative payment models, including ACOs, to make them even more effective.

ACOs are here to stay, but they will likely adapt over time to be more value-driven, with a focus on a narrower patient segment, greater responsibility for patient outcomes, and improved integration of specialist services. Orthopaedic surgeons can thrive in such a system, but they must be actively involved to help drive positive change within it. By doing so, orthopaedic surgeons can ensure that they are able to deliver high-value musculoskeletal care to a diverse patient population, while also being compensated fairly.

REFERENCES

1. Centers for Medicare & Medicaid Services: NHE Fact Sheet. Available at: https://www.cms.gov/Research-Statistics-Data-and-Systems/Statistics-Trends-and-Reports/NationalHealthExpendData/NHE-Fact-Sheet#:~:text=NHE%20grew%204.6%25%20to%20%243.6,16%20percent%20of%20total%20NHE. Accessed December 1, 2020.

2. Porter ME: Value-Based Health Care Delivery: Core Concepts. *Harvard Business School.* January 15, 2020. Available at: https://www.isc.hbs.edu/Documents/pdf/2020-intro-vbhc-porter.pdf. Accessed January 31, 2021.

3. Tikkanen R, Abrams MK: U.S. Health Care from a Global Perspective, 2019: Higher Spending, Worse Outcomes? The Commonwealth Fund. January 30, 2020. Available at: https://www.commonwealthfund.org/publications/issue-briefs/2020/jan/us-health-care-global-perspective-2019. Accessed December 1, 2020.

4. Porter ME: What is value in health care? *N Engl J Med* 2010;363(26):2477-2481.

5. Navathe AS, Emanuel EJ, Venkataramani AS, et al: Spending and quality after three years of Medicare's voluntary bundled payment for joint replacement surgery. *Health Aff (Millwood)* 2020;39(1):58-66.

6. Siddiqi A, White PB, Mistry JB, et al: Effect of bundled payments and health care reform as alternative payment models in total joint arthroplasty: A clinical review. *J Arthroplasty* 2017;32(8):2590-2597.

7. Barnett ML, Wilcock A, McWilliams JM, et al: Two-year evaluation of mandatory bundled payments for joint replacement. *N Engl J Med* 2019;380(3):252-262.

8. Haas DA, Zhang X, Kaplan RS, Song Z: Evaluation of economic and clinical outcomes under centers for medicare & medicaid services mandatory bundled payments for joint replacements. *JAMA Intern Med* 2019;179(7):924-931.

9. Centers for Medicare & Medicaid Services: Accountable Care Organizations (ACOs), 2020. Available at: https://www.cms.gov. Accessed December 1, 2020.

10. HealthCare.gov. Health Maintenance Organization (HMO), 2020. Available at: https://www.healthcare.gov/glossary/health-maintenance-organization-hmo/. Accessed December 1, 2020.

11. Christianson JB, Wholey DR, Sanchez SM: State responses to HMO failures. *Health Aff (Millwood)* 1991;10(4):78-92.

12. Stanford GSB Staff: Managed Care: What Went Wrong? Can It Be Fixed? Stanford Graduate School of Business, 1999. Available at: https://www.gsb.stanford.edu/insights/managed-care-what-went-wrong-can-it-be-fixed. Accessed December 1, 2020.

13. Tu T, Muhlestein D, Kocot SL, White R: *The Impact of Accountable Care: Origins and Future of Accountable Care Organizations*. Leavitt Partners, 2015. Available at: https://www.brookings.edu/wp-content/uploads/2016/06/impact-of-accountable-careorigins-052015.pdf. Accessed December 1, 2020.

14. Centers for Medicare & Medicaid Services: Medicare Physician Group Practice Demonstration, 2020. Available at: https://innovation.cms.gov/medicare-demonstrations/medicare-physician-group practice-demonstration. Accessed December 7, 2020.

15. Kaplan RS, Jehi L, Ko CY, Pusic A, Witkowski M: Health care measurements that improve patient outcomes. *NEJM Catal Innov Care Deliv* 2021;2(2).

16. Fisher ES, Staiger DO, Bynum JP, Gottlieb DJ: Creating accountable care organizations: The extended hospital medical staff. *Health Aff (Millwood)* 2007;26(1):w44-w57.

17. Berwick DM, Nolan TW, Whittington J: The triple aim: Care, health, and cost. *Health Aff (Millwood)* 2008;27(3):759-769.

18. Burke T: Accountable care organizations. *Public Health Rep* 2011;126(6):875-878.

19. Centers for Medicare & Medicaid Services: Shared Savings Program: About the Program, 2020. Available at: https://www.cms.gov/Medicare/Medicare-Fee-for-Service-Payment/sharedsavingsprogram/about. Accessed December 10, 2020.

20. Centers for Medicare & Medicaid Services: Next Generation ACO Model, 2020. Available at: https://innovation.cms.gov/innovation-models/next-generation-aco-model. Accessed December 1, 2020.

21. American Hospital Association: Accountable Care Organizations, 2020. Available at: https://www.aha.org/accountable-care-organizations-acos. Accessed December 10, 2020.

22. Sullivan G, Feore J: *Physician-Led Accountable Care Organizations Outperform Hospital-Led Counterparts*. Avalere Health, 2019. Available at: https://avalere.com/press-releases/physician-led-accountable-care-organizations-outperform-hospital-led-counterparts. Accessed December 10, 2020.

23. Continuum: What Is the Medicare Shared Savings Program (MSSP)? 2020. Available at: https://www.carecloud.com/continuum/medicare-shared-savings-program-mssp/. Accessed December 11, 2020.

24. Porter ME, Lee TH: The Strategy That Will Fix Health Care. *Harvard Business Review*, 2013. Available at: https://hbr.org/2013/10/the-strategy-that-will-fix-health-care. Accessed December 20, 2020.

25. Porter ME, Kaplan RS: How to Pay for Health Care. *Harvard Business Review*, 2016. Available at: https://hbr.org/2016/07/how-to-pay-for-health-care. Accessed December 20, 2020.

26. Liao JM, Shan EZ, Zhao Y, Shah Y, Cousins DS, Navathe AS: Overlap between medicare's comprehensive care for joint replacement program and accountable care organizations. *J Arthroplasty* 2021;36(1):1-5.

27. Bernstein DN, Reitblat C, van de Graaf VA, et al: Is there an association between bundled payments and "cherry picking" and "lemon dropping" in orthopaedic surgery? A systematic review. *Clin Orthop Relat Res* 2021;479(11)2430-2443.

28. Bone and Joint Initiative USA: The Burden of Musculoskeletal Diseases in the United States. Musculoskeletal Diseases and the Burden They Cause in the United States Website, 2020. Available at: https://www.boneandjointburden.org/. Accessed December 10, 2020.

29. Haskins J: Desperately Seeking Surgeons. Association of American Medical Colleges (AAMC), 2019. Available at: https://www.aamc.org/news-insights/desperately-seeking-surgeons. Accessed December 1, 2020.

30. Levine WN, Gibson WK: Should Physician Advocacy Be a Core Component of Medical Professionalism? *Healio*, 2020. Available at: https://www.healio.com/news/orthopedics/20200110/should-physician-advocacy-be-a-core-component-of-medical-professionalism. Accessed Decemeber 1, 2020.

31. Bernstein DN, Fear K, Mesfin A, et al: Patient-reported outcomes use during ortho-paedic surgery clinic visits improves the patient experience. *Musculoskeletal Care* 2019;17(1):120-125.

Tools for High-Value Orthopaedic Care Delivery

Elizabeth Duckworth, MD, MBA • Eugenia Lin, MD
Olivia Manickas-Hill, BA • Prakash Jayakumar, MD, PhD

INTRODUCTION

The shift toward value-based health care in the United States, since the enactment of the Patient Protection and Affordable Care Act (ACA) in 2010, has sparked a demand for tools and technologies to support stakeholders engaged in realizing this goal. Government agencies, regulatory bodies, professional groups, commercial insurers, pharmaceutical and biomedical device companies, and health care provider organizations are increasingly recognizing the need for such tools to better prepare them for delivering a range of value-oriented functions. This chapter defines concepts and unmet needs that provide the inspiration for tools and technologies enabling value-based health care delivery. A description of current state-of-the-art and future patient-facing, surgeon-facing, and systems-level tools contributing to an essential toolkit for high-value orthopaedic practices is also provided.

OVERVIEW OF HIGH-VALUE MODELS OF CARE DELIVERY

In orthopaedics, the largest transformation toward value-based reimbursement to date has been the Centers for Medicare & Medicaid Services (CMS) implementation of the Comprehensive Care for Joint Replacement (CJR) model in April 2016. Mandating hospitals across the country to accept bundled payment for a surgical episode of care around total hip and total knee arthroplasty, the CJR model places a greater emphasis on accountability for quality and costs of care by promoting coordination between hospitals, physicians, and postacute care providers. The CJR model and other value-oriented initiatives signal the requirement for tools and technologies, such as robust electronic health records and outcome measurement platforms, to deliver optimal care while also offering a lens on performance and benchmarking fit for value.[1] Accountability for quality and costs of care for Medicare patient populations has also been realized in the engagement of groups of hospitals, practices, and clinicians within accountable care organizations.[2]

None of the following authors or any immediate family member has received anything of value from or has stock or stock options held in a commercial company or institution related directly or indirectly to the subject of this chapter: Dr. Duckworth, Dr. Lin, Olivia Manickas-Hill, and Dr. Jayakumar.

Value-based practice and payment reform in orthopaedics is now expanding beyond surgical procedures toward management of the condition over a full cycle of care, the original vision in the seminal work, *Redefining Health Care*.[3] With this in mind, tools for high-value care can be key drivers for the development of alternative condition-based bundled payment models across orthopaedic care (**Figure 1**).

CONCEPTS AND UNMET NEEDS FOR DEVELOPING HIGH-VALUE TOOLS
Value-Based Health Care

Value-based health care is defined as care that achieves health outcomes benefiting patients relative to the costs of care.[4] Importantly, this definition relies on the direct measurement of outcomes that matter to the individual over a full cycle of care. These outcomes should include a range of quality metrics from patients' perspectives of their physical, emotional, and social health and well-being to clinically

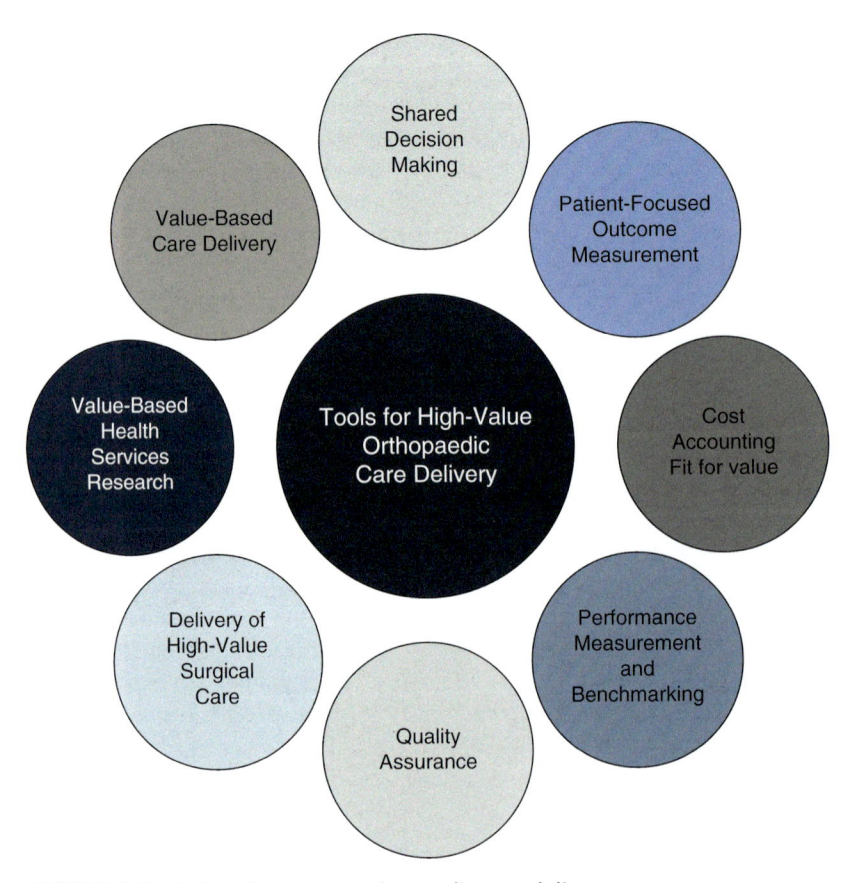

FIGURE 1 Tools for high-value orthopaedic care delivery.

effective outcomes including those related to hospitalization, complications, rehabilitation, and recurrences.[5] The denominator includes the total cost of care for managing a patient's condition and should incorporate direct and indirect costs spanning the gamut of inpatient, outpatient, rehabilitation, drugs and devices, physician services, equipment, and facility costs, as well societal costs through loss of productivity.[5] Considering the costs of a full cycle of care may also support increased spending on higher value preventive services while disincentivizing the shift in costs from one type of service or provider of services to another.[4]

Patient-Centered Care

Patient-centered care is defined as care that respects and responds to individual patient preferences, values, and needs, while ensuring patients remain at the center of their care and clinical decision making.[6] This concept includes the effect of care on patient-specific factors (physical, psychological, and social health and well-being) alongside the individual's experience of care.[7] Communication, trust, and empathy form some of the cornerstones of patient-centered care and enable patients to more effectively engage in their health care ecosystem. Shared decision making (SDM) is the expert communication of clinical information including management options to help clinicians and patients arrive at informed treatment decisions aligned with the patient's preferences, values, and needs. This concept combines several patient-centered elements and is increasingly being adopted in orthopaedics.[8] Patient-centered care has been embraced by the American Academy of Orthopaedic Surgeons via its appropriate use criteria, which utilize validated tools to extrapolate the appropriateness of an intervention within different patient and treatment combinations.[9]

Integrated Care

Integrated care is defined as care that is coordinated across professionals, facilities and support systems; continuous over time and between visits; tailored to patients' needs and preferences; and based on shared responsibility between patients and caregivers while systematically measuring outcomes.[10] In this regard, there has been growing interest in comprehensive, team-based, condition-focused approaches to orthopaedic care in the form of integrated practice units (IPUs).[11] IPUs are structurally and functionally organized around conditions (rather than specific providers or procedures) over a full care cycle, involving a range of treatment strategies.[11] The full range of treatments (including surgical and nonsurgical care) are delivered by a dedicated multidisciplinary team working within a common organizational unit, accountable for outcomes and costs of care under a bundled payment arrangement.[12] Relatively few IPUs exist in current clinical practice; however, several institutions have adopted integrated care pathways (ICPs) that offer a specific, time-dependent regimen used to standardize care during a course of treatment.[11] Vertically integrated institutions such as Geisinger Health and Kaiser Permanente have embraced ICPs for joint replacement surgery and seen reductions in length of hospital stay, complications, redundancy in ancillary services, and waste through enhanced interdisciplinary coordination.[12,13] ICPs have also been applied extensively in geriatric and nongeriatric fracture management and resulted in decreased complications, length of stay, time to surgery, and costs of care.[14] Integrated care may also be considered comprehensive care by design because it aims to provide for the holistic needs of patients; one common example is the combined medical, surgical, and rehabilitation care provided by orthogeriatric teams in managing geriatric trauma patients.[15] The benefits of a more complete integrated, biopsychosocial approach is increasingly being recognized in orthopaedics, especially in relation to the comprehensive management of osteoarthritis.[16] The concepts of value-based health care, patient-centered care, and integrated care demand the development of practical, safe, and effective tools and technologies for delivering high-value orthopaedic care.

PATIENT-FACING TOOLS DESIGNED FOR HIGH-VALUE ORTHOPAEDIC CARE

Tools enabling the capture of patient-generated health data are integral to value-based health care. Patient-generated health data is defined as health-related data created, recorded, and gathered from patients (or family members or other caregivers) to help establish a patient's health status.[17] This type of information derived from patients is distinct from objectively reported data by clinicians or clinical systems.

Patient-Reported Outcome Measures

Patient-reported outcome measures (PROMs) are validated measures of physical, psychological, and social health and well-being reported by the patient that have revolutionized orthopaedic clinical research and are now being increasingly used in clinical practices across orthopaedic subspecialties.[18] PROMs enable quantification of a patient's perceptions of their health and responses to medical interventions with respect to function, symptoms, and quality of life.[19] The introduction of national registries incorporating PROMs has had a meaningful effect in several countries through the evaluation of patient outcomes for different surgical techniques, analysis of positive predictors of these outcomes, and comparison across orthopaedic and non-orthopaedic conditions.[20,21] The American Board of Orthopaedic Surgery collects PROMs as part of the Part II Board Certification process and the CMS incentivizes PROMs collection through quality reporting and bonus payment initiatives.[22,23] Effective PROMs should demonstrate reliability (how well the tool repeatedly assesses the same item), validity (whether the tool measures the content it intends to measure), and responsiveness (the tool's sensitivity to change over time) while also being user-friendly and easy to interpret (the degree to which qualitative and clinical meaning can be assigned to a PROMs quantitative scores or change in scores).[24,25] Measuring PROMs before and after a treatment intervention provides an opportunity to objectively measure the effect of an intervention on the patient's health from their perspective. This effect has traditionally been quantified using fixed-scale measures developed from classic test theory. In recent decades, there has been increased use of computer adaptive tests (CATs), developed using item response theory, which enables follow-up questions to be administered based on the patient's response to a prior question.[26] Although fixed-scale PROMs require patients to answer most, if not all, questions to arrive at a valid score, CATs generally involve fewer but more tailored questions, and therefore result in more precise and efficient capture of patient outcomes. The most commonly used CATs are the Patient Reported Outcome Measurement Information System (PROMIS) measures developed by the National Institutes of Health. Development of PROMIS was prompted by the need for a valid, reliable, and generalizable set of measures that could be applied across clinical conditions, providing comprehensive coverage of different levels of a relevant health domain, while maintaining efficiency and reducing burden on responders.[18,27] The PROMIS instruments score health domains using a common metric, normalized to the US general population. Over a 5-year period from 2014 to 2018, the volume of orthopaedic studies leveraging PROMIS increased sixfold, with most studies examining the domains of physical function, pain interference, and depression.[28]

PROMs provide a range of functions from tracking, screening, and segmentation of patient phenotypes, to enabling decision support and SDM.[29] For instance, PROMs have been used in anterior cruciate ligament reconstruction and total joint arthroplasty (TJA) to aid surgeons in determining whether surgical intervention will benefit the patient by comparing a patient's individual recovery to an expected recovery curve.[30,31] Some institutions have committed to gathering PROMs for all patients across the spectrum of orthopaedic care, with the goal of longitudinally tracking outcomes of their population.[26] Broadly, within orthopaedics, PROMs fall under the categories of health, health-related quality of life, and quality of life. Under health, PROMs range from disease-specific, region-specific, or condition-specific PROMs, as well as psychosocial PROMs.[32,33] The American Academy of Orthopaedic Surgeons has compiled a list of approved, open-access PROMs from a 2015 Quality Outcomes Data Work Group to evaluate PROMS for general health and condition or PROMs specific to an anatomic region.[34]

Patient-Reported Experience Measures

Patient-reported experience measures (PREMs) broadly capture patient perceptions of their experience with health care.[35] PREMs range from measures of patient satisfaction with various structural and functional aspects of health care such as waiting times, access to facilities, and ability to navigate services, to (perhaps more importantly) the quality of communication and interpersonal interactions with clinicians and clinical teams.[36] PREMs capturing satisfaction with clinician-patient communications and trust in providers, alongside confidence with the level of information received and involvement in care, are shown to have a positive association with PROMs in patients undergoing hip and knee arthroplasty.[37] In the United States, the Consumer Assessment of Healthcare Providers and Systems (CAHPS) provide a suite of PREMs developed by the Agency for Healthcare Research and Quality, aiming to reflect key areas of overall patient experience related to structural, functional and interpersonal aspects of care. Since 2013, part of the value-based payment for hospitals initiated by CMS reflects the results of the hospital version of the Consumer Assessment of Healthcare Providers and Systems (known as H-CAPS).[7]

Patient Activation Measures

Patient activation measures (PAMs) are tools that measure an individual's understanding, competence, and willingness to participate in care decisions and processes; rather, the knowledge, skills, and confidence a person has in engaging with their health and health care ecosystem.[6] Active engagement of patients in their care has been demonstrated to improve health outcomes, patient experience, and lower health care costs.[38] PAMs enable providers to understand both an individual patient's level of activation and, more broadly, the levels of activation among various segments of their population. In particular, the Patient Activation Measure-13 (PAM-13) and the shorter PAM-10 have been used in orthopaedic care.[39]

Patient Decision Aids

SDM empowers patients to become active participants in their health and care by enabling both physician and patient to contribute to medical decision making. This approach depends on expert communication and education delivered by physicians that encourages patients to comfortably disclose their preferences, needs, and values to make informed treatment decisions.[8,40] Studies have shown SDM leads to better patient satisfaction, improved decision quality, more appropriate use of health care resources by patients, and better outcomes.[41-43] Based on a Cochrane review, SDM does not have a significant effect on the duration of the clinician-patient encounter, nor does it place additional burden on an already busy clinic schedule, adding only 2.55 minutes per encounter. Studies also suggest that these additional few minutes need not involve the physician but can be managed by midlevel health professionals.[44]

Patient decision aids (PDAs) are tools designed to facilitate SDM by helping patients understand relevant evidence-based information, empowering patients to better understand potential benefits and harms, and to aid communication between patients and clinicians.[45] Importantly, PDAs are distinct from patient education materials (which are also useful tools) in that they more actively direct patients toward making an informed choice among multiple treatment options. Some PDAs also help align treatment options with patient preferences rather than providing information about specific treatments or treatment plans after they have already been set in place.[46] In orthopaedic care, PDAs have been studied most frequently in patients with persistently painful preference-sensitive conditions (ie, where multiple valid treatment options exist) such as degenerative disease of the spine and osteoarthritis of the hip and knee.[47] PDAs can take multiple forms, including written booklets, videos, and interactive online tools and can be provided to patients before, during, or after an initial encounter with an orthopaedic practitioner. PDAs may also be effective in empowering patients to make informed decisions at a given point in time as well as providing ongoing guidance along different phases of a care pathway. Evidence suggests that orthopaedic patients with hip osteoarthritis and degenerative disease of the spine recall only 38% and 45% of verbal information respectively, after outpatient clinic visits with a provider, and as little as 18% of information 6 weeks after surgery.[48,49] PDAs could help address this knowledge and retention gap by providing patients with supportive resources on demand.

SDM-Related Outcome Metrics

SDM-related outcome measures (SROMs) can be used as part of an orthopaedic service's SDM initiative alongside implementation of PDAs. Somewhat similar to PROMs, these tools provide a measure of effect from the patient's perspective in relation to various elements of the decision-making process (eg, preparation for decision-making [Preparation for Decision-Making Scale], Decision Quality and level of SDM [Decision Quality Index, CollaboRATE survey], decisional conflict [Decision Conflict Scale, SURE 4-item screener], decisional regret [Decision Regret Scale], and decision support [Decision Support Analysis Tool, DSAT-10]), as well as numerical rating scales for various aspects of satisfaction with the consultation such as clinician-patient interaction.[50] Further validated tools (eg, OPTION) have also been developed to independently observe, measure, and score the extent and quality of SDM delivered by clinicians. Tools and checklists for the development and application of PDAs are also provided by the International Patient Decision Aids Standards (IPDAS) initiative.[51]

CLINICAL APPLICATIONS FOR VALUE AND PERFORMANCE MEASUREMENT

A key component of these patient-facing tools, aside from their psychometric characteristics (validity, reliability, responsiveness), is the capability for users to interpret and apply them in real-world clinical settings and the potential for utilization as performance measures in gauging value. The ability to understand how the scores are generated by such tools is crucial to apply these metrics at the clinical and systems levels. The minimal clinically important difference (MCID) is the smallest change in a treatment outcome (eg, PROM scores) that a patient would identify as important and that would indicate a change in the patient's management or health status.[52] MCID thresholds of many commonly used PROMs are available in the orthopaedic literature and can be used to benchmark performance and assess clinically meaningful improvement.[53] Differences smaller than the MCID are unlikely to matter to patients. MCID can be calculated using statistical methods (eg, the distribution method) based on typically selecting a threshold at 0.5 standard deviation within the distribution of outcome scores, or a subjective approach (eg, the anchor method), aligning scores to anchor questions reflecting patient satisfaction and patient perceptions around functional improvement.[54] The anchor method is generally preferred, given that it more closely reflects patient perceptions of improvement, aligns with expectations, and helps to better define substantial clinical benefit (SCB) thresholds. SCB reflects an improvement in outcomes thought by the patient to be considerable. This may be particularly relevant in assessing the effect of interventions, such as TJA, which has a strong record in improving symptoms and function, and for which minimal clinical improvement should really be the standard outcome.[55] SCB may also be useful in the treatment of sports injuries involving high-performing athletes and those with functional expectations on the higher end of the spectrum.[56] Another tool for enabling clinically meaningful interpretation of patient-generated outcomes data is the patient acceptable symptom state, defined as an absolute threshold for symptoms experienced with a specific condition beyond which patients consider themselves well and therefore satisfied with treatment.[57] Although MCID and SCB can be defined using an existing PROMs dataset or with the simple addition of a single anchor question, these thresholds do not account for the fact that it is easier to achieve a larger magnitude of change in patients who have extreme baseline values, nor do they provide an indication of a patient's successful return to activities of daily living, work, and recreation, or satisfaction with their level of improvement.[58] Although the patient acceptable symptom state requires additional scoring, it can be used to determine success of an intervention in patients who do not have preoperative PROMs, is less sensitive to baseline symptom levels, and provides a useful tool for setting expectations around the potential outcomes of treatment.[59] The use of these thresholds is gaining interest along with the development of PROMs as performance measures, defined as standardized tools, administered at designated time points, with an established risk-adjusted scoring methodology.[60]

Surgeon-Facing Tools

Clinical risk assessment tools (CRATs) provide validated metrics that can be utilized by surgeons to better understand the risks associated with a given treatment option. In orthopaedics, CRATs such as the Risk Assessment and Predictor Tool (RAPT), have commonly been used to predict discharge disposition home or to a rehabilitation facility following TJA.[61] More recently, data have been gathered to power a similar risk assessment tool in geriatric patients with hip fractures.[62] The largest drawback to CRATs is their varying levels of accuracy.[63] Work continues to develop models involving higher levels of accuracy, with the goal of reducing costly postacute care.[64] The Modified Frailty Index was introduced by the Canadian Study of Health and Aging and uses comorbidities (eg, hypertension, diabetes mellitus, vascular disease) to more comprehensively evaluate a patient's health status to predict postoperative complications.[65] This tool is shown to be predictive of increased mortality after femoral neck fractures as well as life-threatening complications and reoperation following total hip and total knee arthroplasty.[66,67]

Web-based orthopaedic personalized predictive tools provide personalized predictions of clinical outcomes based on the analysis of large volumes of data utilizing algorithmic mathematical modeling and predictive analytics.[68] A 2019 study identified 31 discrete web-based orthopaedic personalized predictive tools designed to provide personalized prediction in various orthopaedic settings.[69] These tools were designed for use in a variety of orthopaedic subspecialties including trauma, spine, TJA, and oncology; three-fourths of these tools had been developed since 2010.[69]

System-Level Tools: Core Platforms for Health Records and Patient Outcomes—Electronic Medical Records and Data Analytics Engines

A robust, interoperable, and user-friendly electronic health record is a core tool that can provide advanced management capabilities for value-oriented health care systems. These technologies can enable a more holistic longitudinal view of patients and improve care navigation (coordination and continuity of care) by multidisciplinary teams while reducing variation and waste. The functionalities of these platforms now extend beyond simple repositories of health information, toward the administration and collection of PROMs, PREMs, and other forms of data including social determinants of unmet health and social needs. Electronic medical records (EMRs) provide access to this information at points of care and enable decision support. They may also provide functions beyond frontline applications at the patient level, enabling a more population-based health view with a lens on the health of their patient community. EMRs should also be interoperable and aligned with a strong data analytics engine, advanced enterprise data warehouse or cloud capabilities alongside dynamic real-time reporting and analytics.

With the coronavirus disease 2019 (COVID-19) pandemic and a widening gap in access and affordability of care, structural and health-related social needs are found to be associated with health outcomes. In a move to address health needs upstream, there has been a recent call for systematic screening for social determinants of health, such as housing or food insecurity. Various effective screening tools exist, such as the Protocol for Responding to and Assessing Patients' Assets, Risks, and Experiences, or PRAPARE, which is used and developed by the National Association of Community Health Centers.[70] In an effort to align national outcome measurements, CMS compiled validated questions in an abbreviated screening tool known as the Accountable Health Communities Health-Related Social Needs Screening Tool.[71] These population-based health tools equip organizations to address health-related social needs and, although not without its technical challenges, could be extremely effective if integrated into EMRs. This functionality could enable practices to identify and address the needs of patients through collaboration with community services, primary care networks, and other services upstream.

As behavioral health and health-related social needs become incorporated into discussions between clinicians and patients, EMRs and billing code development follows suit. A wider range of ICD-10 codes and "Z" codes, traditionally being used by behavioral health providers such as social workers and other allied health care professionals, are increasingly being implemented in primary and specialty care. EMR innovation must include access to data at population levels to improve the health of communities, whether through the incorporation of psychosocial PROMs or concordant billing codes.

PATIENT PORTALS

Patient portals enabling education, channels for communication, and continuity of care may be part of the EMR or stand alone, enhancing engagement of individuals in the care delivery process. Patient portals are secure websites that allow patients to access personal health information online using a secure username and password.[72] Such portals facilitate longitudinal care by providing patients with easy access to records such as doctor's visits, medication lists, and laboratory results, as well as a secure means of communication with health care providers to request prescription refills, ask questions, and schedule appointments. Although research into the use of patient portals is relatively new, it has been associated with improving adherence to medications, facilitating effective patient-clinician communication, and enabling the discovery of medical errors.[73] Patient portals can also be used to send and record PROMs and PREMs, and several major EMRs have integrated patient portals with the capability to design, distribute, and collect customizable questionnaires.[74] The Partners Healthcare Patient Gateway at Massachusetts General Hospital/Brigham and Women's Health in Boston, Massachusetts is a platform that includes PROMs such as the Knee injury and Osteoarthritis Outcome Score among other orthopaedic and nonorthopaedic PROMs that patients can complete before, during, or after their visit.[75] In this system, physicians can help patients interpret their progress over time. The eventual goal is to build a robust database that can aid in clinical decision-making.

OUTCOME MEASUREMENT PLATFORM

A range of commercial and research-grade (eg, RecCAP) patient outcome measurement platforms exist, enabling electronic capture of PROMs and other forms of patient-generated health data. Digitization enables functionalities (eg, data visualization and analysis) and efficiencies (eg, time saving, automation) beyond manual paper entry. Most electronic PROM platforms support remote delivery, allowing patients to complete questionnaires by text, email, smartphone, tablet or their desktop computers at home.[76] In addition, these electronic platforms offer integration into EMR systems, which enable real-time review with patients and other clinical team members during clinic appointments and tracking of results over time.[77] Outcome measurement platforms have enabled the creation of large collections of PROMs data.

JOINT REPLACEMENT REGISTRIES

Data from PROMs are perhaps most valuable in aggregate and outcome measurement platforms and have enabled the creation of large collections of PROMs data. In the United States and across the world, these orthopaedic data are most typically aggregated in joint replacement registries, which provide insights into clinical outcomes at scale.[78] The United States, with its multipayer infrastructure, has both regionally focused registries, such as the Michigan Arthroplasty Registry Collaborative Quality Initiative (MARCQI), and broader registries, such as the Function and Outcomes Research for Comparative Effectiveness in Total Joint Replacement (FORCE-TJR) registry and American Joint Replacement Registry (AJRR) developed in partnership with the American Association of Orthopaedic Surgeons in 2009.[79,80] These registries also capture a range of clinical outcomes, including readmission rates, complications, and implant survival.[77]

ADVANCED COST ACCOUNTING PLATFORMS

Time-driven activity-based costing (TDABC), introduced by Kaplan and Anderson in 2004, provides a data-driven, targeted estimate of costs based on resources used by patients for their condition over a cycle of care.[81] Using costs for supplied resources (generating a cost per minute of all aspects of a health care professional's time), and practical capacity (actual productive time spent on each capacity-supplying resource), the method has enabled the definition of actual costs of care for orthopaedic conditions such as hip and knee osteoarthritis.[82] TDABC can be considered a versatile tool for defining and increasing awareness of costs from the "bottom-up" compared to traditional cost accounting (eg, using ratio of costs to charges [RCC] and relative value units [RVU]), which takes a "top-down" approach and defines costs based on charges and revenues. Although these legacy approaches are familiar and easier to perform, they risk an overestimation of total costs.[81] In orthopaedic care, TDABC has estimated the costs of TJA and ankle fracture care to be 48% to 59% of traditional accounting estimates.[83,84] Recent studies have used TDABC to identify implants and personnel to be the largest cost drivers in total hip, total knee, and total shoulder arthroplasty.[82,85] However, TDABC has limitations: it often excludes substantial indirect overhead costs, although one proposed model has been to standardize the most frequently used indirect overhead costs (maintenance, information technology, hospital administration, and billing) in the model.[86]

CURRENT AND FUTURE TECHNOLOGIES FOR HIGH-VALUE ORTHOPAEDIC CARE

Digital Phenotyping and Passive Patient-Generated Health Data

Digital phenotyping is the moment-by-moment quantification of human phenotypes in situ using data related to activity, behavior, and communications obtained from personal digital devices, such as smartphones and wearable sensors. It offers a technology capable of passively capturing patient-generated health data.[87] Personalized health information measured within an individual's usual settings may provide metrics for tracking, decision support, and enhancing patient-centered care. A review of scope demonstrates an acceleration of work in this area over the past 5 years, particularly in the context of orthopaedic surgery.[88] The measurement of and synthesis of activity, biometric, and communications data may provide suitable biomarkers of clinically meaningful health outcomes. Future work is geared to utilize this data alongside PROMs for the prediction of outcomes, risk profiling, SDM, and surgical optimization.

Artificial Intelligence, Machine Learning, Deep Learning

Artificial intelligence (AI) is broadly defined as a branch of computer science that simulates intelligent behavior in computers. In health care, AI offers the promise of enhanced predictive, diagnostic, and decision-making capabilities through three key domains: (1) advanced data discovery and extraction, (2) improved diagnostics and prediction, and (3) enhanced clinical and decision support.[89] These tools aim to decrease overall spending by reducing time, resource utilization, manpower, and computational power.[89] Data discovery and extraction has been successfully applied to work flows via natural language processing tools used for physician dictation as well as to clinical outcomes via stratification of patients by risk potential and prediction of adverse events.[90] AI has improved diagnostics and prediction across several domains of orthopaedic care, including improved image acquisition and disease detection compared with conventional imaging for detecting long bone and fragility fractures, differentiating between benign and malignant bone tumors, determining prognosis for patients with cancer, determining the risk of mortality after arthroplasty, and mapping disease progression for developmental dysplasia of the hip and degenerative disease of the spine and lower extremities.[91,92] In the domain of supporting clinical decision making, AI in combination with PROMs and demographic data have been applied to SDM in knee osteoarthritis, anterior cruciate ligament deficiency, and complex degenerative spinal disease. More specifically, AI has been leveraged to provide patient-specific risk-benefit ratios and prediction of health outcomes following arthroplasty.[93] Finally, AI is being applied to increase procedural efficiency in the operating room by guiding surgical teams through orthopaedic procedures with the goal of reducing variation in techniques in the operating room.

AI has already had widespread effect across multiple domains of orthopaedic care; however, significant ethical, legal, policy, and practice considerations remain. The ethical challenges in using AI stem from the varying levels of risk to patient privacy and confidentiality related to data transfer and sharing, consent, and patient autonomy. In addition, there remain unknown factors over the potential for robots to autonomously adapt and alter the course of a procedure.[94] Current regulatory frameworks and ethical guidelines need to keep pace with the progress in technology.[95] Regulatory and professional bodies should provide guidance on interventions aligned with AI solutions, include meaningful endpoints (those driving changes beneficial to clinicians and patients), appropriate benchmarks (assuring these are dynamic based on evolving sets of real-world data and performance), and longitudinal audit mechanisms (incorporating postmarket surveillance of a solution evolving over time as AI-driven algorithms learn).[95] On an individual level, surgeons should understand the population characteristics used to develop algorithms and work with programmers to calibrate their outputs to match the needs of the patient populations being treated.[96] Future training of orthopaedic providers must focus on the interaction between clinicians, patients, and technology. There is also a need to demonstrate the effect of AI on value with high-quality cohort and randomized controlled trials using PROMs, cost-effectiveness analyses, and rapid quality improvement studies. AI has been leveraged for orthopaedics in multiple studies[97] (**Table 1**).

Machine learning (ML) is a process by which a computer improves its own performance (eg, via the analysis of image files) by continuously incorporating new data into an existing statistical model (**Table 2**). ML encompasses automatic procedures of incremental function optimization, which can be conducted under supervised or unsupervised learning. Supervised learning requires a human to manually input large volumes of data that are paired to a correct output function (eg, a correct diagnosis made using a radiologic image). In contrast, for unsupervised learning, the correct inputs are not known or given, and instead inferred by an algorithm on the basis of the relationship between the input data points.[92] These techniques can be applied to individual-level and population-level data.[98] Since 2010, the volume of orthopaedic literature citing ML has increased tenfold in areas ranging from disease detection (eg, spine pathology, osteoarthritis, fracture, anterior cruciate ligament/posterior cruciate ligament injury) and clinical assessment (eg, shoulder strength, skeletal bone age, gait analysis) to treatment efficacy (eg, optimal injection point, prosthesis control).[99-105] These studies have utilized medical imaging, both biomechanical and patient generated, spanning a range of ML techniques.

Deep learning (DL) is as a form of AI that enables computers to learn from experience and understand systems in terms of information hierarchies.[106] As the

TABLE 1 Artificial Intelligence Applied to Orthopaedics

Study	Application	Notes
Thong et al (2016)	Optimization of 3D spine model vectors for the automatic detection of adolescent idiopathic scoliosis	—
Olczak et al (2017)	Identification of fractures from radiographic images	—
Chen et al (2017)	ML-based predictions for physician order entry show that prioritizing small amounts of recent data is more effective than using larger amounts of older data toward future clinical predictions	Concept decaying clinical data based on practice patterns is critical to appreciate
Kruse et al (2017)	Prediction of hip fractures from dual x-ray absorptiometry	—
Cilla et al (2017)	Use of ML to optimize short-stem THA design to produce optimal mechanical performance	—
Konda (2018)	An AI system (PersonaCARE) helps manage NYU's middle age and geriatric fracture population based on all of the principles of value-based health care	—
Kamuta et al (2019)	Determined that a bundled care model for hip fractures is an unsustainable value-based model	—
Ramkumar et al (2019)	Predicted length of state, inpatient costs, and patient disposition for lower extremity joint replacement	First introduction of patient-specific payment model
Shah et al (2019)	Automatic measurement and segmentation of articular cartilage thickness in healthy knees on MRI	—
Harris et al (2019)	Prediction of 30-day complications and mortality following TJA	Utilized the National Surgical Quality Improvement Program database
Greenstein et al (2019)	ANN utilization of in-house EMR data to predict skilled nursing facility utilization following TJA	—

(Continued)

TABLE 1 Artificial Intelligence Applied to Orthopaedics (Continued)

Study	Application	Notes
Fontana et al (2019)	ML to preoperatively predict with fair to good accuracy which patients may achieve minimally clinically important differences postoperatively in TJA	Study was the subject of *Clinical Orthopaedics and Related Research's* "Editor's Spotlight"
Thirukumaran et al (2019)	Use of NLP to identify orthopaedic surgical site infections	—
Galbusera et al (2019)	Valuable review of AI and ML in spine research	Recommended reading

3D = three-dimensional, AI = artificial intelligence, ANN = artificial neural network, EMR = electronic medical record, ML = machine learning, MRI = magnetic resonance imaging, NLP = natural language processing, NYU = New York University, THA = total hip arthroplasty, TJA = total joint arthroplasty

Data from Myers TG, Ramkumar PN, Ricciardi BF, Urish KL, Kipper J, Ketonis C: Artificial intelligence and orthopaedics: An introduction for clinicians. *J Bone Joint Surg Am* 2020;102:830-840.

computer gathers knowledge through cycles of learning and experience, requirements are minimal to none for ongoing manual input. This process allows the computer to learn complicated concepts.[106] DL in orthopaedics to date has mostly been applied to imaging data with a focus on predicting pathology in adolescent idiopathic scoliosis, spondylolisthesis, spinal column and long bone fractures, hip osteoarthritis, and skeletal bone age.[107-112] A major advantage of DL is efficiency and handling of large volumes of complex structured and unstructured data. It is critical for human users to understand and have access to the analytics behind the outputs, alongside controls to ensure safe handling and accurate interpretation of data.[113,114]

Real-Time Location Systems

Real-time locating systems (or real-time location systems) (RTLS) are local systems that can identify and track assets in real (or near-real) time.[115] This functionality

TABLE 2 Advantages and Disadvantages of Machine Learning

Advantages	Disadvantages
Trends and patterns are identified easily	High level of error susceptibility
Continuous improvement	Complex computing requires processing power
Allows adaptation without human intervention	Adequate and appropriate data required
Handles highly complex datasets	Results still require interpretation

could support the development of orthopaedic multidisciplinary teams, enhance efficiencies in clinic workflow, and automating TDABC and other activity-based methods of cost accounting for increasing value. Such systems are composed of fixed readers that receive wireless signals from small unique tags attached to objects of interest. This network of readers can determine if the tagged object is located within a confined indoor or outdoor space. RTLS can provide location information to hospital information systems, admission/discharge/transfer systems, radiology information systems, and operating room systems via an open application programming interface.[116] Both physical components of RTLS, the reader and the tag, can be outfitted with additional features including those for communication (eg, push/call buttons, indictor status buttons, voice-to-voice capability, buzzers, LED lights, LCD screens), additional data gathering (eg, temperature and motion sensors), and writeable memory to log and store data.[117] RTLS systems can provide location at a variety of resolutions (**Table 3**) and be designed around a range of technologies (eg, infrared, ultrasonography, camera vision, Bluetooth, radiofrequency identification, GPS, WiFi, and cellular) that each have their benefits and drawbacks.[118,119] Prior to selecting a given RTLS solution, a practice must consider

TABLE 3 Real-Time Locating Systems Resolution

Resolution	Description	Example
Presence-based locating	RTLS returns tag location as present in a given area	A bed is detected on a floor of a hospital
Room level locating	RTLS returns tag location as present in a specific room	Nurse presses a panic button and her exact room location is reported by the system
Subroom level locating	RTLS returns tag location as present in a specific part of a room	A location engine detects how much time a doctor spent at each bedside in a two-bed hospital room
Choke point locating	RTLS returns a tag location as present at a specific choke point	A patient bed is located at the entry/exit point of a room and its previous location at other entry/exit points demonstrates its location of travel
Associating	RTLS returns a tag location as being in proximity to another tag	A piece of durable medical equipment is located next to a specific patient bed
Precise locating	RTLS returns a tag location as being precisely located on a map of the world/detailed indoor map	A tag on a surgical equipment set is located in the central processing department of a large trauma center

Data from Kamel Boulos MN, Berry G: Real-time locating systems (RTLS) in healthcare: A condensed primer. *Int J Health Geogr* 2012;11:25.

its own unique needs and physical and information technology infrastructure. For example, it will likely be challenging to rely on a cellular-based system in an older hospital complex with numerous concrete walls and subterranean floors. Finally, use of RTLS to monitor staff and/or patients requires clear disclosure and practices must be prepared to address privacy concerns prior to investing in RTLS.

SUMMARY

There are an increasing array of data-driven tools and technologies to support clinicians in practicing high-value orthopaedic care. Although these tools and capabilities are at various stages of development and adoption, the fundamental elements of value (outcomes that matter to patients and true costs of care) can start to be incorporated in orthopaedic practices using grassroots approaches, such as the use of paper-based or freely available research-grade software to administer PROMs. Advancement and availability of tools and technologies for driving value-based health care is inevitable and it will be just as important for culture change to adopt these capabilities to harness the full power of these solutions in high-value orthopaedic practices.

REFERENCES

1. Centers for Medicare & Medicaid Services: Comprehensive care for joint replacement model. Available at: https://innovation.cms.gov/innovation-models/cjr. Accessed January 14, 2021.

2. Centers for Medicare & Medicaid Services: Accountable care organizations (ACOs). Available at: https://www.cms.gov/Medicare/Medicare-Fee-for-Service-Payment/ACO. Accessed January 15, 2021.

3. Porter ME, Teisberg EO: *Redefining Health Care: Creating Value-Based Competition on Results.* Harvard Business School Press, 2006.

4. Porter ME: What is value in health care? *N Engl J Med* 2010;363(26):2477-2481.

5. Wei DH, Hawker GA, Jevsevar DS, Bozic KJ: Improving value in musculoskeletal care delivery: AOA critical issues. *J Bone Joint Surg Am* 2015;97(9):769-774.

6. Institute of Medicine (US) Committee on Quality of Health Care in America: Crossing The Quality Chasm: A New Health System For The 21st Century, 2001. Available at: https://www.med.unc.edu/neurosurgery/wp-content/uploads/sites/460/2018/10/Crossing-the-Quality-Chasm.pdf. Accessed May 3, 2023.

7. Harwood JL, Butler CA, Page AE: Patient-centered care and population health: Establishing their role in the orthopaedic practice. *J Bone Joint Surg Am* 2016;98(10):e40.

8. Elwyn G, Frosch D, Thomson R, et al: Shared decision making: A model for clinical practice. *J Gen Intern Med* 2012;27(10):1361-1367.

9. American Academy of Orthopaedic Surgeons. Preventing Venous Thromboembolic Disease In Patients Undergoing Elective Hip And Knee Arthroplasty: Evidence-Based Guideline And Evidence Report, 2011. Available at: https://www.aaos.org/quality/quality-programs/tumor-infection-and-military-medicine-programs/venous-thromboembolic-disease-in-elective-tka-and-tha-prevention/. Accessed May 3, 2023.

10. Singer SJ, Kerrissey M, Friedberg M, Phillips R: A comprehensive theory of integration. *Med Care Res Rev* 2020;77(2):196-207.

11. Manning BT, Callahan CD, Robinson BS, Adair D, Saleh KJ: Overcoming resistance to implementation of integrated care pathways in orthopaedics. *J Bone Joint Surg Am* 2013;95(14):e100, 1-6.

12. Jimenez Muñoz AB, Duran Garcia ME, Rodriguez Perez MP, Sanjurjo M, Vigil MD, Vaquero J: Clinical pathway for hip arthroplasty six years after introduction. *Int J Health Care Qual Assur Inc Leadersh Health Serv* 2006;19(2-3):237-245.

13. Pearson S, Moraw I, Maddern GJ: Clinical pathway management of total knee arthroplasty: A retrospective comparative study. *Aust N Z J Surg* 2000;70(5):351-354.

14. Kates SL, Mendelson DA, Friedman SM: The value of an organized fracture program for the elderly: Early results. *J Orthop Trauma* 2011;25(4):233-237.

15. Adunsky A, Arad M, Levi R, Blankstein A, Zeilig G, Mizrachi E: Five-year experience with the 'Sheba' model of comprehensive orthogeriatric care for elderly hip fracture patients. *Disabil Rehabil* 2005;27(18-19):1123-1127.

16. Ring D: Editorial comment: Comprehensive orthopaedic care. *Clin Orthop Relat Res* 2018;476(4):694-695.

17. HealthIT.gov: Patient-Generated Health Data. Available at: https://www.healthit.gov/topic/scientific-initiatives/pcor/patient-generated-health-data-pghd. Accessed May 1, 2023.

18. Brodke DJ, Saltzman CL, Brodke DS: PROMIS for orthopaedic outcomes measurement. *J Am Acad Orthop Surg* 2016;24(11):744-749.

19. Patrick D, Guyatt GH, Acquadro C: Patient-reported outcomes, in Higgins JPT, Green S, eds: *Cochrane Handbook for Systematic Reviews of Interventions Version 510 The Cochrane Collaboration*, 2011. Available at: http:www.handbook.cochrane.org. Accessed May 3, 2023.

20. Lindgren JV, Wretenberg P, Karrholm J, Garellick G, Rolfson O: Patient-reported outcome is influenced by surgical approach in total hip replacement: A study of the Swedish hip arthroplasty register including 42,233 patients. *Bone Joint J* 2014;96-B(5):590-596.

21. Jameson SS, Mason J, Baker P, et al: A comparison of surgical approaches for primary hip arthroplasty: A cohort study of patient reported outcome measures (PROMs) and early revision using linked national databases. *J Arthroplasty* 2014;29(6):1248-1255.e1.

22. The American Board of Orthopaedic Surgery: Certification examinations part II: Patient reported outcomes. Available at: https://www.abos.org/certification-exams/part-ii/. Accessed May 2, 2023.

23. Stulberg J: The physician quality reporting initiative – A gateway to pay for performance: What every health care professional should know. *Qual Manag Health Care* 2008;17(1):2-8.

24. Ruzbarsky JJ, Marom N, Marx RG: Measuring quality and outcomes in sports medicine. *Clin Sports Med* 2018;37(3):463-482.

25. Dacombe PJ, Amirfeyz R, Davis T: Patient-reported outcome measures for hand and wrist trauma: Is there sufficient evidence of reliability, validity, and responsiveness? *Hand (N Y)* 2016;11(1):11-21.

26. Baumhauer JF, Bozic KJ: Value-based healthcare: Patient-reported outcomes in clinical decision making. *Clin Orthop Relat Res* 2016;474(6):1375-1378.

27. Horn ME, Reinke EK, Couce LJ, Reeve BB, Ledbetter L, George SZ: Reporting and utilization of Patient-Reported Outcomes Measurement Information System® (PROMIS®) measures in orthopedic research and practice: A systematic review. *J Orthop Surg Res* 2020;15(1):553.

28. Black N: Patient reported outcome measures could help transform health care. *BMJ* 2013;346:f167.

29. Andrawis J, Akhavan S, Chan V, Lehil M, Pong D, Bozic KJ: Higher preoperative patient activation, associated with better patient-reported outcomes after total joint arthroplasty. *Clin Orthop Relat Res* 2015;473(8):2688-2697.

30. Berliner JL, Brodke DJ, Chan V, SooHoo NF, Bozic KJ: John Charnley award: Preoperative patient-reported outcome measures predict clinically meaningful improvement in function after THA. *Clin Orthop Relat Res* 2016;474(2):321-329.

31. Papuga MO, Beck CA, Kates SL, Schwarz EM, Maloney MD: Validation of GAITRite and PROMIS as high-throughput physical function outcome measures following ACL reconstruction. *J Orthop Res* 2014;32(6):793-801.

32. Gagnier JJ: Patient reported outcomes in orthopaedics. *J Orthop Res* 2017;35(10):2098-2108.

33. MOTION Group: Patient-reported outcomes in orthopaedics. *J Bone Joint Surg Am* 2018;100(5):436-442.

34. American Academy of Orthopaedic Surgeons: Patient reported outcome measures. Available at: https://www.aaos.org/quality/research-resources/patient-reported-outcome-measures/. Accessed May 3, 2023.

35. NSW Agency for Clinical Innovation: About patient reported measures. Available at: https://aci.health.nsw.gov.au/statewide-programs/prms/about. Accessed May 3, 2023.

36. Weldering T, Smith SM: Patient-reported outcomes (PROs) and patient-reported outcome measures (PROMs). *Health Serv Insights* 2013;6:61-68.

37. Black N, Varaganum M, Hutchings A: Relationship between patient reported experience (PREMs) and patient reported outcomes (PROMs) in elective surgery. *BMJ Qual Saf* 2014;23(7):534-542.

38. Hibbard JH, Greene J: What the evidence shows about patient activation: Better health outcomes and care experiences; fewer data on costs. *Health Aff (Millwood)* 2013;32(2):207-214.

39. Grogan Moore ML, Jayakumar P, Laverty D, Hill AD, Koenig KM: Patient-reported outcome measures and patient activation: What are their roles in orthopedic trauma? *J Orthop Trauma* 2019;33(suppl 7):S38-S42.

40. Smith MA: The role of shared decision making in patient-centered care and orthopaedics. *Orthop Nurs* 2016;35(3):144-149.

41. Slover J, Shue J, Koenig K: Shared decision-making in orthopaedic surgery. *Clin Orthop Relat Res* 2012;470(4):1046-1053.

42. Bozic KJ, Belkora J, Chan V, et al: Shared decision making in patients with osteoarthritis of the hip and knee: Results of a randomized controlled trial. *J Bone Joint Surg Am* 2013;95(18):1633-1639.

43. Stacey D, Hawker G, Dervin G, et al: Decision aid for patients considering total knee arthroplasty with preference report for surgeons: A pilot randomized controlled trial. *BMC Musculoskelet Disord* 2014;15:54.

44. Stacey D, Légaré F, Col NF, et al: Decision aids for people facing health treatment or screening decisions. *Cochrane Database Syst Rev* 2014;2014(1):CD001431.

45. Adam JA, Khaw FM, Thomson RG, Gregg PJ, Llewellyn-Thomas HA: Patient decision aids in joint replacement surgery: A literature review and an opinion survey of consultant orthopaedic surgeons. *Ann R Coll Surg Engl* 2008;90(3):198-207.

46. Molenaar S, Sprangers M, Postma-Schuit F, et al: Feasibility and effects of decision aids. *Med Decis Making* 2000;20(1):112-127.

47. Ibrahim SA, Blum M, Lee GC, et al: Effect of a decision aid on access to total knee replacement for black patients with osteoarthritis of the knee: A randomized clinical trial. *JAMA Surg* 2017;152(1):e164225.

48. Langdon IJ, Hardin R, Learmonth ID: Informed consent for total hip arthroplasty: Does a written information sheet improve recall by patients? *Ann R Coll Surg Engl* 2002;84(6):404-408.

49. Saigal R, Clark AJ, Scheer JK, et al: Adult spinal deformity patients recall fewer than 50% of the risks discussed in the informed consent process preoperatively and the recall rate worsens significantly in the postoperative period. *Spine (Phila Pa 1976)* 2015;40(14):1079-1085.

50. Barr PJ, Elwyn G: Measurement challenges in shared decision making: Putting the 'patient' in patient-reported measures. *Health Expect* 2016;19(5):993-1001.

51. Elwyn G, O'Connor A, Stacey D, et al: Developing a quality criteria framework for patient decision aids: Online international Delphi consensus process. *BMJ* 2006;333(7565):417.

52. Crosby RD, Kolotkin RL, Williams GR: Defining clinically meaningful change in health-related quality of life. *J Clin Epidemiol* 2003;56(5):395-407.

53. Maltenfort M, Díaz-Ledezma C: Statistics in brief: Minimum clinically important difference – Availability of reliable estimates. *Clin Orthop Relat Res* 2017;475(4):933-946.

54. Glassman SD, Copay AG, Berven SH, Polly DW, Subach BR, Carreon LY: Defining substantial clinical benefit following lumbar spine arthrodesis. *J Bone Joint Surg Am* 2008;90(9):1839-1847.

55. Katz NP, Paillard FC, Ekman E: Determining the clinical importance of treatment benefits for interventions for painful orthopedic conditions. *J Orthop Surg Res* 2015;10:24.

56. Nwachukwu BU, Chang B, Fields K, et al: Defining the "substantial clinical benefit'" after arthroscopic treatment of femoroacetabular impingement. *Am J Sports Med* 2017;45(6):1297-1303.

57. Muller B, Yabroudi MA, Lynch A, et al: Defining thresholds for the patient acceptable symptom state for the IKDC subjective knee form and KOOS for patients who underwent ACL reconstruction. *Am J Sports Med* 2016;44(11):2820-2826.

58. Carragee EJ: The rise and fall of the "minimum clinically important difference." *Spine J* 2010;10(4):283-284.

59. Mannion AF, Loibl M, Bago J, et al: What level of symptoms are patients with adult spinal deformity prepared to live with? A cross-sectional analysis of the 12-month follow-up data from 1043 patients. *Eur Spine J* 2020;29(6):1340-1352.

60. Safran D: Feasibility and value of patient-reported outcome measures for value-based payment. *Med Care* 2019;57(3):177-179.

61. Gholson JJ, Pugely AJ, Bedard NA, Duchman KR, Anthony CA, Callaghan JJ: Can we predict discharge status after total joint arthroplasty? A calculator to predict home discharge. *J Arthroplasty* 2016;31(12):2705-2709.

62. Arshi A, Iglesias BC, Zambrana LE, et al: Postacute care utilization in postsurgical orthogeriatric hip fracture care. *J Am Acad Orthop Surg* 2020;28(18):743-749.

63. Menendez ME, Schumacher CS, Ring D, Freiberg AA, Rubash HE, Kwon YM: Does "6-clicks" day 1 postoperative mobility score predict discharge disposition after total hip and knee arthroplasties? *J Arthroplasty* 2016;31(9):1916-1920.

64. Goltz DE, Ryan SP, Attarian D, Jiranek WA, Bolognesi MP, Seyler TM: A preoperative risk prediction tool for discharge to a skilled nursing or rehabilitation facility after total joint arthroplasty. *J Arthroplasty* 2021;36(4):1212-1219.

65. Rockwood K, Andrew M, Mitnitski AB: A comparison of two approaches to measuring frailty in elderly people. *J Gerontol A Biol Sci Med Sci* 2007;62(7):738-743.

66. Patel KV, Brennan KL, Brennan ML, Jupiter DC, Shar A, Davis ML: Association of a modified frailty index with mortality after femoral neck fracture in patients aged 60 years and older. *Clin Orthop Relat Res* 2014;472(3):1010-1017.

67. Shin JI, Keswani A, Lovy AJ, Moucha CS: Simplified frailty index as a predictor of adverse outcomes in total hip and knee arthroplasty. *J Arthroplasty* 2016;31(11):2389-2394.

68. Bernstein DN, Fear K, Mesfin A, et al: Patient-reported outcomes use during orthopaedic surgery clinic visits improves the patient experience. *Musculoskeletal Care* 2019;17(1):120-125.

69. Curtin P, Conway A, Martin L, Lin E, Jayakumar P, Swart E: Compilation and analysis of web-based orthopedic personalized predictive tools: A scoping review. *J Pers Med* 2020;10(4):223.

70. National Association of Community Health Centers: PRAPARE implementation and action toolkit. Available at: http://www.nachc.org/research-and-data/prapare/toolkit/. Accessed January 10, 2021.

71. Centers for Medicare and Medicaid Services: The accountable health communities health-related social needs screening tool. Available at: https://innovation.cms.gov/files/worksheets/ahcm-screeningtool.pdf. Accessed May 3, 2023.

72. Office for the National Coordinator for Health Information Technology: What is a patient portal? Available at: https://www.healthit.gov/faq/what-patient-portal. Accessed May 3, 2023.

73. Dendere R, Slade C, Burton-Jones A, Sullivan C, Staib A, Janda M: Patient portals facilitating engagement with inpatient electronic medical records: A systematic review. *J Med Internet Res* 2019;21(4):e12779.

74. Massachusetts Medical Society: Patient-reported outcome measures: current state and MMS principles. Available at: http://www.massmed.org/proms. Accessed May 3, 2023.

75. Partners Healthcare: About patient reported outcome measures (PROMs). Available at: http://caredecisions.partners.org/partners-care-decisions/patient-reported-outcome-measures-proms/. Accessed May 3, 2023.

76. Borowsky PA, Kadri OM, Meldau JE, Blanchett J, Makhni EC: The remote completion rate of electronic patient-reported outcome forms before scheduled clinic visits-a proof-of-concept study using patient-reported outcome measurement information

system computer adaptive test questionnaires. *J Am Acad Orthop Surg Glob Res Rev* 2019;3(10):e19.00038.

77. Makhni EC: Meaningful clinical applications of patient-reported outcome measures in orthopaedics. *J Bone Joint Surg Am* 2021;103(1):84-91.

78. Rolfson O, Karrholm J, Dahlberg LE, Garellick G: Patient-reported outcomes in the Swedish hip arthroplasty register: Results of a nationwide prospective observational study. *J Bone Joint Surg Br* 2011;93(7):867-875.

79. Hallstrom B, Singal B, Cowen ME, Roberts KC, Hughes RE: The Michigan experience with safety and effectiveness of tranexamic acid use in hip and knee arthroplasty. *J Bone Joint Surg Am* 2016;98(19):1646-1655.

80. Ayers DC, Fehring TK, Odum SM, Franklin PD: Using joint registry data from FORCE-TJR to improve the accuracy of risk-adjustment prediction models for thirty-day readmission after total hip replacement and total knee replacement. *J Bone Joint Surg Am* 2015;97(8):668-671.

81. Kaplan R, Anderson S: Time-driven activity-based costing. *Harv Bus Rev* 2004;82(11):131-138, 150.

82. Menendez ME, Lawler SM, Shaker J, Bassoff NW, Warner JJP, Jawa A: Time-driven activity-based costing to identify patients, incurring high inpatient cost for total shoulder arthroplasty. *J Bone Joint Surg Am* 2018;100(23):2050-2056.

83. Palsis JA, Brehmer TS, Pellegrini VD, Drew JM, Sachs BL: The cost of joint replacement: Comparing two approaches to evaluating costs of total hip and knee arthroplasty. *J Bone Joint Surg Am* 2018;100(4):326-333.

84. McCreary DL, White M, Vang S, Plowman B, Cunningham BP: Time-driven activity-based costing in fracture care: Is this a more accurate way to prepare for alternative payment models? *J Orthop Trauma* 2018;32(7):344-348.

85. DiGioia AM, Greenhouse PK, Giarrusso ML, Kress JM: Determining the true cost to deliver total hip and knee arthroplasty over the full cycle of care: Preparing for bundling and reference-based pricing. *J Arthroplasty* 2016;31(1):1-6.

86. Pathak S, Snyder D, Kroshus T, et al: What are the uses and limitations of time-driven activity-based costing in total joint replacement? *Clin Orthop Relat Res* 2019;477(9):2071-2081.

87. Insel TR: Digital phenotyping: Technology for a new science of behavior. *J Am Med Assoc* 2017;318(13):1215-1216.

88. Jayakumar P, Lin E, Galea V, et al: Digital phenotyping and patient-generated health data for outcome measurement in surgical care: A scoping review. *J Pers Med* 2020;10(4):282.

89. Jayakumar P, Moore MLG, Bozic KJ: Value-based healthcare: Can artificial intelligence provide value in orthopaedic surgery? *Clin Orthop Relat Res* 2019;477(8):1777-1780.

90. Rajkomar A, Oren E, Chen K, et al: Scalable and accurate deep learning with electronic health records. *NPJ Digit Med* 2018;1:18.

91. Harris AHS, Kuo AC, Weng Y, Trickey AW, Bowe T, Giori NJ: Can machine learning methods produce accurate and easy-to-use prediction models of 30-day complications and mortality after knee or hip arthroplasty? *Clin Orthop Relat Res* 2019;477(2):452-460.

92. Cabitza F, Locoro A, Banfi G: Machine learning in orthopedics: A literature review. *Front Bioeng Biotechnol* 2018;6:75.

93. Sambare T, Uhler L, Bozic KJ: Shared decision making: Time to get personal. Available at: https://catalyst.nejm. Accessed May 1, 2023.

94. Makhni EC, Makhni S, Ramkumar PN: Artificial intelligence for the orthopaedic surgeon: An overview of potential benefits, limitations, and clinical applications. *J Am Acad Orthop Surg* 2021;29(6):235-243.

95. O'Sullivan S, Nevejans N, Allen C, et al: Legal, regulatory, and ethical frameworks for development of standards in artificial intelligence (AI) and autonomous robotic surgery. *Int J Med Robot* 2019;15(1):e1968.

96. Parikh RB, Obermeyer Z, Navathe AS: Regulation of predictive analytics in medicine. *Science* 2019;363(6429):810-812.

97. Myers TG, Ramkumar PN, Ricciardi BF, Urish KL, Kipper J, Ketonis C: Artificial intelligence and orthopaedics: An introduction for clinicians. *J Bone Joint Surg Am* 2020;102(9):830-840.

98. Bayliss L, Jones LD: The role of artificial intelligence and machine learning in predicting orthopaedic outcomes. *Bone Joint J* 2019;101-B(12):1476-1478.

99. Spampinato C, Palazzo S, Giordano D, Aldinucci M, Leonardi R: Deep learning for automated skeletal bone age assessment in X-ray images. *Med Image Anal* 2017;36(suppl):41-51.

100. Lemoyne R, Mastroianni T, Hessel A, Nishikawa K: Implementation of machine learning for classifying prosthesis type through conventional gait analysis. *Annu Int Conf IEEE Eng Med Biol Soc* 2015;2015:202-205.

101. Pogorelc B, Gams M: Diagnosing health problems from gait patterns of elderly. *Annu Int Conf IEEE Eng Med Biol Soc* 2010;2010:2238-2241.

102. Phinyomark A, Osis ST, Hettinga BA, Kobsar D, Ferber R: Gender differences in gait kinematics for patients with knee osteoarthritis. *BMC Musculoskelet Disord* 2016;17:157.

103. Atkinson EJ, Therneau TM, Melton LJ, et al: Assessing fracture risk using gradient boosting machine (GBM) models. *J Bone Miner Res* 2012;27(6):1397-1404.

104. Silver AE, Lungren MP, Johnson ME, O'Driscoll SW, An KN, Hughes RE: Using support vector machines to optimally classify rotator cuff strength data and quantify postoperative strength in rotator cuff tear patients. *J Biomech* 2006;39(5):973-979.

105. Jamaludin A, Lootus M, Kadir T, et al: ISSLS prize in bioengineering science 2017: Automation of reading of radiological features from magnetic resonance images (MRIs) of the lumbar spine without human intervention is comparable with an expert radiologist. *Eur Spine J* 2017;26(5):1374-1383.

106. Goodfellow I, Bengio Y, Courville A: *Deep Learning*. MIT University Press, 2016.

107. Thong W, Parent S, Wu J, Aubin CE, Labelle H, Kadoury S: Three-dimensional morphology study of surgical adolescent idiopathic scoliosis patient from encoded geometric models. *Eur Spine J* 2016;25(10):3104-3113.

108. Forsberg D, Sjöblom E, Sunshine JL: Detection and labeling of vertebrae in MR images using deep learning with clinical annotations as training data. *J Digit Imaging* 2017;30(4):406-412.

109. Olczak J, Fahlberg N, Maki A, et al: Artificial intelligence for analyzing orthopedic trauma radiographs. *Acta Orthop* 2017;88(6):581-586.

110. Al-Helo S, Alomari RS, Ghosh S, et al: Compression fracture diagnosis in lumbar: A clinical CAD system. *Int J Comput Assist Radiol Surg* 2013;8(3):461-469.

111. Xue Y, Zhang R, Deng Y, Chen K, Jiang T: A preliminary examination of the diagnostic value of deep learning in hip osteoarthritis. *PLoS One* 2017;12(6):e0178992.

112. Giordano D, Kavasidis I, Spampinato C: Modeling skeletal bone development with hidden Markov models. *Comput Methods Programs Biomed* 2016;124:138-147.

113. Cabitza F, Rasoini R, Gensini GF: Unintended consequences of machine learning in medicine. *J Am Med Assoc* 2017;318(6):517-518.

114. Caruana R, Lou Y, Gehrke J, Koch P, Sturm M, Elhadad N: Intelligible models for healthcare: Predicting pneumonia risk and hospital 30-day readmission, in *Proceedings of the 21th ACM SIGKDD International Conference on Knowledge Discovery and Data Mining*. August 2015, pp 1721-1730. Accessed May 3, 2023.

115. Kamel Boulos MN, Berry G: Real-time locating systems (RTLS) in healthcare: A condensed primer. *Int J Health Geogr* 2012;11:25.

116. Dimond D: The optimal RTLS solution for hospitals. *J Healthc Inf Manag* 2009;23(2):4-5.

117. Malik A: *RTLS For Dummies*. Wiley Publishing, 2009.

118. Liu H, Darabi H, Banerjee P, Liu J: Survey of wireless indoor positioning techniques and systems. *IEEE Trans Syst Man Cybern Part C Appl Rev* 2007;37(6):1067-1080.

119. Curran K, Furey E, Lunney T, Santos J, Woods D, McCaughey A: An evaluation of indoor location determination technologies. *J Location Based Serv* 2011;5(2):61-78.

CHAPTER 13

Payer Perspective on Value-Based Health Care in Orthopaedics

Daniel B. Murrey, MD, MPP • Christopher Naso, MPH
Brandy Keys, MPH

INTRODUCTION

Patients rarely pay the majority of their medical care costs alone. Payers, either as a government entity or a private company representing themselves, employers, or other stakeholders, are key participants in the move to value-based care. They can be either facilitators or barriers to this change, and as such, physicians must learn to partner effectively with them. By better understanding their needs and perspectives more fully, physicians will be better able to forge a positive working relationship that delivers mutual success.

ROLE OF THE PAYER

To understand the perspective of payers on value-based health care, it is important to first understand the role of payers in the healthcare system. Payers serve as organizing entities connecting those who fund the cost of medical care, typically employers, individuals, or health plans, with those who provide health care services across a defined geographic area. They do this via four distinct functions, each of which may be performed by the payer itself or delegated to another entity (**Table 1**): (1) network development, which develops a network of high-quality providers and negotiate rates; (2) network management for quality assurance and utilization review, which determines whether claims meet clinical necessity and quality-based contractual criteria; (3) claims management, which processes claims that can be done by a third-party administrator, health plan, or other risk entity; and (4) serving as a risk-bearing entity, which takes ownership for all or a portion of costs and may base payment on quality metrics and health outcomes.

TABLE 1 Roles of the Payer

Value Segment	Description	Rationale
Network development	Identifying, selecting and contracting with providers for patient access to comprehensive health care services	Access A third-party entity with knowledge of the health-care provider marketplace can create a network for patients to have access to comprehensive health services. Cost/Access By representing multiple patients, a third-party entity can negotiate cost reductions for health services, which can also be associated with access in circumstances where higher out-of-pocket costs change the medical behavior of patients. Quality A third-party entity can select providers to participate in the network based on historical quality and health outcome performance.
Network management	Quality assurance and utilization review of providers in a patient's network	Cost/Access A third-party entity can work to ensure that providers and corresponding health services are offered at an affordable price. Quality A third-party entity can monitor standards of clinical necessity and appropriateness of care to ensure that a certain level of quality is provided, and health outcomes achieved for patients throughout the network.
Claims management	Processing, analyzing, and paying claims to providers	Cost The claims process is designed to determine what a third-party entity will pay to a provider based on the negotiated contract to offset out-of-pocket costs for patients.
Risk-bearing entity	Spreading actuarial risk evenly across a patient population to mitigate expenses	Cost To ensure affordable premiums, a third-party entity offers insurance to a patient population large enough to offset any variability and unforeseen high-expense provider visits. Quality To ensure value for patients in the network, a third-party intermediary can base its payment on achieving certain quality metrics and health outcomes.

TYPES OF PAYERS

The marketplace is largely made up of federal and commercial insurers, with other entities such as workers' compensation and personal liability insurance playing a smaller role. The largest federal payer is Medicare, which has two forms: traditional Medicare and Medicare Advantage. Historically, traditional Medicare has primarily paid fee-for-service (FFS) claims on a fixed fee schedule that is adjusted annually. In more recent years, Medicare has increasingly introduced value-based reporting or performance adjustments through programs such as Merit-Based Incentive Payment Systems as well as experimental pilots in bundle arrangements such as Comprehensive Care for Joint Replacement (CJR) and Bundled Payments for Care Improvement Advanced (BPCI Advanced) models. Patients are enrolled in traditional Medicare on achieving eligibility but may opt into a Medicare Advantage program run by a commercial payer. In this instance, Medicare pays the commercial payer a capitated fee for those patients and the commercial payer is responsible for managing the group for that fee, subject to bonuses or penalties based on quality and access. Medicaid differs from state to state but is usually paid in a manner similar to traditional Medicare, albeit typically at lower rates, but a few states are experimenting with value-based models. Some states manage Medicaid themselves based on their own fee schedule while others contract with commercial payers to manage it. Commercial payers, such as United, Cigna, CVS Aetna, Humana, and Blue Cross Blue Shield (BCBS) plans, are private companies who create plans for employers and individuals who are not eligible for or participating in a government plan.

Commercial insurers differ in significant ways from federal payers. For traditional Medicare and most Medicaid plans, the payer plays all four roles using a fixed fee schedule (not negotiated, although there is variability by region and by different criteria across providers) and are obligated to maintain a network open to any participating provider willing to abide by their rules. Conversely, commercial payers must negotiate rates with each provider within the network and are driven by market demand to include providers based on affordability, access needs, quality, and network stability.

In addition, commercial payers most often are not the risk-bearing entity. Most national commercial plans (eg, United, CVS Aetna, Cigna) derive the bulk of their business by performing the first three functions on behalf of larger self-insured employers (usually with more than 250 employees), whereas the employer bears the cost of care plus administrative fees charged by the payer. BCBS plans tend to have a larger proportion of individual policies (risk held by insurer, sometimes called fully insured) and small business plans (risk split between business and insurer, sometimes called partially insured), but also derive a significant portion of their business from these self-insured businesses.

National commercial payers play an important role for companies that work across multiple states. The payer's national footprint allows employers to offer common benefits to all employees via a single carrier, rather than cobbling together multiple state plans. Some BCBS plans have also entered multistate business through mergers to create Anthem (14 BCBS plans) and HCSC (5 BCBS plans).

Multistate or national payers create uniformity of benefits and administration required by regulatory compliance for the employers and have negotiated to create national provider networks that support those companies irrespective of where they grow. The revenue from large employers is great enough and the risk pool is large enough that they can afford the ups and downs of claims experience and would rather do so than pay extra to the insurer for mitigating that risk.

However, when a national payer is not the risk-bearing entity but simply manages the network and payment administration for a large employer that is self-insured, their incentives to reduce total cost of care (TCOC) are diminished or may even by eliminated. They are often paid by a percentage of the total spending, so reducing cost could actually lower their revenues. Their main incentive is to retain the employer's business by simply being more affordable or having a better network than other national payers, not actually to reduce total spending. This dynamic has allowed the cost of commercial plans to employers to increase steadily so that more employers are willing to consider advancing affordability through bundled payments and site-of-service incentives or restricting choice through tiered networks and health maintenance organizations (HMOs).

HMOs limit the choice of provider to only those in-network whereas preferred provider organizations offer better pricing if an in-network provider is chosen but out-of-network care is still covered. Staff-model HMOs such as Kaiser Permanente also own or directly employ some or all of their provider network, including physician groups and facilities, combining traditional insurance functions with care delivery systems in a single vertically integrated organization.

Medicare Advantage takes Medicare risk and shifts it to a commercial payer for them to manage. That payer can then either manage the risk themselves or subdelegate it to an independent practice association (IPA), physician group, or health system. Delegation may be conditioned on using certain networks and/or achieving standards for quality and access. Currently, United Healthcare, Humana, and various BCBS entities administer most Medicare Advantage plans. In general, commercial payers have not subdelegated portions of risk based on disease category, such as musculoskeletal disease. When they subdelegate, they would typically delegate either all of the professional fee component (physician payments) or the global fee to an IPA entity with a primary care base sufficient to manage that care and spending. Specialists either continue to see their patients at the Medicare rate or can negotiate with the IPA like any other payer to accept a rate different than standard Medicare to be in-network for that IPA and continue to receive their business. In some instances, the IPA will subdelegate specialty risk to a specialist group or network who then has to service that patient population for a fixed fee.

BALANCING ACCESS, AFFORDABILITY, QUALITY, AND NETWORK STABILITY

Payers must balance affordability of their network with stability of the network. Eliminating a provider because they will not agree to lower rates creates dissatisfaction among patients who must switch doctors and/or frustration if there is a limited provider selection in the network. That dissatisfaction is reported back to the employer who was trying to use health insurance as a tool to retain employees, so the default is to satisfy employees by keeping open networks rather than pushing for lower costs. Preferred provider organization plans have traditionally been used to satisfy this desire by enabling employees to see both in-network and out-of-network providers, but with higher associated costs.

After many years of employee wage and benefits shifting to cover increased health care costs rather than increased wages, the average worker has seen wage stagnation relative to health care coverage that still continues.[1,2] Eventually, the pendulum must swing back to enhance wage growth at the expense of health care cost inflation. Payers use designations such as Blue Distinction® or "centers of excellence" to create tiered networks that still allow choice but reward patients for choosing providers who deliver higher quality, more affordable care.

In markets such as Southern California, where HMOs have been long established, patients and employers are increasingly opting for them, particularly staff model HMOs that have undergone significant care redesign. With greater affordability relative to other market options, Kaiser Permanente has seen steadily increasing market share there even with limitations to patient choice of provider.[3]

These circumstances are further influenced by local market dynamics, such as market concentration and historical business and contractual arrangements between employers, payers, and providers. The American Medical Association issues a yearly report, "Competition in Health Insurance: A Comprehensive Study of the U.S. Markets," that outlines the market power of health insurance companies in all states. In 2020, the American Medical Association found that BCBS of Alabama had more than 85% of the commercial market share in Alabama, BCBS of Michigan had more than 65% of the commercial market share in Michigan, and Anthem had more than 60% of the commercial market share across all metropolitan statistical areas in Kentucky.[4] These are some of the more highly concentrated markets in the country. Payers in these dominant circumstances have little market incentive to strive for value-based care contracting because employers need their network to access care for their employees and providers need their network to attain patients, and it is difficult for other payers to compete for market share. Opportunities in these highly concentrated markets may be limited but may best be found among competitors of the dominant payer. Competitor payers may be more likely to take on the work needed for value-based care activities to break into the market. Alternatively, direct-to-employer provider models and employer-led collaboratives such as Pacific Business Group on Health that focus on cost and quality considerations may be the best alternative in these circumstances.

Market dynamics associated with providers and employers also play a role in the ability to engage in value-based care contracts locally. The Center on Health Insurance Reforms at Georgetown University conducted an analysis on six mid-size healthcare markets with recent provider consolidation: Detroit, Michigan; Syracuse, New York; Northern Virginia; Indianapolis, Indiana; Asheville, North Carolina; Colorado Springs, Colorado.[5] Two of these six markets represent some of the conflicting agendas that can undermine the push to value.

Northern Virginia Market Case Study

A case study has shown the Northern Virginia market to have several environmental factors.[6] The region has a large city government workforce and is heavily unionized, more individuals are moving away from the city to the suburbs because of high housing costs, and brokers and employee benefit managers have been slow to embrace new models of care delivery and network design. These factors have contributed to a lack of desire by employers to pursue many cost containment strategies, such as narrow networks and alternative payment models. A narrow network places strain on employers and should be considered a last resort.

Other models, such as accountable care organizations (ACOs), faced similar reluctance with employers because ACOs were seen as a tepid endorsement of a narrow network, given that employees would be unaware of what was happening. Payers in Northern Virginia found it difficult to push for new approaches if a hospital or healthcare system had significant clout. The process is different with hospitals: value-based health care may be promoted, but the financial bottom line must be met. One challenge is maintaining the appearance of an ACO without joining one.

Both payers and providers found it challenging to break old referral patterns. Complacency was noted among payers, as they are not prepared to use penalties, and the incentives are not yet large enough to generate change in referral patterns. Payers and purchasers explained that the dominant health system's reach across the region and market clout made excluding them from plan networks or pushing patients to use other facilities through tiering strategies impractical. From the provider perspective, the risk-sharing arrangements have no favorable terms and there is no economic incentive.

Stakeholders are exploring a variety of strategies in this market. Employer strategies include shifting employees to higher cost-sharing, high-deductible plans, and reference-based pricing. A payer sets a maximum price it is willing to pay for a given episode of care. If the facility charges more, the patient must pay the difference. This generally narrows the variability of prices in a market and encourages patients to comparison shop. Payer strategies include encouraging delivery of health services outside the hospital setting. This includes encouraging procedures in ambulatory settings and offering 24-hour clinical hotlines to reduce emergency department use. Provider strategies include acquiring physician practices, ambulatory care centers, and other nonhospital facilities to recapture revenue.

Indianapolis Market Case Study

Environmental trends in the market in Indianapolis, Indiana, include horizontal and vertical consolidation among the main hospital systems, market concentration by the largest payer, and largely administrative service-only contracts across payers.[7] These factors have contributed to an increase in costs and relatively little uptake of alternative payment models and novel network design approaches.

After one hospital's acquisition of a sleep laboratory, the laboratory immediately began charging the hospital's negotiated rate, which was typically higher than that of the laboratory when it was an independent provider. After acquisition, physicians refer patients within their health system rather than to lower-cost providers. Employers have long demanded broad networks for employees. With many administrative service-only contracts between payers and employers, higher list prices mean higher administrative fees for payers. It is not in the payers' interests to keep prices down because they make more money when prices increase steadily.

ACOs and/or bundled payments have not been actively pursued because of existing discount-based tactics and insufficient clout among small payers to push providers to take on more risk. Employers noted that previous strategies such as high-deductible health plans and employee wellness programs could no longer constrain cost growth because the burden was unsustainable for employees. Although interested in ACOs, employers also lacked the resources to engage in direct contracting, noting that the effort required is too extensive, and that interference from providers about direct contracting has thus prevented any progress.

Employer strategies discussed in the Indianapolis study include narrow or tiered networks, reference pricing, centers of excellence, engaging in direct contract negotiations with providers, and guiding enrollees to lower-cost care settings such as clinics that are onsite or nearby (this includes a capitated rate to deliver primary care services, and for some, a referral service that connects patients to a care manager, as well as lower-priced laboratory, imaging, and other services).

Codependent variables in the market include (1) employers ask the major payers to reduce costs by developing narrow network products; (2) payers seek reassurance from employers that there will be a market for those products; and (3) clinicians want to know that, if they make price concessions to be part of a narrow network, patient volume will increase, filling available beds.

Advantages of Value-Based Health Care

Other studies have described the challenges the healthcare system faces and the ways in which value-based health care could address them. Instead of building a complete system from nothing, a transition is necessary from the current market. Healthcare markets vary widely in their current readiness and capacity for this transition, and most tend to move incrementally and slowly. Providers must carefully weigh their own readiness before pursuing these deals and work together with payers to determine the next phase of transition along the continuum of value-based options.

Often, physicians have a conservative initial reaction to these initiatives, opting to double down on what they know and do well: traditional FFS arrangements. However, this risks having patients redirected to others who agree to engage when the treating physician does not, and over time, the physician's market relevance becomes threatened. In addition, value-based health care offers significant opportunity for those providing better quality or more affordable care to receive recognition. Rather than basing payment on negotiating leverage in the marketplace, physicians are paid for being better than their competitors, which aligns incentives to improve patient care. Incentives to provide care that produces the best outcomes for patients can also greatly enhance physician satisfaction working in these models.

VALUE-BASED HEALTH CARE CONTINUUM

Value-based contracting initiatives for specialists can be viewed on a continuum of risk and complexity, ranging from initiatives that require minimal effort and no risk to those that require the physicians to become not only providers but also the payer for care in a population (**Tables 2** and **3**). US markets vary considerably in the degree to which payers enter these arrangements. Physicians should start by understanding where the payers in their market are on this continuum and determine if this is their preferred point of entry. Once successful at performing on contracts at that entry point, physicians can work with payers to move up the continuum of risk and complexity.

The American Society of Actuaries defines different types of risk in value-based contracting; these include (1) utilization risk – the risk of changes in utilization (volumes) and payment changes, relative to operating cost changes (variable costs); (2) technical risk – the risk of structuring technical of a contract to match the population and circumstances; (3) insurance risk – the risk of normal variation in

---

TABLE 2 Alternative Payment Models: Types of Risk in Value-Based Contracting

Type of Risk	Level of Control
Performance: The risk related to inefficiency, suboptimal quality, and high cost of care.	High – The most controllable aspect for providers because it directly applies to the provision of care delivery and health outcomes associated with that care. Applicable to all front-line providers.
Technical: The risk of appropriately structuring technical elements of a contract to match the population and circumstances. Utilization: The risk of changes in utilization (volumes) and payment changes, relative to operating cost changes (variable costs).	Medium – Less controllable because it involves risk related to appropriate financing (technical, utilization risk) of a practice. For example, are alternative payment model payments able to cover overhead, needed care redesign, and other necessary expenses? Does the contractual agreement factor in exclusion criteria that are outside the control of the provider? Applicable to the financing arm of a provider entity.
Insurance: The risk related to the normal variation in demand for medical services over time, and differences in utilization within segments of insured populations.	Low – Least controllable aspect for providers because it relates to the normal and unexpected variation of population-level demand for health services. Applicable to those willing to take on insuring a population.

Adapted from Navigating the Value-Based Care Landscape, A Musculoskeletal Guide. American Academy of Orthopaedic Surgeons, 2020. Available at: https://www.aaos.org/globalassets/quality-and-practice-resources/practice-management/value-based-care-guide.pdf. Accessed May 23, 2023.

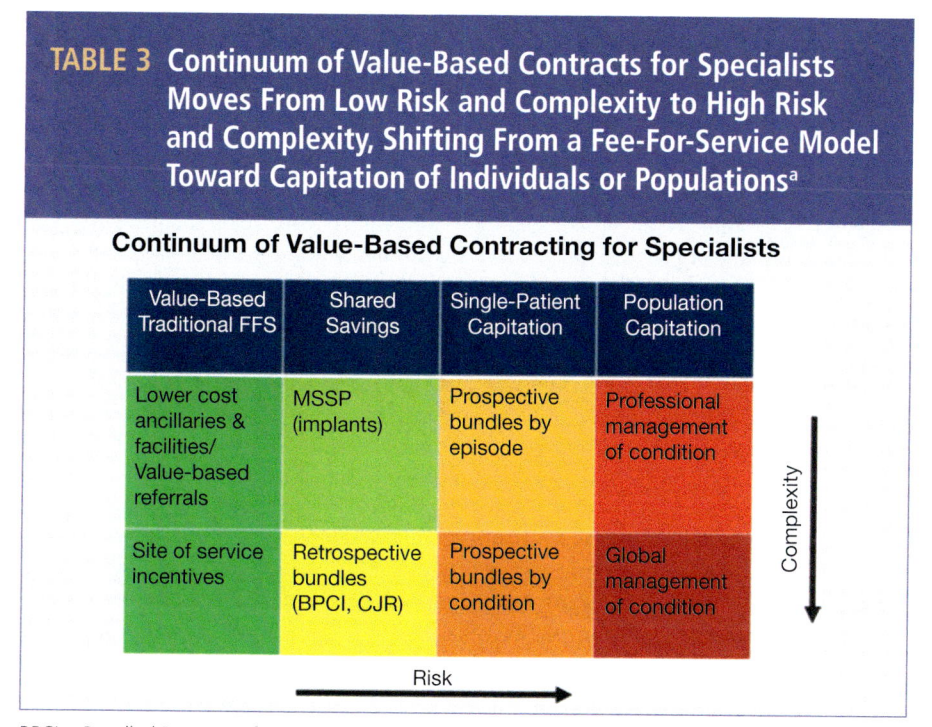

TABLE 3 Continuum of Value-Based Contracts for Specialists Moves From Low Risk and Complexity to High Risk and Complexity, Shifting From a Fee-For-Service Model Toward Capitation of Individuals or Populations[a]

Continuum of Value-Based Contracting for Specialists

Value-Based Traditional FFS	Shared Savings	Single-Patient Capitation	Population Capitation
Lower cost ancillaries & facilities/ Value-based referrals	MSSP (implants)	Prospective bundles by episode	Professional management of condition
Site of service incentives	Retrospective bundles (BPCI, CJR)	Prospective bundles by condition	Global management of condition

Risk →

Complexity ↓

BPCI = Bundled Payments for Care Improvement, CJR = Comprehensive Care for Joint Replacement, MSSP = Medicare Shared Savings Program

[a]The continuum from green to yellow to red to deep red represents a continuum of increasing risk and increasing complexity.

demand for medical services over time; and (4) suboptimal risk – the risk of inefficiency, suboptimal quality, and high cost of care.[8]

To guide musculoskeletal providers in deciding what types of risk to take on in various value-based contracts and alternative payment models, the American Academy of Orthopaedic Surgeons has created a framework for determining which types of risk are easier and those that are advanced.[9]

The function and potential opportunities of eight formats of health care models, describing how they work and what opportunities they may offer to both the surgeon and the payer, are described in the next paragraphs. Specialists should understand the different types of value-based contracting arrangements that exist.

HEALTH CARE MODELS

Value-Based FFS

In the traditional FFS world, it is considered a disadvantage to have lower negotiated rates with commercial payers. However, in a value-based world where referrals may be redirected to lower-cost providers, it can become an advantage. If a practice has lower professional fee rates or lower rates for ancillary services such as imaging, therapy, and surgery centers, patients and some referring physicians may preferentially use that practice. Some insurers have published price comparisons online that clearly demonstrate the cost difference between using different surgeons or even the same surgeon at a different hospital or ambulatory surgery center.[10] In addition, in 2020, CMS pushed regulation to increase price transparency among providers, which will likely make this information more broadly available to patients.[11]

Practicing value-based FFS health care does not require special contract negotiations, but it does benefit from raising awareness among patients and referring doctors that who they choose can significantly affect how much services cost. Because many surgeons already have lower rates than their competitors, assuming comparable quality, they are already value-based FFS health care, but may not be taking advantage of that. In this context, validating the quality of care while promoting affordability can create a good starting argument for physicians to enter more advanced contract structures with payers.

Incentivized Value-Based FFS

In an incentivized value-based FFS, commercial payers provide higher professional fees to shift site of service to surgical facilities that cost less, especially ambulatory surgical centers (ASCs), assuming quality is maintained. These arrangements are typically contingent on significant outpatient-eligible cases being done in high-cost settings historically as well as existence of low-cost facilities in market. The increased professional fee to physicians is easily offset by the lower facility cost for reduction of TCOC.

Incentivized value-based FFS can be an attractive option for orthopaedic surgeons for many reasons. There is no downside risk and physicians get an automatic increase to professional fees as long as quality is maintained. Additional facility revenue may be realized for physician-owners of ASCs. Higher professional fees and ASC profits are attractive but to gain these incentives, surgeons must reorganize their schedules and block out time to account for inpatient and ASC blocks that can be inconvenient or affect workflow. Physicians must also consider backlash from hospitals for shifting cases and take steps to mitigate a breakdown in relationships.

From a payer perspective, incentivized value-based FFS may be useful in markets where the cost differentials are significant. Pilot models are not yet widespread and payers may wish to create more accountability so that these incentives will reduce TCOC if utilization or quality profile worsens.

Shared Savings for Expenses

As part of a broad Medicare program designed to promote the creation of ACOs between facilities and provider groups, Medicare Shared Savings Programs (MSSPs) are the next step in the continuum of value-based contracting for specialists. Multiple pathways are available that allow sharing savings created by reduced expense between providers that would otherwise be disallowed by anti-kickback statutes. For orthopaedics, these models are frequently used as a way for hospitals to engage surgeons in implant cost reduction strategies and reward them.

MSSP models are typically simple for orthopaedic surgeons to administer and maintain, although the opportunity is generally short-lived and unidimensional. A common example for orthopaedists is implant standardization programs. A cohort of surgeons agrees to limit implant choice to one or two vendors, and these vendors offer the hospital discounts on those implants for the volume shift. A portion of those savings go to the hospital, but a portion may be redirected to participating surgeons or their service line. The ability to share those savings is usually restricted to 1 to 2 years. After that, the savings are locked in but no longer shared.

CMS sees MSSP arrangements as a useful way for facilities to lower costs of implants and other physician-preferred items without violating Stark laws. MSSPs are meant to be an entry point to cooperation and coordination among providers; therefore, payers may be encouraged to enter these relationships, which lead to the acceptance of more risk in the future.

Retrospective Bundled Payments

Orthopaedics has been on the leading edge of Medicare retrospective bundled payment models. CJR and BPCI models are retrospective bundled payment models and the programs most familiar to orthopaedic surgeons given their widespread implementation. With retrospective bundled payment models, Medicare or a commercial payer analyzes historical episode costs (usually 3 days preoperative and 90 days postoperative) bundling facility, clinician and postacute charges. These data are used to create a target price, which may be a percentage of an entity's historical charges or of the market average. Savings are shared if the average cost of future episodes is below the target price. If the cost is above the target price, the clinician and/or facility must repay the overage per the terms of the arrangement. Targets are typically repriced with a new lower target after 2 to 3 years.

Retrospective bundled payment models are simple for payers to administer, thus there may be more options available to orthopaedic surgeons. These arrangements incentivize preoperative conditioning and individualized postoperative planning, and the clinician can typically identify early low-hanging fruit to improve on unmanaged care. As with value-based FFS models, procedures can be shifted for commercial payers to lower cost sites of care if appropriate to reduce facility fees. If Medicare allows the procedure in ASCs, similar site-of-care optimization may be achieved. Active postacute care treatment can reduce use of skilled nursing and inpatient rehabilitation facilities.

One drawback is slow feedback, which limits the effect of incentives. When payouts are received 6 to 9 months after an episode, directly linking optimizations back to outcomes is difficult. Perhaps the biggest criticism of retrospective bundled payment models is their unsustainability. It is difficult to continue finding new savings that outweigh the costs of redesign and may result in a "race to the bottom," in which health care entities must cut costs year after year to avoid repayment. If a model is not adequately risk-adjusted, this could lead to "cherry-picking" patients who are healthier. In addition, retrospective bundles do not address the decision to perform surgery and the appropriateness of care.

Payers may find these arrangements easiest to administer based on current payment infrastructure. Iterative repricing resets the base target price for the episode of care in the market and should lower total spending over time, which appeals to payers. However, early results have shown mixed reviews on the effectiveness of these programs.[12]

Prospective Bundled Payment for Episodes

Further along the continuum of value-based contracting for specialists, single-patient capitation models introduce more risk and increase in complexity. Some commercial payers are beginning to engage in prospective bundled payments for episodes where the bundled price is negotiated between the payer and the physician group or facility (ie, the initiator of the bundle). The initiator negotiates fees with or without incentives with each facility and clinician (eg, anesthesiologist, surgeon, physician assistant, physical therapist) and is free to redesign care outside of typical authorization rules. Freedom to redesign can create incentives for outcomes that drive lower cost. For example, postoperative nausea and/or pain control results in incentives for the anesthesiologist. If the contract requires full risk, then the initiator can also reinsure against actuarial risk or set stop-loss limits in the contract.

Prospective episodic bundles incentivize preoperative conditioning and individualized postoperative planning, in which orthopaedic surgeons may already be extensively involved. Bundle initiators get a portion of TCOC savings, not just a professional fee. Compared with retrospective bundles, prospective bundles typically are not repriced as often because a commercial bundle with lower cost providers has sustained benefit relative to higher-cost providers in the market.

Downside risk is perhaps the greatest barrier to engaging in prospective episodic bundles. The bundle initiator is responsible for payment of any complications and readmissions in these models; therefore, appropriate risk mitigating steps must be considered during contracting. Although some influence on the decision to perform surgery and the appropriateness of care may be reflected in these models, FFS is still the basis of payment calculation.

Prospective bundles with commercial payers have been shown to create significant savings per case with positive effects on both quality-of-care outcomes and patient experience. By creating a more navigated patient experience, expectations are well established preoperatively, reducing patient anxiety and creating a safety net that reduces the likelihood of a patient inadvertently ending up in the emergency department or another facility without the physician's knowledge. In addition, the intentional nature of the care pathway tends to produce more consistent results. Cost savings of 15% to 30% to the employer while reducing complications by one-half has been reported.[13]

Prospective Bundled Payment for Conditions

Bundles by condition are considerably more complex in design than episodic models, and most are still in development instead of implementation. The bundled price is negotiated between payer and physician group, IPA, or health system on a per-patient basis for treatment of a condition (eg, moderate/severe lower extremity osteoarthritis) rather than an episode (eg, total joint arthroplasty). Cost of all care for the initiating diagnosis is included for a timeframe that captures meaningful outcomes during both surgical or nonsurgical care periods. Individual patient modifiers can be used to account for risk adjustment. The bundle initiator must negotiate with all downstream providers for relevant patient care.

From the perspective of orthopaedic surgeons, prospective condition-based bundles account for the appropriateness of the decision to perform surgery and reflect long-term outcomes. The bundle initiator gets a portion of TCOC savings over an extended period instead of a single procedure. Additionally, these models support development of specialized integrated care teams by patient condition. Ideally, the care team would be rewarded both for making the surgical episode more efficient, similar to an episode bundle, but also for reducing the occurrence of surgery that is unlikely to bring meaningful improvement to patients.

Although payers may be attracted to the incentive to reduce unnecessary use, there are several challenges with condition-based prospective bundles. The first challenge is the difficulty for payers to reliably attribute and carve out claims by patient by condition, particularly among those with multiple comorbidities. The second challenge is choosing initiators among caregivers in related specialties without alienating the network needed for other plans. Risk adjustment can also be challenging. Finally, there is a risk of double payment if the bundle initiator accepts payment but the patient receives care by a different provider who is approved in the plan for other conditions. For the surgeon, such programs require significant coordination with other clinicians, and significant experience and analysis to negotiate pricing and control leakage. The bundle initiator is responsible for all complications and some or all leakage management and therefore can experience substantial losses without adequate systems in place.

Subcapitation for Professional Services for a Condition in a Population

The final category in the continuum of value-based contracting for specialists is capitation for a defined population of patients. Capitation is a single payment per patient for a defined period and may include professional services only or global capitation inclusive of facility and ancillary spending. Typically, this is seen in a Medicare Advantage plan where a commercial payer accepts delegated risk from Medicare and then an IPA or primary care provider group accepts delegation from the commercial payer to cover the Medicare Advantage population at a capitated rate below that of the commercial payer. Subsequently, a specialty group could accept subcapitation, delegation of capitated rate for treatment of an array of diseases (eg, musculoskeletal) for a fixed fee to cover professional services for that patient population. Incentives are based on Medicare Star ratings and access scores.

Again, orthopaedic surgeons will appreciate how this model accounts for appropriateness of the decision to perform surgery and reflect long-term outcomes. The subcapitation group can also benefit from redesign for efficient use of professional resources and may receive additional incentives for quality and access.

Significant experience and analysis required to negotiate pricing and control leakage may be a barrier to entry for orthopaedic surgeons. Lack of participation in facility or postacute redesign limits the subcapitation group's effect to upside savings and innovation. Responsibility for leakage of patients to other professional providers may also be significant concern, particularly in competitive or saturated markets.

Medicare and commercial payers rarely enter subcapitated arrangements directly with specialists; however, risk-bearing IPAs and primary care provider groups may do so. In situations where the specialty group has a record for high quality and affordability, the risk-bearing group may be interested in subcapitation with an orthopaedic group to divert risk and provide network stability, but risks their bonuses from Medicare if the subcapitated group fails to perform on quality or access.

Subcapitation for Global Services for a Condition in a Population

Subcapitation for global services for a condition in a population of patient is the most complex and risky form of value-based contracting for a specialty group. In this case, the group is responsible not just for professional services but for all care of musculoskeletal conditions. Assembling a full-service network, controlling leakage, managing utilization and access, and negotiating with ancillary providers all play a role in success. Again, commercial payers and Medicare have not typically entered into such arrangements directly with specialists, but some highly experienced risk-bearing IPAs and primary care provider groups have. Significant experience with the analysis of population data and contract negotiation for their care is paramount for the surgeon when considering this type of risk.

Current Forms of Health Care Models and Regional Variation

Payers have different profiles for what types of value-based arrangements they are willing to enter and can readily administer. Traditional Medicare has mostly used a combination of incentives for reporting or various types of retrospective shared savings models such as MSSP, CJR, and BPCI (**Table 4**). These allow them to maintain existing claims processing infrastructure and distribute a lump-sum payment for savings accrued long after the episode is complete.

Commercial payers also enter retrospective bundles for the same reason, building on the Medicare models that have been developed and benefiting from their existing claims payment systems. Some have also experimented with pilots of prospective bundles and also site-of-service incentives to shift care to lower-cost settings (**Table 5**).

Medicare Advantage plans and a few commercial plans are based on capitation arrangements. The risk-bearing entity pays most providers a negotiated FFS rate, preferentially using those who practice value-based FFS, and may enter into shared savings arrangements. Once a record is established with the specialist group, the risk-bearing entity may then agree to enter a subcapitation arrangement for either professional or global risk (**Table 6**).

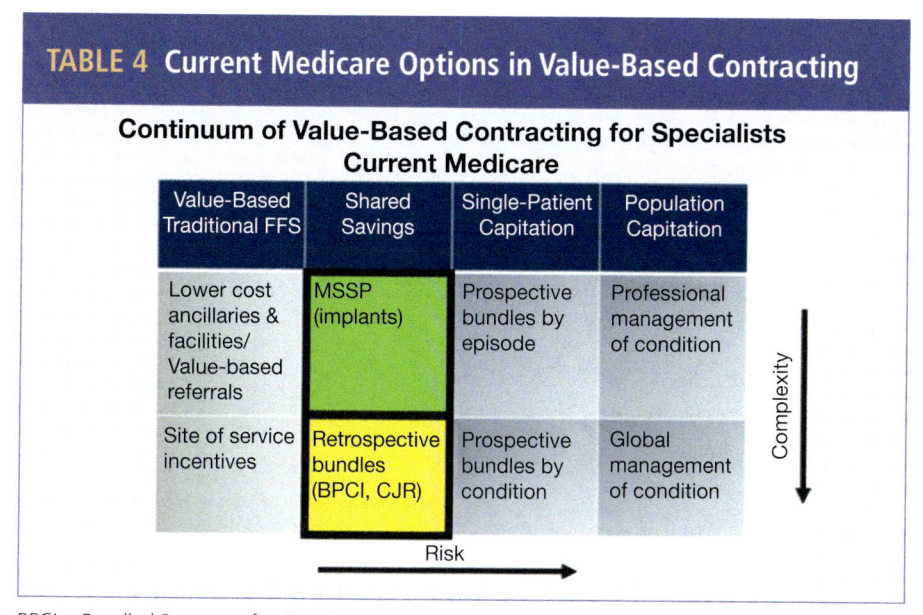

TABLE 4 Current Medicare Options in Value-Based Contracting

Continuum of Value-Based Contracting for Specialists
Current Medicare

BPCI = Bundled Payments for Care Improvement, CJR = Comprehensive Care for Joint Replacement, MSSP = Medicare Shared Savings Program

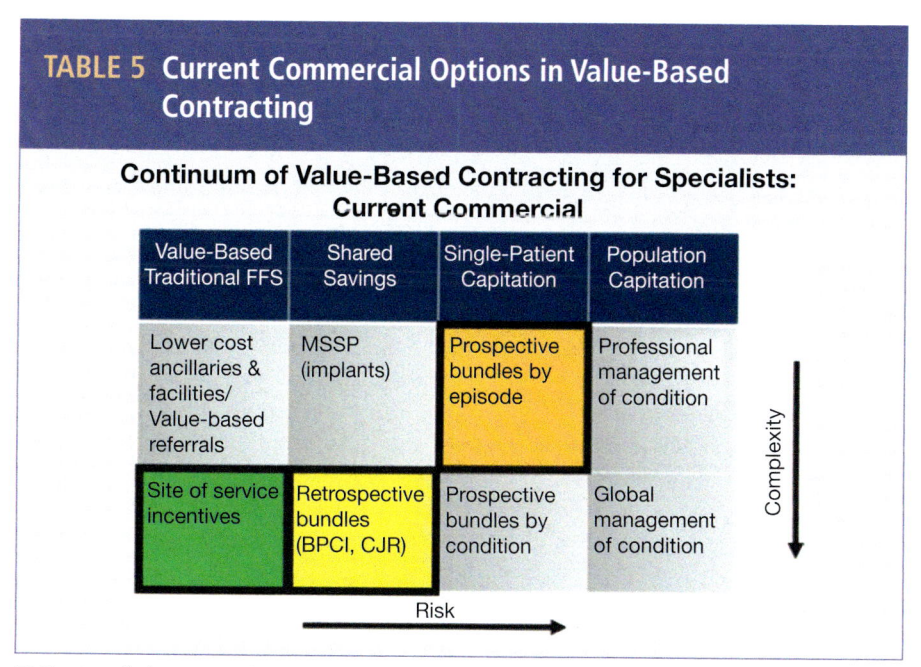

TABLE 5 Current Commercial Options in Value-Based Contracting

Continuum of Value-Based Contracting for Specialists:
Current Commercial

BPCI = Bundled Payments for Care Improvement, CJR = Comprehensive Care for Joint Replacement, MSSP = Medicare Shared Savings Program

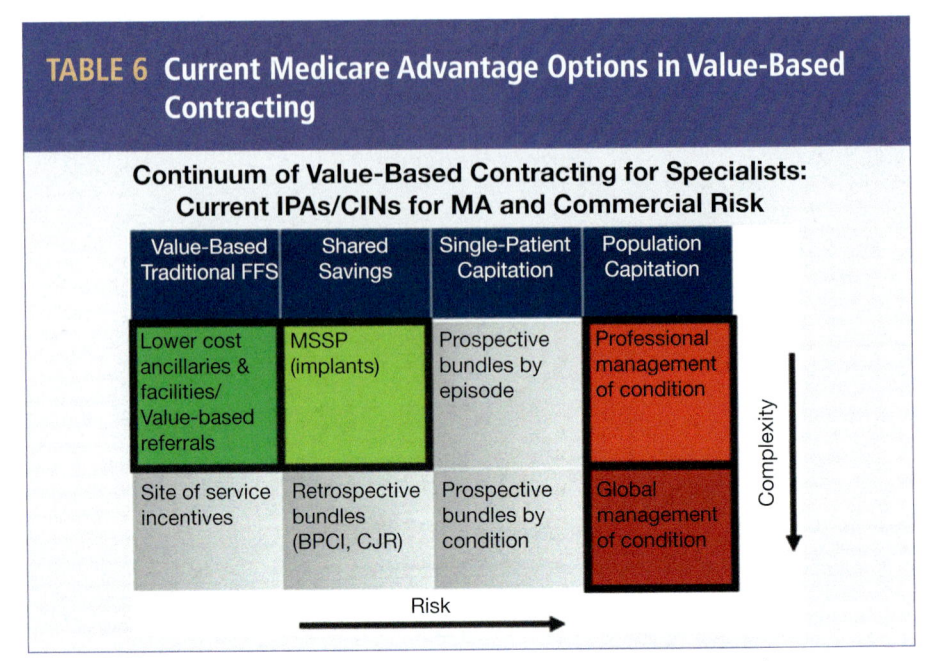

TABLE 6 Current Medicare Advantage Options in Value-Based Contracting

Continuum of Value-Based Contracting for Specialists: Current IPAs/CINs for MA and Commercial Risk

Value-Based Traditional FFS	Shared Savings	Single-Patient Capitation	Population Capitation
Lower cost ancillaries & facilities/ Value-based referrals	MSSP (implants)	Prospective bundles by episode	Professional management of condition
Site of service incentives	Retrospective bundles (BPCI, CJR)	Prospective bundles by condition	Global management of condition

Complexity ↓

Risk →

BPCI = Bundled Payments for Care Improvement, CIN = clinically integrated network, CJR = Comprehensive Care for Joint Replacement, IPA = independent practice association, MA = Medicare Advantage, MSSP = Medicare Shared Savings Program

DEMONSTRATING VALUE AND NEGOTIATING WITH PAYERS

Demonstrating value in the context of negotiating with payers requires evidence of both quality and affordability that exceeds that of others in the market. Although commercial payers do not have a standard way of assessing quality or affordability, CMS has introduced gradually expanding requirements over the past decade, initially requiring only reporting of and more recently requiring participation in risk-based models.

Beginning with the Physician Quality Reporting System and now its replacement, the Merit-based Incentive Payment System, these systems mostly capture process measures because they can be easier to develop and may rely on elements already being captured in medical records without the need for additional outcome collection tools. Facility-reported and physician-reported outcomes are also collected and reported. Although process and outcome metrics can be useful, value is ultimately discerned by the patient and not the healthcare system. Therefore, the most concrete way to demonstrate opportunities to increase value is by providing patient-reported outcome metrics. The National Quality Forum[14] has determined that outcome measures do not assess the processes of care, but the actual results: the state or change in patient care is measured rather than the steps taken during the delivery of care. Outcome measures of particular interest to payers are those reducing the likelihood of incurring additional costs, either through overutilization or patient harm.

CMS has steadily demanded reporting designed to adhere to these principles[15] (**Table 7**). They have been used as an important way to evaluate the quality of clinicians, ultimately resulting in potential bonuses and penalties.

TABLE 7 Examples of Quality Reporting Metrics Used by the Centers for Medicare & Medicaid Services

Category	Examples	Description	Value Rationale
Process measure	Evaluation or interview for risk of opioid misuse (quality ID 414)	Patients prescribed opiates for longer than 6 weeks evaluated for risk of opioid misuse using a brief validated instrument or patient interview documented at least once during opioid therapy in the medical record.	Demonstrates adherence to process, which may reduce overuse of opioids.
	Falls: Screening for future fall risk (quality ID 318)	Patients 65 years and older screened for future fall risk during the measurement period.	Demonstrates adherence to process, which may reduce risk of fracture.
Outcome measure	Surgical site infection (quality ID 357)	Patients age 18 years and older who had a surgical site infection after a procedure.	Low rates indicate care that reduces preventable patient harm and may decrease length of stay.
	Unplanned hospital readmission within 30 Days of principal procedure (quality ID 356)	Patients with an inpatient readmission to the same hospital for any reason or an outside hospital (if known to the surgeon), within 30 days of the principal surgical procedure.	Low rates indicate care that reduces preventable patient harm and cost associated with additional hospital admissions.
Patient-reported outcome measure (PROM)	Functional status change for patients with knee impairments (quality ID 217)	Measures risk-adjusted change in functional status for patients aged 14 years or older and with knee impairments.	Illustrates patient perspective of their change in health status.
	Leg pain after lumbar fusion (quality ID 473)	Measures leg pain rated by the patient, who underwent lumbar fusion. Leg pain is rated on the visual analog scale pain scale at approximately 1 year (9-15 months) postoperatively.	Illustrates patient perspective of their health status and well being.

Data from Centers for Medicare & Medicaid Services: Measure Inventory. Measures Inventory Tool, n.d. https://cmit.cms.gov/CMIT_public/ListMeasures.

Because commercial payers do not have a standard for quality reporting, any work done to comply with CMS requirements should be reused when soliciting commercial contracts. Commercial payers are competing to acquire and retain employer-based business so metrics that matter to an employer will matter to them: patient satisfaction, complication rates, readmission rates, return to work rates, patient reported functional outcomes, and cost. Although collection of quality measures is resource intensive, particularly collection of patient-reported outcome measures, the data can be used for compliance with government programs such as Merit-Based Incentive Payment Systems, the BPCI Advanced Model, and state-run Medicaid quality payment initiatives. They can also be the basis for getting the attention of commercial payers who, unlike CMS, are not required to work the same way with all network physicians.

Commercial payers selectively pursue value-based contracting based on whether a provider is likely to be successful, where they perceive significant opportunities for enhanced value exists, and whether the effort and risk required by the payer justifies the activity. For the surgeon to get the payers' attention and prove that they are capable of managing value-based arrangements successfully requires evidence of success, or at least evidence of preparation. The easiest way to convince a payer of success is to show the surgeon's results on previous risk-based contracts. However, it should be recognized that success in CJR or BPCI, which is largely predicated on reducing postacute utilization, may not translate to a commercial bundled payment where success is predicated on reduced in-hospital spending or shifting site of service. However, it still shows the ability to change physician behavior given proper incentives.

In the absence of a record of success, evidence of focus on quality improvement and self-examination through collection of patient-reported outcome metrics and a quality improvement committee shows the willingness to invest in infrastructure and the time needed to transform care. In addition, a market-leading reputation for quality, broad geographic coverage, and designation as a center of excellence can be persuasive. Market conditions must also be favorable for a payer to invest time and energy in a value-based arrangement. Surgeons perceive value creation in terms of how much could be saved on a given episode of care by changing site of service and eliminating low-value care. However, being able to present an analysis that demonstrates a significant reduction in episode costs is only part of the equation. Payers orient toward the cost for a given population rather than an individual episode; therefore, having significant scale is also important. The TCOC reduction relative to total budget is typically the measure that is most effective.

A payer can only focus on only so many things. Creating new programs such as these use a great deal of resources both to create the programs and manage them. In addition, having multiple programs in a market can result in duplicative payments or incentives that undermine the savings. Payers must determine that a given program will work for the surgeon but can also be scaled over additional procedures or markets without disrupting existing programs. From a surgeon's perspective, saving $3,000 on each of the 100 joint replacements performed each year creates tremendous value, reducing spending by

$300,000. However, if the payer has a billion-dollar budget for a region, focusing on a tiny fraction of spending may not be worthwhile unless it is likely to be scaled and have a lasting effect.

SUMMARY

Payers are responsible for creating networks and negotiating payment rates, managing payments, and in some cases, bearing financial risk for the claims. They also must represent the interests of employers they represent and seek to retain membership for themselves. Value-based contracting arrangements affect each of those functions, potentially narrowing networks, creating incentive payments, adding factors such as quality and access to payment calculations, and shifting risk to providers. For surgeons to enter into these agreements with payers, they must convince themselves and their payer partners that they can successfully manage each of those aspects in a new way that enhances patient outcomes, experience, and affordability without unintended negative consequences. A continuum of progressively more complex value-based care arrangements can allow surgeons and the delivery systems in which they work to enhance their capabilities and build trusting partnerships with payers for mutual long-term success.

REFERENCES

1. Rae M, Copeland R, Cox C: Tracking the Rise in Premium Contributions and Cost-Sharing for Families with Large Employer Coverage. Peterson-KFF Health System Tracker, 2019. Available at: https://www.healthsystemtracker.org/brief/tracking-the-rise-in-premium-contributions-and-cost-sharing-for-families-with-large-employer-coverage/#Total%20family%20health%20spending%20for%20large%20group%20enrollees,%202003-2018. Accessed June 2, 2023.

2. Claxton G, Damico A, Rae M, Young G, McDermott D, Whitmore H: Health benefits in 2020: Premiums in employer-sponsored plans grow 4 percent; employers consider responses to pandemic. *Health Aff (Millwood)* 2020;39(11):2018-2028.

3. Kaiser Family Foundation: Market Share and Enrollment of Largest Three Insurers – Small Group Market. Available at: https://www.kff.org/other/state-indicator/market-share-and-enrollment-of-largest-three-insurers-small-group-market/?currentTimeframe=0&sortModel=%7B%22colId%22:%22Location%22,%22sort%22:%22asc%22%7D. Accessed May 23, 2023.

4. American Medical Association: 2022 Update: competition in health insurance, a comprehensive study of U.S. markets. Table A-1. Market concentration (HHI) and largest insurers' market shares, as of Jan. 1, 2021. Available at: https://www.ama-assn.org/system/files/competition-health-insurance-us-markets.pdf. Accessed May 23, 2023.

5. Corlette S: New Georgetown CHIR Report Finds Ability of Insurers, Employers to Respond to Provider Consolidation is Limited. Available at: https://ccf.georgetown.edu/2019/10/25/new-georgetown-chir-report-finds-ability-of-insurers-employers-to-respond-to-provider-consolidation-is-limited/. Accessed March 22, 2023.

6. Hoadley J, Corlett S, Hoppe O, Center on Health Insurance Reforms: Assessing Responses to Increased Provider Consolidation. Case Study Analysis: The Northern Virginia Health Care Market, 2018. Available at: https://chirblog.org/wp-content/

uploads/2020/02/GtownCHIR_ProviderConsolidation_NorthernVA_Nov2018.pdf. Accessed June 2, 2023.

7. Corlett S, Keith K, Hoppe O: Center on Health Insurance Reforms. Assessing Responses to Increased Provider Consolidation. Case Study Analysis: The Indianapolis Health Care Market, 2019. Available at: https://chirblog.org/wp-content/uploads/2020/02/GtownCHIR_ProviderConsolidation_Indianapolis_Jun2019.pdf Accessed May 23, 2023.

8. Society of Actuaries: Provider Payment Arrangements, Provider Risk, and Their Relationship with the Cost of Health Care. Available at: https://www.soa.org/globalassets/assets/Files/Research/Projects/research-2015-10-provider-payment-report.pdf. Accessed March 22, 2023.

9. American Academy of Orthopaedic Surgeons: Navigating the Value-Based Care Landscape, A Musculoskeletal Guide, 2020. Available at: https://www.aaos.org/globalassets/quality-and-practice-resources/practice-management/value-based-care-guide.pdf. Accessed May 23, 2023.

10. Blue Cross Blue Shield: Find a doctor and cost estimator tools. Available at: https://www.bluecrossnc.com/find-doctor-and-cost-estimator Accessed June 2, 2023.

11. Centers for Medicare and Medicaid Services: CMS Completes Historic Price Transparency Initiative. Available at: https://www.cms.gov/newsroom/press-releases/cms-completes-historic-price-transparency-initiative. Accessed March 22, 2023.

12. Navathe AS, Emanuel EJ, Venkataramani AS, et al: Spending and quality after three years of medicare's voluntary bundled payment for joint replacement surgery. *Health Aff (Millwood)* 2020;39(1):58-66.

13. Murrey DB: *Creating Physician-Owned Bundled Payments*. NEJM Catalyst, 2016. Available at: https://catalyst.nejm.org/doi/full/10.1056/CAT.16.0592

14. National Quality Forum: The Right Tools for the Job. Available at: https://www.qualityforum.org/Measuring_Performance/ABCs/The_Right_Tools_for_the_Job.aspx. Accessed March 22, 2023.

15. Centers for Medicare & Medicaid Services: Measures Inventory Tool. Available at: https://cmit.cms.gov/cmit/#/MeasureInventory. Accessed June 2, 2023.

Ambulatory Surgery Centers and Physician-Owned Hospitals

Paul Rizk, MD • Rory R. Wright, MD, FAAOS

INTRODUCTION

Although ambulatory surgery centers (ASCs) and physician-owned hospitals (POHs) are now commonplace in the US healthcare system, they have had a significant effect on the evolution of value in medicine in a relatively short period of time. Historically, most, if not all, surgical procedures were performed in a hospital setting, largely a result of tradition, training, and Medicare's payment methodology. The creation and growth of ASCs and POHs were developed to improve outcomes and create a more convenient and efficient practice environment.

ORIGINS OF ASCs AND POHs

Early proponents of ASCs and POHs wanted to increase value for patients by improving quality, accessibility, and affordability of surgery for patients.[1,2] The subsequent effect can be distilled into benefits that accrued to payers, providers, and most importantly, patients. The concept of "health care value" has been defined as health outcomes achieved relative to the cost of achieving those outcomes. This definition of value[3] (**Table 1**) complements the concept of shared value put forth by Porter and Kramer:[4] that business decisions and social policies must benefit both society and corporations. This also embodies the core philosophy of ASCs and POHs in delivering the best outcomes for the patient and in the process, establishing the best practice environment for surgeons.

TABLE 1 Framework of Value Regarding Quality and Cost of Ambulatory Surgery Centers

Quality		
Structure of orthopaedic procedure	Process of orthopaedic procedure	Outcome of orthopaedic procedure
Cost		
Preoperative	Intraoperative	Postoperative
	Perspective 1: Patient Perspective 2: Clinician/Hospital Perspective 3: Payer Perspective 4: Society	

THE ASC

History, Policy, and Legislation

Before discussing the effect that ASCs have in creating value for patients, their short yet complex history must be examined because the growth and development of ASCs have shaped the function of the US healthcare system. Originally, the ASC concept was completely novel, and early innovators had to overcome practical hurdles to realize and promote the spread and standardization of ASCs. Reimbursement, licensing, and regulation needed to be formalized with commercial and governmental payers. Regulatory progress followed, but was slower, and ultimately defined the role of the ASC in the US healthcare environment.

The concept of ambulatory surgery finds roots in the work of Robert Campbell and Andrew Fullerton, surgical pioneers at the Royal Victoria Hospital in Belfast, Northern Ireland, who first described outpatient surgery for an inguinal hernia in the *British Medical Journal* in 1899[5] and *Lancet* in 1904.[6] This change in the early 1900s was spurred by the development of short-acting anesthetic agents that allowed the possibility of rapid recovery from surgery. Pioneers skirted around the idea of ambulatory surgery until the early 1960s, when health care professionals and legislators called for an improvement in accessibility, safety, and affordability of surgery.[1]

The ASC made its US debut in 1966 and 1967 in California and Washington, DC, respectively, following several years of discussion and physician development. These first two entities were associated with hospitals, but Wallace Reed, MD, and John Ford, MD, began to lobby for a stand-alone facility, which ultimately was realized on February 12, 1968 as a "Surgicenter." Although initial reports were promising and patient satisfaction was high, insurance companies refused reimbursement because the relevant policy at the time required admission to the hospital for 18 hours postoperatively. Payer hesitation to approve ambulatory surgery was rooted in concern for safety, but ultimately stunted the growth of ASCs.

In the early 1970s, with new American Society of Anesthesiologists guidelines for safety, the number of ASCs began to rapidly expand (**Figure 1**). At the national and state level, legislation allowed expansion and financial stability as malpractice lawsuits decreased and proof of safety increased. By 1979, more than 100 ASC facilities were operating in the United States. In the 1980s, the number of facilities continued to increase, with Medicare developing and updating Current Procedural Terminology codes and payment rates, ultimately still in current use. With the Centers for Medicare & Medicaid Services (CMS) on board with ASC utilization and payments, expansion continued in the 1990 and 2000s, reaching 5,400 ASCs in 2015.[1]

Currently, ASCs are subject to regulatory standards at the state and federal levels, with independent accreditation. Federally, ASCs must be certified under Medicare Conditions for Coverage and demonstrate compliance with state law. Medicare also restricts the scope of procedures at ASCs while it requires reporting of quality measures and maintenance of emergency preparedness plans.[3,7] The regulation of scope of practice lies in the Medicare CMS inpatient-only procedure list and ASC approval list. This significantly restricted ASCs, but in 2018, total knee arthroplasty (TKA) was removed from the inpatient-only procedure list, but still had to be performed in a hospital. Total hip arthroplasty (THA) was removed in 2020 and TKA was added to the ASC covered list. By January 1, 2021, Medicare-funded musculoskeletal procedures were permitted to be performed at an ASC, eventually extending to all procedures.

At the state level, 43 states require licensure to operate an ASC and the remaining seven require some form of accreditation similar to Medicare certification.

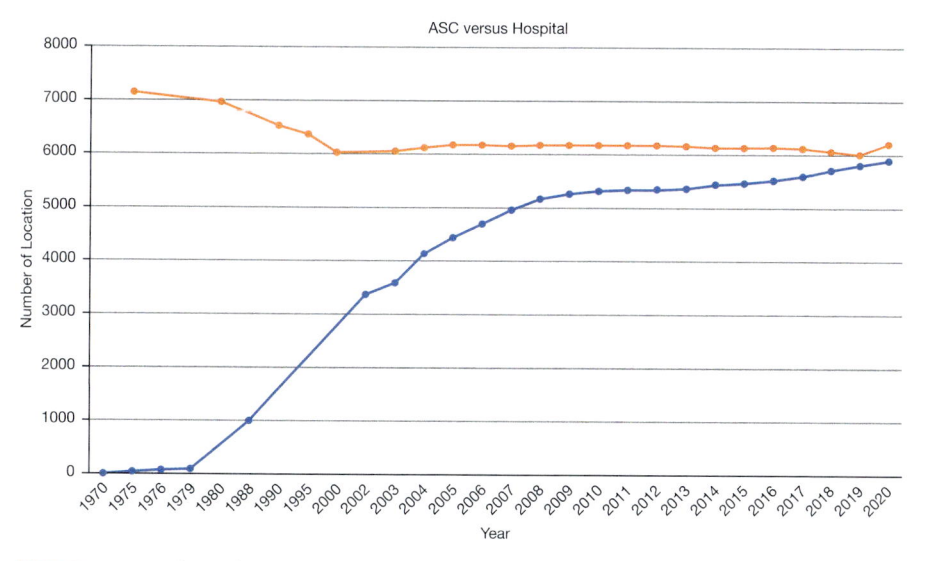

FIGURE 1 Number of ambulatory surgical centers versus hospitals in the United States over the past 40 years. (Data from https://www.medpac.gov.)

Independent bodies that accredit ASCs include Accreditation Association for Ambulatory Health Care, the American Association for the Accreditation of Ambulatory Surgery Facilities, the American Osteopathic Association, and The Joint Commission. There are 18 states that do not require ASC accreditation at this time.[7] Although this timeline illustrates how regulatory policy has lagged behind the advancement of outpatient surgery, it is encouraging to see legislation catch up to ASC innovation and advancement of outpatient care.

Quality

With the explosive growth of ASCs and the need to demonstrate and standardize system processes for outpatient surgery, various centers developed criteria and protocols. Driven by the foundational pursuit of increased efficiency, decreased cost to patients and the healthcare system, and preservation of the safety of patients, the protocols focused primarily on maintaining the quality of outcomes as well as the ability to safely ambulate, successfully manage pain with oral medications, spontaneously void, and to tolerate a diet prior to same-day discharge. In 2009, Berger et al[8] demonstrated the implementation of a regimented perioperative protocol for outpatient surgery sufficient for outpatient TKA or unicompartmental knee arthroplasty with few readmissions, emergency room visits, or complications. Another published protocol for optimization of patients as candidates for same-day discharge preoperatively was from Moore et al[9] where patients underwent preoperative laboratory, telephone screening questionnaire, and physical examination to stratify patients into one of three categories. Each category placed a patient on an assessment schedule with preoperative anesthesia evaluation for optimization of modifiable risk factors for surgery. These protocols, among many others, highlighted relevant factors such as older age, later surgery end time, greater number of patient reported allergies, risk assessment and prediction tool score, and STOP-BANG sleep apnea score that affected the likelihood of a patient being discharged on the day of surgery.[9] Additionally, protocols such as these illustrated the importance of preoperative evaluation and contributed to the value of outpatient surgery through improvement of perioperative efficiency, safety, pain management, and well-defined postoperative management. It is important to acknowledge that the widespread implementation of outpatient surgical care pathways not only delivered consistent patient outcomes in the ASC, but the downstream effect led to quality improvement in the hospital setting as well; this occurred as a result of both competition and transfer of lessons learned in the ASC setting. In standardizing perioperative optimization, patient education begins early, and expectations are set creating the opportunity to achieve higher postoperative patient satisfaction and better patient-reported outcomes. This strategy allows the perioperative team to fine-tune daily workflow knowing that patients meet a specific set of criteria and that the objectives for each patient are largely the same.[10] Optimization of perioperative evaluation, patient education, expectations, and workflow improvement act in concert to improve the overall value of the orthopaedic procedure in question.

Through their development over decades, ASCs have undergone a rigorous vetting process to demonstrate equal, if not better, outcomes when compared with the traditional inpatient setting. Quality comparisons include the rate of readmission, complications, and adverse events. In expanding ASC breadth, efficacy in the hospital outpatient department was established first. An American College of Surgeons—National Surgical Quality Improvement Program analysis evaluated hospital stays and categorized patients into outpatient (less than one midnight) versus inpatient (more than one midnight). Using a propensity score matching and multivariate analysis, adverse events and readmissions were evaluated and it was found that the only increased risk for outpatient joint arthroplasty procedures was for a blood transfusion when compared with inpatient procedures. Otherwise, there were no increases in minor (pneumonia, wound dehiscence, urinary tract infection, or renal insufficiency) or serious (return to operating room, wound-related infection, thromboembolic event, renal failure, heart attack, cardiac event, stroke, or unplanned intubation, sepsis, or death) adverse events. This study, among many others, demonstrated that arthroplasty procedures could be performed safely in the outpatient setting.[9] Another study prospectively evaluated inpatient (more than 24 hours, admitted as inpatient status) versus outpatient (in this study, this includes both patients who are discharged the same day of surgery and those who are placed in an observation status and discharged the following day) TKA and found equivalent Knee Society scores, functional scores, and ranges of motion between cohorts at a mean of 24 months postoperatively. Outpatient TKA was also found to have similar quality of recovery.[11]

Within the realm of outcomes, and given a significant part of the burgeoning performance improvement movement in arthroplasty, patient-reported outcome measures (PROMs) have been used to further evaluate patient outcomes associated with inpatient, outpatient, and ASC procedures. Prospectively, a single surgeon evaluated 43 TKA inpatients and outpatients with a diary, complications, emergency department visits, and PROM results. Patient reports showed that quality of recovery was similar between groups and no outcome scores had statistically significant differences. There were no statistical differences between groups in complications or return to the emergency department.[12] A study of Medicare patients evaluated TKA patients who spent 3 to 4 nights in a hospital with patients who had shortened or extended-stay outpatient procedures. At 2 years, the outpatient and 1- to 2-day- stay groups reported less pain and stiffness.[13]

Notwithstanding PROM evaluation, overall patient satisfaction is also equivalent if not superior in outpatient surgery. A prospective study of 43 inpatient and 43 outpatient TKA patients evaluated 12-Item Short Form Health Survey scores, Hospital Consumer Assessment of Healthcare Providers and Systems, custom tools, and the National Health Service Friends and Family Test. Outpatients had superior quality of recovery postoperative day 1 measured by the Quality of Recovery-9 tool, had overall lower opioid requirement, and better reported pain levels. There was a correlation between well-controlled pain and satisfaction score. Ultimately, outpatient TKA resulted in no difference in PROM and satisfaction when compared with inpatient TKA.[12] ASC outcomes, whether clinical or patient reported, indicate that outpatient surgery via ASCs is a positively driving force in adding/improving value in orthopaedic surgery.

Cost

Implementation and development of ASCs demanded rationalization for the capitalization of new infrastructure, drawing off staff from other health care settings, and specialization of staff for a smaller variety of procedures. To make the change justifiable, there must be a large volume of patients who undergo the procedure and it must be reimbursed at a reasonable and sustainable rate. It is thoroughly documented that there is projected to be an increased volume of orthopaedic procedures, especially THA and TKA, and this trend is projected to continue as the population ages. This provides a significant amount of demand that, when combined with increased accessibility and lower price, makes the procedure readily available to more of the population, thus mobilizing latent demand. Because ASCs do not require the same infrastructure and services as a fully equipped hospital, fixed institutional costs are lower.

When comparing ASCs and hospitals, there are several reasons why patients are shifting surgical care to ASCs. Results from the Surgical Care Consumer Choice Survey found that patients consider travel time, recommendations, experience, ease of scheduling, and convenience of parking. However, the most important factor driving the shift from hospitals to ASCs is cost. Patients rate cost as the most influential factor of all of the aforementioned reasons combined.[14] Part of the cost savings of surgical intervention at an ASC is due to reduced Medicare and commercial carrier facility reimbursement, or cost to the payer. Further decreased cost due to the culture and mission of ASCs creates an even greater cost efficiency equation for patients. Many of the supply chain savings delivered by this culture are passed on to the consumer. Hospitals, by the nature of this competition, are or will be driven to improve efficiency and offer lower prices to patients for similar procedures. At this time, the differences in price are quite pronounced. Two studies evaluated the differences in price between outpatient and inpatient surgery for TKA and THA, and found that at 2 years, costs associated with the outpatient and the 1- to 2-day-stay groups were $8,527 and $1,967 lower than the 3- to 4-day-stay group, respectively.[11] Another study found average costs per patient were $11,677 for the ambulatory group and $19,361 for the inpatient group.[15]

Evaluation of the cost and outcomes of total shoulder arthroplasty, THA, TKA, and spine surgery performed at ASCs have been widely reported in the literature.[12,16,17] Studies have estimated that overall commercial payer savings for a primary TKA can be $8,500 or 30% per case when performed at an ASC compared with inpatient surgery.[16] At the procedural level, there is abundant evidence confirming the decreased cost associated with procedures performed at ASCs when compared to those same procedures performed in an inpatient setting. When the same service is offered at a lower cost, there is a direct increase in the value, which is resulting in increased utilization of ASCs.

In addition to being the driving factor for patients, cost is lower in ASCs when compared with those of both the hospital outpatient department and inpatient surgery environments. The cost component of value can be broken down by cost to payer (CMS decreases payment for the ASC, commercial insurers follow suit), patient (lower price overall decreases out of pocket cost to patients), and society (as CMS pays less for the same procedure, the cost of health care decreases and the overall value to society improves, increasing the availability of surgery for the population). Each of these aspects stems from the cost of the procedure, which is the primary focus of the ASC; delivering high-quality care with efficiency, decreased supply chain costs, and increased specialization.

Finally, physician ownership serves as the primary ownership model for ASCs: 64% of ASCs are solely physician owned, with that percentage increasing to 90% when including partial physician ownership.[18] Physician ownership within an ASC significantly affects both the cost and quality metrics when calculating the value provided by ASCs. Physician leadership of an ASC drives additional cost savings in the ASC environment by leveraging behavioral economics among investors and promoting the elimination of unwarranted variation among clinicians. Because the physician has a direct understanding of the implementation of resources in the healthcare setting, the internal perspective that yields the highest effect from the lowest cost leads to a lower cost margin. Physician innovation and focus on patient care also emphasizes the low cost but highly effective interventions for patients, which is mirrored in POHs. Furthermore, the clinical perspective of physicians significantly influences quality as physician ownership focuses resources to address patient experience and overall outcomes. Therefore, the physician owner-leader serves to significantly shift the cost/quality benefit in ASCs in a favorable direction for the consumer/patient.

The 2019 CMS Procedure Price Lookup demonstrates the differences in cost for some orthopaedic procedures (**Figure 2**).

Clearly, surgical procedures performed at an ASC are superior in the cost aspect of the value equation.

On a regional or system level, critics suggest that ASCs have an overall negative effect on the health care system and drive up costs for general hospitals. The argument follows that because ASCs select patients with less complex conditions for surgery, the overall cost at general hospitals is driven upward. The selection of patients with less complex conditions is intuitive because ASCs must service patients who can undergo surgical intervention and recover reasonably quickly, but the increased burden to general hospitals does not follow. Furthermore, modification to the diagnosis-related group (DRG) 470 (inpatient reimbursement methodology) coding increased reimbursement for patients whose conditions are more complex and encounter complications, offsetting some of the cost that is associated with complex patients. The shift of patients with less complex conditions to the ASC setting unlocks resources and staff that are better equipped to treat patients whose conditions are more complex and ill patients in the hospital setting. Furthermore, with increased efficiency, ASCs introduce an element of competition

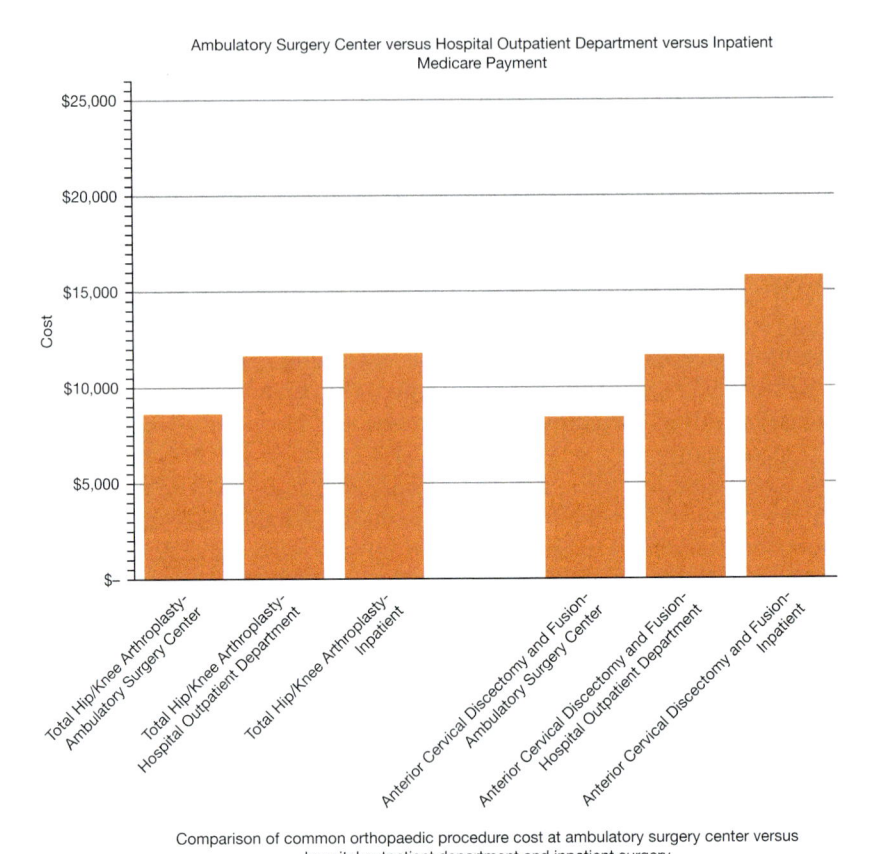

Comparison of common orthopaedic procedure cost at ambulatory surgery center versus hospital outpatient department and inpatient surgery

FIGURE 2 Medicare payment for orthopaedic procedures. (Data from Centers for Medicare & Medicaid Services [CMS] CMS Databook 2020.)

to the health care arena that drives innovation, cost reduction, and overall value improvement. Financial evaluation of ASCs in Arizona, California, and Texas from 1997 to 2004 examined the effects on revenue, costs, and profit margins of hospitals that offered the same services in the same region. This study used an empirical method with three regression models, each focused on one of the following dependent variables: net patient revenue (revenue), total operating expenses (cost), and profit margins (margins). The measures of quantity of output were number of admissions, number of outpatient visits, number of outpatient surgeries, and average length of hospital stay. This study found that the number of ASCs in operation for 2 years or longer was positively associated with both revenue and cost at the general hospital level. In addition, no association was noted between hospital margins and the number of specialty hospitals after 2 years of operation, suggesting that the introduction of specialty hospitals only has a transitory effect on the profits of larger, general hospitals. On a granular level, the analysis was able to estimate the effect one ASC had on a general hospital on opening, finding that there was a decrease of 0.226% and 0.143% of revenue and cost, respectively, to general hospitals. Ultimately, this illustrates a measurable, yet marginal effect of ASCs opening and competing with general hospitals. Examining ASCs from a value perspective, an increase can be implied in overall value for the local health care system with ASCs due to competitive pressures, increased efficiency, and decreased costs without a large, long-term negative effect on general hospitals.[19] With Medicare altering the reimbursement structure for outpatient services to match lower cost, this net improvement in value can be seen as positively affecting society, payers, and the patient.

The POH

POHs gradually evolved over time with significant, notable establishments marking the early growth of POH in the United States. Drs. Charles and William Mayo established the Mayo Clinic group, which developed the Mayo Property Association. Kaiser Permanente and Geisinger Health are integrated health systems that focus on quality care and excellence (Kaiser Permanente physicians become stockholders in The Permanente Medical Group after 3 years of work. The Permanente Medical Group operates 39 hospitals and other offices under the Permanente umbrella). POHs grew in popularity and prevalence with mixed effect due to physician referral patterns and concern over physicians having a financial conflict of interest resulting in governmental regulation and oversight playing a significant role in growth over the past 40 years. In 1988, the first Stark law was passed, which prohibited a physician from referring a Medicare patient to a clinical laboratory if the physician or family member had financial interest in that laboratory. This was expanded in 1993 with the Omnibus budget reconciliation act, or Stark II law, which expanded the prohibition to other designated health services. Importantly, an exception in Stark II law allowed for physician ownership of and referral to a hospital facility in which the physician had an equity position if it met the conditions of the "whole hospital exemption"; that is, if the physician's financial interest was in the whole hospital as opposed to a specific department or division. It is under this exemption that POHs saw significant growth in the late 1990s and early 2000s. The rapid growth of POHs was halted in 2003 when federal legislation imposed an 18-month moratorium preventing physicians from investing in new specialty hospitals if Medicare patients were referred to those hospitals. Over the next several years, multiple legislative attempts were made to permanently ban physician ownership of hospitals. In 2008 and 2009, CMS enacted payment reductions for procedures commonly performed in specialty hospitals to reduce financial incentive.[20] CMS made changes to the DRG methodology, which affected all hospitals similarly, but were designed to primarily decrease incentive for specialty hospitals that focused on these groups of procedures. CMS divided the DRG 470, which pays for lower extremity total joint arthroplasty, into three groups: major complication or comorbidity, complication or comorbidity, and no complication or comorbidity. There were variable payments based on how many complications the patient incurred during their stay. Patients who had more complications received a higher reimbursement, following a rationalization that the hospital deserved to be paid more because a greater number of services were provided. This negatively incentivized good outcomes as healthy patients who recovered without incident received a lower reimbursement. This was poorly executed and a further misstep because no hospital wanted complications given that transparency in outcomes was becoming more important and publicized. In 2010, the Patient Protection and Affordable Care Act was signed into law. Section 6001 of the law permanently restricted any POH from expanding the number of hospital beds or procedure or operating rooms, as well as ending the whole-hospital exception to the Stark laws. This grandfathered the existing POHs but stopped the completion of those under development and all future POHs. The law was challenged in 2018, and lawmakers supportive of POHs continue to attempt to have section 6001 of the ACA modified, pending hearings in the Supreme Court.[21]

Quality

The superior quality of care at POHs is demonstrated in theory and in studies. Theoretically, the benefit of specialization, a documented and well-described economic concept, suggests that specialization improves quality and efficiency with the overall efficiency of POH and allows for greater adherence to quality-of-care guidelines. Increased quality implicitly decreases charges due to fewer adverse events and preventable errors and avoidable deviation from established clinical practice guidelines. POH are better at following evidence-based clinical practice guidelines and have fewer errors, leading to better outcomes, and indirectly, lower cost.[22] Core competencies and learning allow for improvement of managerial efficiency and homogeneity, leading to task competence in the POH setting. Comparisons between POHs and non-POHs have been drawn throughout the history of POHs, and it appears that POHs are not outliers in terms of patient served, quality of care, or cost to the healthcare system.[23] A study evaluating the concern for overutilization in POHs found largely similar outcomes when evaluating nonsurgical treatments before surgery and the time from initial appointment to the day of surgery. Importantly, length of stay was significantly shorter for patients undergoing both TKA and THA at a POH.[24] Furthermore, another evaluation of POHs versus non-POHs found that although rates of 30-day readmission did not differ significantly between the two types of hospitals, POHs had a lower risk-adjusted complication score, and POHs outperformed non-POHs in all patient-satisfaction categories, including overall hospital rating.[25]

CMS data evaluating HCAHPS scores and five-star ratings shows a clear advantage in quality and patient satisfaction with POH (**Figure 3**).

In the hospital value-based performance rating system, POHs also outperformed non-POHs in multiple score cutoffs. POHs outpace non-POHs at the 50th percentile, the CMS benchmark, whereas POHs continue to broaden the performance gap in the 60th and 75th percentiles (**Figure 4**).

Patient satisfaction is another area of excellence that affects the value of orthopaedic practice by delivering higher quality of care as experienced by patients. A study of 150,000 Medicare patients who underwent TKA or THA at orthopaedic

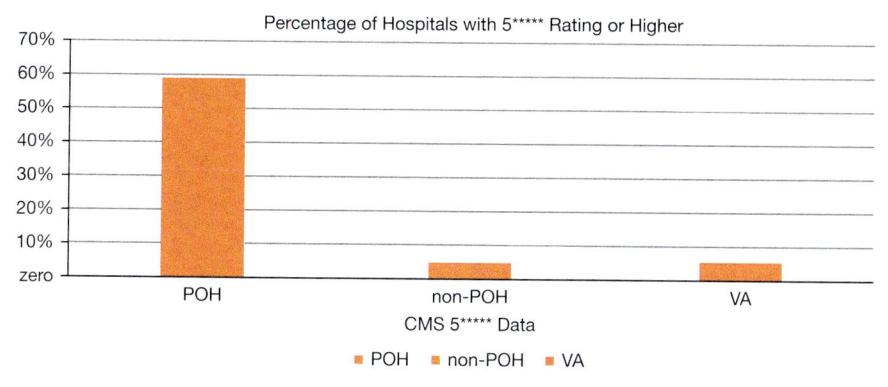

FIGURE 3 Percentage of hospitals with five-star rating or higher from the Centers for Medicare & Medicaid Services (CMS) Databook 2020. POH, physician-owned hospital. (Data from Centers for Medicare & Medicaid Services [CMS] CMS Databook 2020.)

POHs experienced lower rates of adverse outcomes and joint revision compared with patients who underwent similar procedures at general hospitals.[26] Another study of 3,818 hospitals found that hospitals with orthopaedic specialization were associated with improved patient outcomes after adjustment for procedure volume and patient characteristics.[27] CMS data on TKA or THA performed in 45 POHs and 2,657 general non-POHs in 2014 evaluated cost data, patient satisfaction scores, risk-adjusted complication, and 30-day readmission scores for TKA or THA. This study confirmed that non-POHs were in the upper quartile (higher cost) for inpatient payments. This supports the decreased cost and improved value of POHs when compared with general hospitals. POHs demonstrated a lower risk of complication and better patient

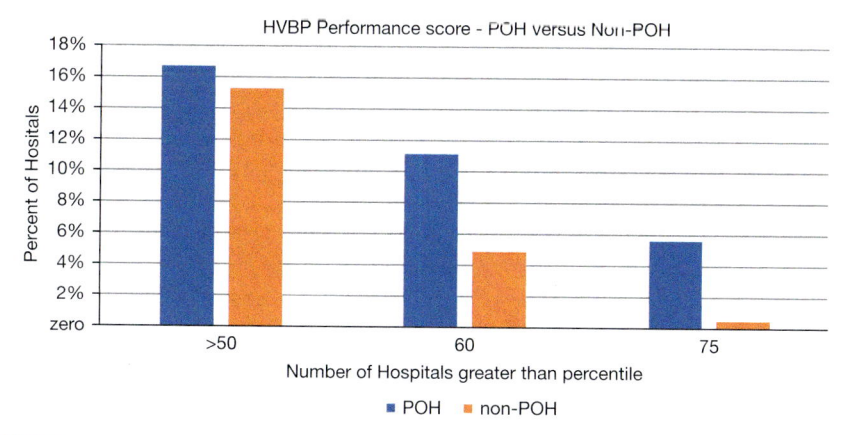

FIGURE 4 Hospital value-based performance (HVBP) performance comparison between physician-owned hospitals (POHs) and non-POHs. (Data from Centers for Medicare & Medicaid Services [CMS] CMS Databook 2020.)

satisfaction.[25] The guiding role of physicians in the management of hospital care allows for more attention to patient-centered care, ensuring consistent patient outcomes, and efficiently directed medical and surgical treatment when compared with non-POHs.

Cost

In evaluating the effect of POHs on the value of orthopaedics, cost again rises to the top of the list of arguments for the continuation and utilization of POHs in orthopaedic surgery. Proponents of POHs argue that physician leadership allows the practice of a hospital to focus primarily on patient care and to optimize workflow. Several studies have investigated the cost effectiveness and overall effects of POHs in various respects. POHs received lower mean Medicare payments than did non-POHs for THA and TKA procedures. When controlling for hospital demographic variables, status as a non-POH was an independent risk factor for being in the upper quartile (higher cost) of all inpatient payments for Medicare Severity–Diagnosis Related Group (MS-DRG) 470.

One observational study compared POHs and non POHs in metrics including quality of care, costs, and payments. The study utilized data from 2,186 acute care hospitals (219 POHs) in 95 referral regions based on Medicare claims and data. Hospital size, patient demographics, case mixtures, quality of care, and cost of care were all evaluated. All metrics were compiled and linear regression analysis was performed to investigate the variables correlated with POHs. Notable findings from the study were that POHs and non-POHs had no clinical or statistical difference in the mixture of admitted patients based on insurance or minority patients. There was also no statistically significant difference in admitted patient comorbidity or predicted mortality score. Hospital length of stay was shorter at POHs. When comparing payments, payments to POHs are substantially less than mean payments to non-POHs for the same services, resulting in a net savings for national expenditure.[28]

Furthermore, multiple studies evaluating the utilization of POHs demonstrated no increase in the number of surgical procedures despite the presence of POH in that respective market. Schneider et al[29] evaluated Medicare expenditures and outcomes nationally to determine the effect POHs had on non-POHs. No correlation was found between Medicare expenditures per enrollee and the presence of POHs in a market and was confirmed by two subsequent studies demonstrating the same lack of effect.[29,30]

Proponents of POHs also suggest that other monetary contributions to society produce a imbalanced effect, namely in the non–tax exempt status of POHs. ASCs and POHs in contradistinction to most hospitals are rarely structured as not-for-profit organizations and any net earnings from these entities are subject to federal and state tax, which, from a broader standpoint, are then available to fund other pressing societal needs. In taking on patients who are insured and able to pay for medical care, POHs pay property tax, income tax, and sales tax in addition to still providing uncompensated care in certain cases. Some would argue that this societal support is greater than the uncompensated care that non-for-profit community hospitals provide. This overall benefit to the community along with services provided demonstrates the cost effectiveness of the POH at the granular and community level. A direct observation of this effect was reported by Barro et al[31] and showed that specialty hospital entrance into a healthcare market resulted in a reduction in expenditures and a decrease in mortality. This overall effect leads to decreased cost and increased value in the orthopaedic field.

Opponents of POHs argue the effect of POH on the wider healthcare system is negative in the funneling of sicker, more complicated patients to general, non-POHs. A systematic review of 46 studies regarding POHs was carried out to examine the effect on quality and value of POH.[28] This review investigated POH safety, effectiveness, equitability, efficiency, patient centeredness, accessibility, and effect on full-service hospital performance. With respect to safety, the review found that patients who underwent procedures at POHs and ASCs had fewer readmissions and fewer complications. Effectiveness delved into adherence to clinical practice guidelines and quality measures in practice. The effect on general hospitals was evaluated in competitive and patient volume/characteristics. Evaluation of competition found that the entry of specialized hospitals encouraged greater cost efficiency of general hospitals and improved operating margins. Patient volume and characteristics evaluation revealed that there is only a limited degree of shift from general hospitals to POH facilities, but those that did shift were lower cost risk.[32-34]

Another consideration when comparing general and non-POHs with ASCs and POHs is that many specialty hospitals are developed as hospitals within hospitals within a general hospital. Other locations have started POHs as joint ventures with a local health system. These are often freestanding single-specialty affiliate hospitals but are coded as a part of the general hospital. This muddying of the waters makes it increasingly difficult to distinguish specialty from general hospitals moving forward, where previously the only criteria needed for a specialty hospital was a stand-alone/freestanding hospital with a focus on a discrete disease or set of procedures. This behavior demonstrates that general hospitals have changed and adapted to the pressure of POH/specialty hospitals.[20] This also demonstrates that hospitals recognize that physician engagement and alignment with ASC and POH models provides superior value to patients by embracing the significance of increased efficiency and lower cost championed by ASCs and POHs.

A physician's financial interest in the hospital ties directly into each of the previous categories, limiting unwarranted and variable interests and incentivizing physician leadership to improve value. The equation for value, outcomes that matter to patients divided by cost, is further improved at both the numerator and the denominator. The outcome of the value equation is improved by increasing the numerator with improved outcome and decreasing the denominator with decreased cost. Physicians who manage these facilities must maintain the highest level of quality to ensure successful competition with other hospitals, continue to draw patients as patient outcomes and satisfaction become more transparent, and surgeon interest in maintaining value increase. Decreasing cost, as detailed throughout the chapter, is the first priority for patients, thus drawing more patient volume to the institution, and overall improving the amount of value added to the healthcare system by the POH. Multiple measures serve the goal of increasing value, including adoption of evidence-based practices, optimizing supply chain management, reductions in length of stay, reductions in postacute care, presurgical optimization, decreasing postsurgical complications and readmissions, and physician governance with administrative support. Effective adoption and implementation of these and other measures ultimately affects the entire value equation, thereby increasing quality and reducing cost.

SUMMARY

ASCs and POHs have a comprehensive and unique history in the US healthcare system, working toward the mission of improving value and delivering care efficiently to patients while driving the evolution of legislation and regulation along the way. They have changed the landscape and practice of orthopaedic surgery, focusing on value through superior quality and outcomes with decreased costs and complications.

ASCs and POHs consistently improve quality, as evidenced by health care–related outcomes, PROMs, and a history of minimizing complications. Streamlined workflow, efficiency of specialization, physician-directed governance, and a focus on patient outcomes all contribute to sustained, improved value delivered by ASCs and POHs. Cost is also significantly decreased via many of the same strategies. Specialization decreases variety of infrastructure and maximizes utilization of staff and equipment, shorter episodes of care and increased efficiency decrease cost, and this is reflected in lower reimbursement by payors.

Why do ASCs and POHs have the capability to achieve such results? This is a complex question, but the core philosophy of improving outcomes while creating a cost-efficient service provides the foundation for each aspect of the results discussed in this chapter. Inherent design and specialization leverage behavioral economics and limit unwarranted variation in freeing clinicians working in the ASCs or POHs to maximize the benefits of specialization. Again, the equity position a clinician holds in either an ASC or POH model enables alignment of clinical and financial goals needed to improve value delivered to patients.

As the field of orthopaedics, and medicine in general, continues to change with an increasing focus on value, the peak of success can be envisioned as appropriate care that is delivered with reduced risk of untoward events, provides improvement in function and pain throughout the course of a condition, and is affordable. ASCs and POHs will continue to move the field closer to that goal.

REFERENCES

1. History of ASCs. Advancing Surgical Care. Available at: https://www.ascassociation.org/advancingsurgicalcare/asc/historyofascs. Accessed April 28, 2023.

2. Hedley-Whyte J, Milamed DR: The evolution of sites of surgery. *Ulster Med J* 2006;75(1):46-53.

3. Ambulatory Surgery Center: A Positive Trend in Health Care. Ambulatory Surgery Center Association. Available at: https://www.ascassociation.org/advancingsurgicalcare/aboutascs/industryoverview/apositivetrendinhealthcare.

4. Porter M, Kramer M: Strategy and society: The link between competitive advantage and corporate social responsibility. *Harv Bus Rev* 2006;84(12):78-92. Available at: https://hbr.org/2006/12/strategy-and-society-the-link-between-competitive-advantage-and-corporate-social-responsibility. Accessed April 28, 2023.

5. Langton J, Eve F, Campbell R, et al: A discussion on the treatment of hernia in children. *Br Med J* 1899;2(2016):470-474.

6. Campbell R: The operative treatment of hernia in infants and young children, illustrated by 114 consecutive cases. *The Lancet* 1904;163(4193):88-89.

7. Federal Regulations. Ambulatory Surgery Center Association. Available at: https://www.ascassociation.org/federalregulations/overview. Accessed April 28, 2023.

8. Berger RA, Kusuma SK, Sanders SA, Thill ES, Sporer SM: The feasibility and perioperative complications of outpatient knee arthroplasty. *Clin Orthop Relat Res* 2009;467(6):1443-1449.

9. Moore M, Brigati D, Crijns T, Vetter T, Schultz W, Bozic K: Enhanced selection of candidates for same-day and outpatient total knee arthroplasty. *J Arthroplasty* 2020;35(3):628-632.

10. Schneider JE, Miller TR, Ohsfeldt RL, Morrisey MA, Zelner BA, Li P: The economics of specialty hospitals. *Med Care Res Rev* 2008;65(5):531-553.

11. Bovonratwet P, Ondeck NT, Nelson SJ, Cui JJ, Webb ML, Grauer JN: Comparison of outpatient vs inpatient total knee arthroplasty: An ACS-NSQIP analysis. *J Arthroplasty* 2017;32(6):1773-1778.

12. Gauthier-Kwan OY, Dobransky JS, Dervin GF: Quality of recovery, postdischarge hospital utilization, and 2-year functional outcomes after an outpatient total knee arthroplasty program. *J Arthroplasty* 2018;33(7):2159-2164.e1.

13. Edwards PK, Milles JL, Stambough JB, Barnes CL, Mears SC: Inpatient versus outpatient total knee arthroplasty. *J Knee Surg* 2019;32(8):730-735.

14. Heuser E: Overview of Results from the Surgical Care Consumer Choice Survey. Advisory Board, 2016. Available at: https://www.advisory.com/topics/classic/2016/04/what-do-consumers-want-from-surgical-care.

15. No Increased Risk of Complications for Joint Replacement in Ambulatory Surgery Setting. EurekAlert!, 2019. Available at: https://www.eurekalert.org/pub_releases/2019-03/hfss-nir031319.php.

16. Huang A, Ryu JJ, Dervin G: Cost savings of outpatient versus standard inpatient total knee arthroplasty. *Can J Surg* 2017;60(1):57-62.

17. Gregory JM, Wetzig AM, Wayne CD, Bailey L, Warth RJ: Quantification of patient-level costs in outpatient total shoulder arthroplasty. *J Shoulder Elbow Surg* 2019;28(6):1066-1073.

18. Badlani N: Ambulatory surgery center ownership models. *J Spine Surg* 2019;5(suppl 2):S195-S203.

19. Carey K, Burgess JF, Young GJ: Hospital competition and financial performance: The effects of ambulatory surgery centers. *Health Econ* 2011;20(5):571-581.

20. Babu MA, Rosenow JM, Nahed BV: Physician-owned hospitals, neurosurgeons, and disclosure: Lessons from law and the literature. *Neurosurgery* 2011;68(6):1724-1732.

21. Cole CM: Physician-owned hospitals and self-referral. *Virtual Mentor* 2013;15(2):150-155.

22. Popescu I, Nallamothu BK, Vaughan-Sarrazin MS, Cram P: Do specialty cardiac hospitals have greater adherence to acute myocardial infarction and heart failure process measures? An empirical assessment using Medicare quality measures: Quality of care in cardiac specialty hospitals. *Am Heart J* 2008;156(1):155-160.

23. Blumenthal DM, Orav EJ, Jena AB, Dudzinski DM, Le ST, Jha AK: Access, quality, and costs of care at physician owned hospitals in the United States: Observational study. *BMJ* 2015;351:h4466.

24. Chen AF, Pflug E, O'Brien D, Maltenfort MG, Parvizi J: Utilization of total joint arthroplasty in physician-owned specialty hospitals vs acute care facilities. *J Arthroplasty* 2017;32(7):2060-2064.e1.

25. Courtney PM, Darrith B, Bohl DD, Frisch NB, Della Valle CJ: Reconsidering the affordable care act's restrictions on physician-owned hospitals: Analysis of CMS data on total hip and knee arthroplasty. *J Bone Joint Surg* 2017;99(22):1888-1894.

26. Cram P, Vaughan-Sarrazin MS, Wolf B, Katz JN, Rosenthal GE: A comparison of total hip and knee replacement in specialty and general hospitals. *J Bone Joint Surg Am* 2007;89(8):1675-1684.

27. Hagen TP, Vaughan-Sarrazin MS, Cram P: Relation between hospital orthopaedic specialisation and outcomes in patients aged 65 and older: Retrospective analysis of US Medicare data. *BMJ* 2010;340:c165.

28. Trybou J, De Regge M, Gemmel P, Duyck P, Annemans L: Effects of physician-owned specialized facilities in health care: A systematic review. *Health Policy* 2014;118(3):316-340.

29. Schneider JE, Ohsfeldt RL, Morrisey MA, Li P, Miller TR, Zelner BA: Effects of specialty hospitals on the financial performance of general hospitals, 1997-2004. *Inquiry* 2007;44(3):321-334.

30. Cimasi R, Sharamitaro A, Haynes L, Seiler R: Market impact of specialty hospitals: A study of the profitability of general short-term acute care hospitals post market entry of specialty hospitals. *J Health Care Finance* 2008;35(2):1-53.

31. Barro JR, Huckman RS, Kessler DP: The effects of cardiac specialty hospitals on the cost and quality of medical care. *J Health Econ* 2006;25(4):702-721.

32. Bian J, Morrisey MA: Free-standing ambulatory surgery centers and hospital surgery volume. *Inquiry* 2007;44(2):200-210.

33. Courtemanche C, Plotzke M: Does competition from ambulatory surgical centers affect hospital surgical output? *J Health Econ* 2010;29(5):765-773.

34. Hollingsworth JM, Krein SL, Birkmeyer JD, et al: Opening ambulatory surgery centers and stone surgery rates in health care markets. *J Urol* 2010;184(3):967-971.

Outpatient Total Joint Arthroplasty

Samuel Gray McClatchy, MD
Thomas (Quin) Throckmorton, MD, FAAOS

INTRODUCTION

The safety and success of outpatient total joint arthroplasty (TJA) depend on establishing a multidisciplinary total joint program that requires a team approach. Appropriate patient selection is the most important aspect for performing outpatient TJA successfully. One of the biggest advancements that has led to shorter hospital stays and created the potential for same-day discharge was the development of multimodal pain management protocols. Though most outpatient TJAs are performed on the lower extremity, shoulder arthroplasty may be better suited for the outpatient setting because it is not a weight-bearing joint and has a history of shorter hospital stays, decreased mortality rate, less blood loss, and fewer complications than hip and knee arthroplasty. A growing body of knowledge is demonstrating that outpatient total shoulder arthroplasty (TSA) can be safely performed while significantly reducing costs.

BACKGROUND

Outpatient TJA offers a unique case study for the implementation of value-based health care. The large case volumes associated with TJA allow a more objective comparison of outcomes and cost differences than in many other areas of orthopaedic surgery. Over the past decade there has been a significant shift in TJA from a traditionally inpatient procedure to an outpatient procedure. Some projections show that outpatient TJA is expected to increase by more than 450% over the next decade, with estimates that by 2026 more than half of all TJAs will be performed as an outpatient procedure.[1]

In 1965, health care was transformed with the introduction of Medicare and Medicaid. In 2010, the Patient Protection and Affordable Care Act (ACA) was signed into law, driving significant changes to health policy.[2] The ACA enacted major reforms,

Dr. Throckmorton or an immediate family member has received royalties from Exactech, Inc., Responsive Arthroscopy, and Zimmer; is a member of a speakers' bureau or has made paid presentations on behalf of Pacira; serves as a paid consultant to or is an employee of OsteoCentrics and Zimmer; has stock or stock options held in Exactech, Inc., Gilead, Responsive Arthroscopy, and Shoulder JAM; and serves as a board member, owner, officer, or committee member of American Academy of Orthopaedic Surgeons, American Shoulder and Elbow Surgeons, and ASES Foundation. Neither Dr. McClatchy nor any immediate family member has received anything of value from or has stock or stock options held in a commercial company or institution related directly or indirectly to the subject of this chapter.

broadening coverage through subsidized private insurance programs and incentivizing the adoption of a model where health care providers reduce costs through value-based reimbursement.[3] Specifically, the transition to "value-based care" can be defined as delivering the highest quality care at the lowest possible cost.[3] To achieve this goal, the ACA mandated that a certain percentage of payments from the Centers for Medicare & Medicaid Services (CMS) be tied to value-based initiatives. Bundled payment programs such as the Bundled Payments for Care Improvement (BPCI) and the Comprehensive Care for Joint Replacement (CJR) were created to accomplish this goal.[4,5] These programs primarily target lower extremity joint arthroplasties, a significant portion of CMS expenditures. In 2014, Medicare patients underwent 400,000 lower extremity joint arthroplasties at a health care cost of $7 billion.[5]

As a response to the cost pressures generated by the ACA, surgeons have investigated the possibility of realizing cost savings by moving TJA from the traditional hospital setting to the outpatient environment; this can be done either by same-day discharge from a hospital or by moving the surgical setting to an ambulatory surgery center (ASC). The hip and knee literature has emphasized this difference. Aynardi et al[6] demonstrated a cost savings of $6,798 for outpatient total hip arthroplasty (THA) compared with their inpatient cohort. Another study by Lovald et al[7] showed that 2-year costs of the outpatient total knee arthroplasty (TKA) group were $8,527 less than those for the inpatient group.

The cost savings have been further amplified by alternative payment models such as BPCI and CJR. These programs have been designed to maximize value without sacrificing quality of care by incentivizing hospitals and surgeons to reduce unnecessary expenditures and penalizing or rewarding them based on performance.[8] The early results of these programs have been promising with inpatient procedures; however, the results with outpatient arthroplasty are still pending.[9]

Despite the cost savings, to truly create value with outpatient arthroplasty, surgeons must do so without increasing patient risk or compromising outcomes. The outpatient program should be focused on minimizing complications and maximizing patient safety, followed by decreasing costs. Fortunately, advancements in surgical technique, pain management, and blood loss and recovery protocols have helped make this possible. Recent literature has shown that outpatient TJA is a safe alternative to hospital admission for the appropriate patients.[10,11] Greenky et al[12] reported on Medicare patients undergoing THA and found that outpatient procedures had lower 30-day complication and readmission rates in comparison with inpatient procedures.[12] Similar studies have shown a decrease or no difference in complication and readmission rates with outpatient TKA and TSA as well.[10,13] Although complications have been minimized, patient outcomes have still been maintained. A review by Lovett-Carter et al[14] noted that patient-reported outcomes for outpatient THA were high, and 96% were satisfied with the decision to undergo outpatient surgery.[14]

TRANSITION TO OUTPATIENT TJA

The safety and success of outpatient arthroplasty depends on establishing a multidisciplinary total joint program that requires a team approach. The entire process, including the initial patient encounter, preoperative testing and medical clearance, anesthesia, surgical care, postoperative nursing, and rehabilitation, relies on the development of robust pathways and processes to ensure success. The American Association of Hip and Knee Surgeons recognized six essential elements that require optimization for a successful outpatient arthroplasty program: patient selection, patient education and expectation management, social support, clinical and surgical team expertise, surgery center factors, and evidence-based protocols and pathways.[15]

Appropriate patient selection is the most important aspect for performing outpatient TJA successfully and cannot be overemphasized. Choosing the appropriate patient avoids placing undue risk on the patient in the ambulatory surgery setting or in their own home after surgery. In general, patients should be relatively healthy with few medical comorbidities, independent with adequate social support, and with relatively straightforward pathology to minimize additional surgical time or surgical insult to the patient. For example, difficult revision cases with complex pathology requiring significantly increased surgical resources and time are best performed in the inpatient setting. Medical evaluation from a primary care provider and cardiac and/or pulmonary workup, if appropriate, is critical to avoid unexpected medical complications. Development of and adherence to patient selection protocols allow reliable identification of optimal surgical candidates and those more at risk for medical complications or adverse surgical outcomes that would benefit more from inpatient care. Various scoring systems and patient selection algorithms have been proposed to accomplish this goal.[16-18] Fournier et al[19] described an algorithm for identifying appropriate candidates for outpatient total shoulder arthroplasty. Based on this algorithm (**Figure 1**), patient age and preoperative hematocrit can be used for initial screening, followed by a thorough workup and evaluation for pulmonary or cardiac conditions, and finally a history of thromboembolic disease and anticoagulation. Using this algorithm resulted in a low incidence of complications and no hospital admissions.

The next important aspect of an outpatient arthroplasty program is detailed patient and family education. Preoperative education is needed to outline the expectations and environment for a successful recovery postoperatively upon discharge from the hospital. After discharge, patients should have adequate support available and clear and rapid paths of access to team members of the total arthroplasty program to answer questions and address concerns that arise until they have sufficiently recovered from surgery.[15] Thorough education before surgery can decrease patient anxiety about same-day discharge and recovery postoperatively, and help predict any potential problems/may decrease prolonged stays or hospital admissions postoperatively.[16]

The medical and surgical team should be experienced in TJA and should preferably demonstrate successful same-day discharge in the hospital prior to making the transition to the ASC setting. The anesthesia team and recovery room staff should be involved in the development and implementation of rapid recovery protocols and pain pathways to ensure a safe and expeditious recovery from anesthesia. Because studies have shown the benefits of early ambulation and early physical therapy following TJA,[20] a physical therapist or appropriately trained team member should work with the patient postoperatively and determine their

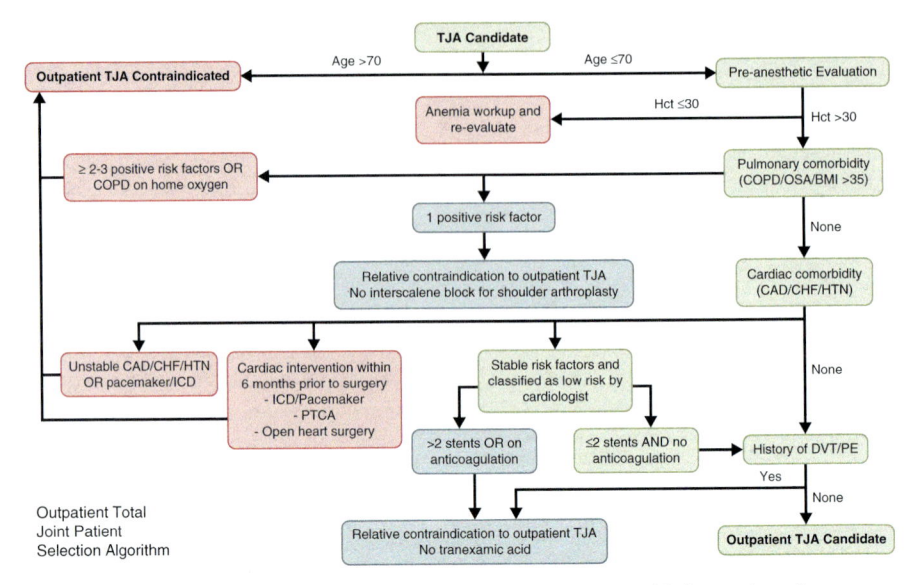

FIGURE 1 Algorithm for patient selection for outpatient total joint arthroplasty (TJA). BMI = body mass index, CAD = coronary artery disease, CHF = congestive heart failure, COPD = chronic obstructive pulmonary disease, HTN = hypertension, ICD = implantable cardioverter-defibrillator, OSA = obstructive sleep apnea, PTCA = percutaneous transluminal coronary angioplasty. (Reproduced with permission from Fournier MN, Brolin TJ, Azar FM, Stephens R, Throckmorton TW: Identifying appropriate candidates for ambulatory outpatient shoulder arthroplasty: Validation of a patient selection algorithm. *J Shoulder Elbow Surg* 2019;28[1]:65-70.)

safety for discharge home from an independence and mobility standpoint. Before discharge, arrangements should also be made for early outpatient physical and/or occupational therapy. The facility also should be adequately equipped to ensure patient safety throughout the procedure and recovery. If a patient is not appropriate for same-day discharge home postoperatively, the facility and staff should be equipped for an overnight stay or transfer to a hospital must be arranged to ensure the patient's safety is maintained. Many ASCs have the capability to observe patients for 23 hours after surgery, but the nursing and other resources necessary for an overnight stay should be put in place before an outpatient TJA program is begun.

ASCs that traditionally perform outpatient-only procedures may not be appropriately equipped, initially, for TJA. Surgery center facilities may have limited storage and sterilization resources. Because TJA is more instrument specific and equipment intensive than traditional outpatient surgeries, a thorough inventory of all equipment needed to perform TJA should be compiled and made available.[17] Although sophisticated inventory management systems are not absolutely necessary, they can assist with monitoring disparate arthroplasty systems and implants. Backup instruments should be available to avoid prolonged anesthesia if a critical instrument is dropped from the sterile field. Case planning and templating pre-operatively are useful to ensure appropriate implants and sizes are available. This planning also can improve intraoperative decision making and surgical time, as well as decrease sterile processing department utilization and costs. Intraoperative complications should be anticipated, and equipment should be available to address such issues if they arise. All of these measures help maximize operational efficiency to optimize a facility's success with outpatient TJA. Additionally, careful attention to room utilization and average surgical times by individual surgeons to make most efficient use of available operating room space is recommended.

The development of evidence-based protocols has been critical to the transition to outpatient arthroplasty.[21,22] These pathways have standardized and improved recovery and safety following TJA.[22-24] One of the biggest advancements that has led to shorter hospital stays and created the potential for same-day discharge is the development of multimodal pain management protocols. Wall[25] first coined the term multimodal pain management in 1988, and described the use of multiple techniques to achieve pain control. Since that time multimodal pain management has developed into a system of using both pharmacologic and nonpharmacologic methods preoperatively, intraoperatively, and postoperatively to control pain.[26] These protocols have led to improved pain control and decreased the need for intravenous pain medication, which in turn have shortened hospital stays and opened the door for same-day discharge.[27] Use of multimodal pain management has also been shown to decrease opioid requirements postoperatively,[28] and recent shoulder literature has shown successful pain control with an opioid-sparing pathway.[29] **Table 1** demonstrates one suggested multimodal pain management protocol.

One of the leading complications following outpatient TJA is blood loss requir-ing a transfusion.[12] Because ASCs do not have immediate transfusion capabilities, this is a costly complication that requires transfer to a hospital for infusion of blood products and potential admission for monitoring. One of the greatest effects on decreasing blood loss in outpatient TJA has come from the adoption of the anti-fibrinolytic drug tranexamic acid. Tranexamic acid has consistently demonstrated its ability to decrease intraoperative blood loss and the need for blood transfusions and is a critical component to safely performing arthroplasty in the outpatient set-ting.[30,31] Traditionally given intravenously or topically, recent studies have shown equivalent efficacy with oral preparations and at a fraction of the cost.[31-33] In addi-tion to tranexamic acid, the use of bipolar sealer in THA has shown significant benefits at safely limiting blood loss without increasing costs.[34-36]

Preoperative hematocrit has been suggested as an independent risk fac-tor for blood transfusion postoperatively.[37,38] Use of preoperative hematocrit requirements as a screening tool for outpatient arthroplasty can further decrease this risk.[39] Yeh et al[39] found that a hematocrit level below 37.2% for age older than 70 years and 36.3% for age younger than 70 years was highly predictive of a postoperative transfusion following TKA. Further, Basora et al[38] identified the odds of requiring transfusion postoperatively increased 3.7-fold for each 3-point decrease from a preoperative hematocrit threshold of 39.0%. Anesthesia

TABLE 1 Multimodal Pain Management Protocol

Medication	Preoperative Dose	Postoperative Dose	Contraindication
Opioid	None	5 to 10 mg oxycodone Q4H as needed for breakthrough pain	Allergy
Acetaminophen	1,000 mg PO or IV once	1,000 mg PO Q8H	Allergy or history of liver disease
NSAID	400 mg celecoxib PO once	200 mg celecoxib PO BID	Allergy, history of CAD, GI bleeding, renal insufficiency, coagulopathy, age older than 80 years or inflammatory bowel disease
Gabapentin	600 mg PO once	300 mg PO Q8H	Allergy, history of dementia or renal insufficiency
Regional block	Single-shot interscalene regional nerve block with 15 to 20 mL of 0.5% ropivacaine	None	Allergy or coagulopathy
Tramadol	None	50 mg PO Q6H	Allergy

BID = twice daily, CAD = coronary artery disease, GI = gastrointestinal, H = hour, IV = intravenous, PO = by mouth, Q = every

pathways using hypotensive spinal anesthesia for lower extremity TJA also have been shown to decrease intraoperative blood loss, speed recovery, and improve pain control postoperatively.[40-42]

Venous thromboembolism (VTE) is a dreaded complication following TJA. VTE prophylaxis postoperatively is necessary, but some agents are expensive and carry increased bleeding risks that are difficult to monitor as an outpatient. Fortunately, multiple studies have shown equivalent effectiveness of aspirin for VTE prevention compared with other oral or injectable agents.[43-45] Aspirin also offers the benefit of being more cost effective and convenient and carries a lower risk of bleeding complications.[45,46] It is the chapter authors' VTE prophylaxis agent of choice in the absence of other significant factors associated with VTE, such as prior thromboembolic event.

TSA has been slower to transition to the outpatient setting than THA and TKA. Inertial forces and changes to regulatory guidelines that have lagged behind THA and TKA are likely contributors. However, pressures from the COVID-19 pandemic have accelerated adoption of outpatient TSA in many parts of the country. However, TSA may be better suited for the outpatient setting because it is not a weight-bearing joint and has a history of shorter hospital stays, decreased mortality rate, lower blood loss, and fewer complications than THA and TKA.[47,48] A growing body of knowledge is demonstrating that outpatient TSA can be safely performed.[10,19,49] Additionally, patients who have undergone TSA have shown a preference for outpatient surgery than an inpatient procedure.[50] TSA also has the benefit of a shorter learning curve, as many protocols for outpatient THA and TKA have already been established and can easily be adopted for use with TSA.

PAYMENT MODELS AND REIMBURSEMENT

With the rising cost of health care and the increasingly strong desire of payers to tie surgical payments to patient outcomes and quality measures, alternative payment models are increasingly becoming more common. The goal of these programs is to incentivize hospitals, physicians, and postacute care providers to reduce costs and improve quality of care.[8] In 2010 the ACA established the Center for Medicare and Medicaid Innovation, with the objective to develop and investigate alternate payment models for reimbursements.[51] Since that time there have been several iterations of payment programs initiated to test bundled payment models to replace traditional fee-for-service models for TJA.

THA and TKA were specifically chosen for these investigational programs because they are the most common inpatient surgeries for Medicare patients and are the largest orthopaedic cost driver and financial burden on the healthcare system. CMS reports that in 2014 there were more than 400,000 lower extremity TJAs at a cost of more than $7 billion.[5] Despite their high incidence and similarities, lower extremity TJAs have high variations in cost. The average Medicare cost per procedure ranges from $16,500 to $33,000.[8] Although implant costs are often thought to be a significant driver in these variations, they are better explained by the usage patterns of postacute care following TJA. Approximately half of the cost of TJA is driven by patient recovery in postacute care facilities, including rehabilitation, skilled nursing facilities, and home health services.

The first bundled payment program including TJA was the BPCI program, which was launched in 2013 and concluded in 2018. It consisted of four models from which participants could choose. The most popular was model 2, which provided bundle payments for the procedure, initial hospitalization, and all related care for up to 90 days from the time of procedure.[52] This program was not arthroplasty specific and included 48 diagnosis-related group codes; however, 75% of participants choose lower extremity joint replacements.[52] Results of the BPCI program were very promising. Murphy et al[53] found that compared with fee-for-service models, BPCI was associated with a statistically significant decrease in costs with no change in adverse events or readmissions. Additionally, programs that were run by physician-owned practices outperformed hospital-run BPCI programs in terms of cost savings.[53]

On April 1, 2016, the CMS implemented the Comprehensive Care for Joint Replacement (CJR) program. CJR is a lower extremity arthroplasty specific program based on early results of the BPCI model. However, the CJR differed from BPCI model 2 in several ways. Enrollment in BPCI was voluntary and also allowed provider groups to assume risk. With the CJR program, participation is mandatory, and claims are reconciled against a target price set by CMS without negotiation. Management of financial risk was also placed solely on the hospitals. Hospitals are responsible for the costs associated with the surgery and the 90-day postoperative period. However, the CJR program does allow hospitals to contract with postacute care facilities or provider groups to share risk and financial incentives. CMS also attempts to link costs to value by including complication rates and Hospital Consumer Assessment of Healthcare Providers and Systems scores as quality metrics.[8] A side-by-side comparison of differences between BPCI and CJR is shown in **Table 2**.

Maniya et al[8] identified four potential negative outcomes of the CJR program. First, penalties to low-volume hospitals may incentivize them to stop offering TJA. Second, penalties may negatively affect patient selection and incentivize hospitals to screen for lower risk patients to decrease cost of care, leaving other patients without access to TJA services. Third, decreased revenue from CMS may place the burden on the private sector and increase costs to private insurances and patients for TJA. Fourth, the dramatic loss of revenue to postacute care facilities may drive them out of the market, decreasing options for patients.

TABLE 2 Side-by-Side Comparison of Differences Between Bundled Payments for Care Improvement and Comprehensive Care for Joint Replacement

	BPCI	CJR
Participation	Voluntary	Mandatory
Region	National	67 selected metro areas
Duration	3 years	5 years
Clinical episodes	48 inpatient, 0 outpatient	2 inpatient, 0 outpatient
Arthroplasty specific	No	Yes
Episode of care length	30/60/90 days	90 days
Responsible group	Hospitals, physicians, extended care facilities	Hospitals
Target price	Participant specific	Combination of provider and regional pricing
CMS discount	2% for 90-day bundle, 3% for remaining models	Variable based on patient quality scores
Reconciliation	Quarterly	Annually
Risk adjustment	MS-DRG only	MS-DRG and hip fracture pathway

BPCI = Bundled Payments for Care Improvement, CJR = Comprehensive Care for Joint Replacement, CMS = Centers for Medicare & Medicaid Services, MS-DRG = Medicare Severity-Diagnosis Related Group

One effort to decrease the risk assumed by hospitals and prevent screening patients due to the CJR program is to adjust reimbursement based on certain non-modifiable factors that increase costs. Currently CMS adjusts reimbursement based on diagnosis-related group codes, geography, and the presence of a fracture; however, these adjustments may underestimate financial risk and be insufficient to account for the true medical complexity of patients.[5,54,55] A study by Cairns et al[56] showed that older age, male sex, and most comorbidities were associated with higher costs, and stratification by these factors resulted in greater accuracy than current CJR adjustment methods.[56]

Early analyses of the effects of the CJR program on participating hospitals have been mixed. Almost all studies have shown a decrease in length of stay and an increased disposition to home for Medicare patients.[57-59] Additionally, some studies have shown decreased readmission rates up to 90 days.[58] Hospital expenses, however, have remained constant, indicating the cost savings likely benefit insurance providers and not participating hospitals.[57] The largest effect from the CJR program appears to affect postacute care facilities, with projections that they may lose $85 million or roughly 6.5% of revenue from lower extremity TJAs.[8]

Based on the successful results of the BPCI program, a BPCI Advanced model began October 1, 2018, and will run through December 31, 2023. Similar to the original BPCI program, BPCI Advanced is a voluntary model and is not arthroplasty specific. However, it does include 12 orthopaedic diagnosis-related group codes. Most notably it includes the addition of total shoulder arthroplasty to the bundled payment model.[60] Another large advancement was the inclusion of select outpatient procedures, which is a deviation from the strictly inpatient-only BPCI and CJR programs. As BPCI Advanced is relatively new, results and analysis of the program remain to be seen.

FUTURE DIRECTIONS

In January 2018, CMS removed TKA from the Medicare inpatient-only list. This is a major change but recognizes the significant shift toward outpatient TJA due to recent advancements and the potential cost savings. However, this change has had some unanticipated negative effects on bundled payment models. Yayac et al[61] noted that due to the change, approximately half of the total knee arthroplasties performed at their institution were reclassified as outpatient by the hospital. Because only inpatient procedures qualify for the BPCI and CJR programs, these procedures were excluded from the bundled payment programs. As a result, average costs for procedures included in the BPCI and CJR programs increased. In future iterations of these models CMS may be able to correct these negative effects. This change is accounted for in the BPCI Advanced model, which included outpatient TKA.

Another negative outcome from the removal of TKA from the inpatient-only list was a steep decrease in facility reimbursement. Theosmy et al[62] showed that outpatient TKA saves hospitals $972 on average compared to an inpatient procedure. However, the Medicare payment for outpatient TKA is $3,157 less per patient. As such, this steep decrease in reimbursement is disproportionate to the cost savings associated with TKA as an outpatient procedure. Davis et al[63] reported similar findings at their institution, where they experienced a $930,463 decrease in reimbursements for TKA over 30 months since implementation. Therefore, these changes have the potential to disincentivize surgeons from performing TKA as a lower cost outpatient procedure, and ongoing advocacy efforts are attempting to address this discrepancy in reimbursements.

Overall, the removal of TKA from the inpatient-only list is an important step that matches the current level of care needed with the services provided. Although THA and TSA are likely to follow, negotiations with CMS must allow an appropriate level of reimbursement so as not to repeat the experience of outpatient TKA.

SUMMARY

Outpatient TJA is a rapidly growing field within orthopaedics and offers unique advantages in the transition to value-based health care. Specifically, the shift from inpatient to outpatient TJA has created great potential for cost savings; however, maintaining patient safety and outcomes prior to making this transition is critical. Fortunately, multiple pathways and protocols have been created to maintain and improve the results demonstrated with inpatient care and assist in the transition to the outpatient setting.

In particular, a convergence of clear physician leadership with motivated administrative and operational leaders is a key component for successful adoption of outpatient TJA. Surgeons can approach colleagues to gain buy-in for the program and lend technical expertise to create, adopt, and implement clinical care pathways. However, financial and contracting expertise is also necessary from an administrative standpoint to approach private insurers and implant vendors, respectively, to negotiate reimbursement rates and implant costs.

TJA has been demonstrated to be a group of high-volume, reproducible procedures with excellent objective outcomes but high cost variability between provider groups and regions. Because they account for a large portion of Medicare expenditures, they are an ideal area for study and process improvement. The bundled payment programs initiated by CMS have been promising; however, this is an evolving area and will continue to develop to find a balance between cost and value. Finally, rapidly developing events, such as the assignment of an outpatient TKA code by CMS, and the potential domino effect extending to outpatient THA and TSA, also bear monitoring. An additional trend to consider is the increasing practice of ASCs contracting directly with employers, rather than insurance companies, as an opportunity to drive higher patient volumes and eliminate administrative processes that are unnecessary and lack value.

REFERENCES

1. Dyrda L: 15 things to know about outpatient total joint replacements and ASCs. *Becker's ASC Review*. January 15, 2021. Available at: https://www.beckersasc.com/orthopedics-tjr/15-things-to-know-about-total-joint-replacements-and-ascs-2021.html. Accessed May 3, 2023.

2. Bauchner H: Medicare and Medicaid, the Affordable Care Act, and US health policy. *J Am Med Assoc* 2015;314(4):353-354.

3. Issar NM, Jahangir AA: The Affordable Care Act and orthopaedic trauma. *J Orthop Trauma* 2014;28(suppl 10):S5-S7.

4. Centers for Medicare & Medicaid Services: Bundled Payments for Care Improvement (BPCI) Initiative: General information. Available at: https://innovation.cms.gov/innovation-models/bundled-payments. Accessed July 20, 2020.

5. Centers for Medicare & Medicaid Services: Comprehensive care for joint replacement model. Available at: https://innovation.cms.gov/innovation-models/cjr Accessed July 20, 2020.

6. Aynardi M, Post Z, Ong A, Orozco F, Sukin DC: Outpatient surgery as a means of cost reduction in total hip arthroplasty: A case-control study. *HSS J* 2014;10(3):252-255.

7. Lovald ST, Ong KL, Malkani AL, et al: Complications, mortality, and costs for outpatient and short-stay total knee arthroplasty patients in comparison to standard-stay patients. *J Arthroplasty* 2014;29(3):510-515.

8. Maniya OZ, Mather RC, Attarian DE, et al: Modeling the potential economic impact of the Medicare comprehensive care for joint replacement episode-based payment model. *J Arthroplasty* 2017;32(11):3268-3273.e4.

9. Edwards PK, Mears SC, Barnes CL: BPCI: Everyone wins, including the patient. *J Arthroplasty* 2017;32(6):1728-1731.

10. Brolin TJ, Mulligan RP, Azar FM, Throckmorton TW: Neer Award 2016: Outpatient total shoulder arthroplasty in an ambulatory surgery center is a safe alternative to inpatient total shoulder arthroplasty in a hospital – A matched cohort study. *J Shoulder Elbow Surg* 2017;26(2):204-208.

11. Shah RR, Cipparrone NE, Gordon AC, Raab DJ, Bresch JR, Shah NA: Is it safe? Outpatient total joint arthroplasty with discharge to home at a freestanding ambulatory surgical center. *Arthroplast Today* 2018;4(4):484-487.

12. Greenky MR, Wang W, Ponzio DY, Courtney PM: Total hip arthroplasty and the Medicare inpatient-only list: An analysis of complications in Medicare aged patients undergoing outpatient surgery. *J Arthroplasty* 2019;34(6):1250-1254.

13. Courtney PM, Froimson MI, Meneghini RM, Lee GC, Della Valle CJ: Can total knee arthroplasty be performed safely as an outpatient in the Medicare population? *J Arthroplasty* 2018;33(7 suppl):S28-S31.

14. Lovett-Carter D, Sayeed Z, Abaab L, Pallekonda V, Mihalko W, Saleh KJ: Impact of outpatient total joint replacement on postoperative outcomes. *Orthop Clin North Am* 2018;49(1):35-44.

15. Meneghini R, Gibson W, Halsey D, Padgett D, Berend K, Della Valle CJ: The American Association of Hip and Knee Surgeons, Hip Society, Knee Society, and American Academy of Orthopaedic Surgeons position statement on outpatient joint replacement. *J Arthroplasty* 2018;33(12):3599-3601.

16. Meneghini RM, Ziemba-Davis M, Ishmael MK, Kuzma AL, Caccavallo P: Safe selection of outpatient joint arthroplasty patients with medical risk stratification: The "outpatient arthroplasty risk assessment score." *J Arthroplasty* 2017;32(8):2325-2331.

17. Toy PC, Fournier MN, Throckmorton TW, Mihalko WM: Low rates of adverse events following ambulatory outpatient total hip arthroplasty at a free-standing surgery center. *J Arthroplasty* 2018;33(1):46-50.

18. Ziemba-Davis M, Caccavallo P, Meneghini RM: Outpatient joint arthroplasty-patient selection: Update on the outpatient arthroplasty risk assessment score. *J Arthroplasty* 2019;34(7 suppl):S40-S43.

19. Fournier MN, Brolin TJ, Azar FM, Stephens R, Throckmorton TW: Identifying appropriate candidates for ambulatory outpatient shoulder arthroplasty: Validation of a patient selection algorithm. *J Shoulder Elbow Surg* 2019;28(1):65-70.

20. Tayrose G, Newman D, Slover J, Jaffe F, Hunter T, Bosco J: Rapid mobilization decreases length-of-stay in joint replacement patients. *Bull Hosp Jt Dis (2013)* 2013;71(3):222-226.

21. Hamilton WG: Protocol development for outpatient total joint arthroplasty. *J Arthroplasty* 2019;34(7 suppl):S46-S47.

22. Berger RA, Sanders SA, Thill ES, Sporer SM, Della Valle C: Newer anesthesia and rehabilitation protocols enable outpatient hip replacement in selected patients. *Clin Orthop Relat Res* 2009;467(6):1424-1430.

23. Goyal N, Chen AF, Padgett SE, et al: Otto Aufranc Award: A multicenter, randomized study of outpatient versus inpatient total hip arthroplasty. *Clin Orthop Relat Res* 2017;475(2):364-372.

24. Gondusky JS, Choi L, Khalaf N, Patel J, Barnett S, Gorab R: Day of surgery discharge after unicompartmental knee arthroplasty: An effective perioperative pathway. *J Arthroplasty* 2014;29(3):516-519.

25. Wall PD: The prevention of postoperative pain. *Pain* 1988;33(3):289-290.

26. Gaffney CJ, Pelt CE, Gililland JM, Peters CL: Perioperative pain management in hip and knee arthroplasty. *Orthop Clin North Am* 2017;48(4):407-419.

27. McLaughlin DC, Cheah JW, Aleshi P, Zhang AL, Ma CB, Feeley BT: Multimodal analgesia decreases opioid consumption after shoulder arthroplasty: A prospective cohort study. *J Shoulder Elbow Surg* 2018;27(4):686-691.

28. Golladay GJ, Balch KR, Dalury DF, Satpathy J, Jiranek WA: Oral multimodal analgesia for total joint arthroplasty. *J Arthroplasty* 2017;32(9 suppl):S69-S73.

29. Leas DP, Connor PM, Schiffern SC, D'Alessandro DF, Roberts KM, Hamid N: Opioid-free shoulder arthroplasty: A prospective study of a novel clinical care pathway. *J Shoulder Elbow Surg* 2019;28(9):1716-1722.

30. Fillingham YA, Ramkumar DB, Jevsevar DS, et al: The safety of tranexamic acid in total joint arthroplasty: A direct meta-analysis. *J Arthroplasty* 2018;33(10):3070-3082.e1.

31. Fillingham YA, Ramkumar DB, Jevsevar DS, et al: The efficacy of tranexamic acid in total hip arthroplasty: A network meta-analysis. *J Arthroplasty* 2018;33(10):3083-3089.e4.

32. Fillingham YA, Kayupov E, Plummer DR, Moric M, Gerlinger TL, Della Valle CJ: The James A. Rand Young Investigator's Award: A randomized controlled trial of oral and intravenous tranexamic acid in total knee arthroplasty – The same efficacy at lower cost? *J Arthroplasty* 2016;31(9 suppl):26-30.

33. Wang F, Zhao KC, Zhao MM, Zhao DX: The efficacy of oral versus intravenous tranexamic acid in reducing blood loss after primary total knee and hip arthroplasty: A meta-analysis. *Medicine (Baltimore)* 2018;97(36):e12270.

34. Suarez JC, Slotkin EM, Szubski CR, Barsoum WK, Patel PD: Prospective, randomized trial to evaluate efficacy of a bipolar sealer in direct anterior approach total hip arthroplasty. *J Arthroplasty* 2015;30(11):1953-1958.

35. Ackerman SJ, Tapia CI, Baik R, Pivec R, Mont MA: Use of a bipolar sealer in total hip arthroplasty: Medical resource use and costs using a hospital administrative database. *Orthopedics* 2014;37(5):e472-e481.

36. Min JK, Zhang QH, Li HD, Li H, Guo P: The efficacy of bipolar sealer on blood loss in primary total hip arthroplasty: A meta-analysis. *Medicine (Baltimore)* 2016;95(19):e3435.

37. Ahmed I, Chan JKK, Jenkins P, Brenkel I, Walmsley P: Estimating the transfusion risk following total knee arthroplasty. *Orthopedics* 2012;35(10):e1465-e1471.

38. Basora M, Tió M, Martin N, et al: Should all patients be optimized to the same preoperative hemoglobin level to avoid transfusion in primary knee arthroplasty? *Vox Sang* 2014;107(2):148-152.

39. Yeh JZY, Chen JY, Bin Abd Razak HR, et al: Preoperative haemoglobin cut-off values for the prediction of post-operative transfusion in total knee arthroplasty. *Knee Surg Sports Traumatol Arthrosc* 2016;24(10):3293-3298.

40. Thompson GE, Miller RD, Stevens WC, Murray WR: Hypotensive anesthesia for total hip arthroplasty: A study of blood loss and organ function (brain, heart, liver, and kidney). *Anesthesiology* 1978;48(2):91-96.

41. Sharrock NE, Salvati EA: Hypotensive epidural anesthesia for total hip arthroplasty: A review. *Acta Orthop Scand* 1996;67(1):91-107.

42. Johnson RL, Kopp SL, Burkle CM, et al: Neuraxial vs general anaesthesia for total hip and total knee arthroplasty: A systematic review of comparative-effectiveness research. *Br J Anaesth* 2016;116(2):163-176.

43. Wilson DG, Poole WE, Chauhan SK, Rogers BA: Systematic review of aspirin for thromboprophylaxis in modern elective total hip and knee arthroplasty. *Bone Joint J* 2016;98-B(8):1056-1061.

44. Hood BR, Cowen ME, Zheng HT, Hughes RE, Singal B, Hallstrom BR: Association of aspirin with prevention of venous thromboembolism in patients after total knee arthroplasty compared with other anticoagulants: A noninferiority analysis. *JAMA Surg* 2019;154(1):65-72.

45. An VV, Phan K, Levy YD, Bruce WJ: Aspirin as thromboprophylaxis in hip and knee arthroplasty: A systematic review and meta-analysis. *J Arthroplasty* 2016;31(11):2608-2616.

46. Mostafavi Tabatabaee R, Rasouli MR, Maltenfort MG, Parvizi J: Cost-effective prophylaxis against venous thromboembolism after total joint arthroplasty: Warfarin versus aspirin. *J Arthroplasty* 2015;30(2):159-164.

47. Farmer KW, Hammond JW, Queale WS, Keyurapan E, McFarland EG: Shoulder arthroplasty versus hip and knee arthroplasties: A comparison of outcomes. *Clin Orthop Relat Res* 2007;455:183-189.

48. Fehringer EV, Mikuls TR, Michaud KD, Henderson WG, O'Dell JR: Shoulder arthroplasties have fewer complications than hip or knee arthroplasties in US veterans. *Clin Orthop Relat Res* 2010;468(3):717-722.

49. Leroux TS, Basques BA, Frank RM, et al: Outpatient total shoulder arthroplasty: A population-based study comparing adverse event and readmission rates to inpatient total shoulder arthroplasty. *J Shoulder Elbow Surg* 2016;25(11):1780-1786.

50. Nelson C, Murphy W, Mulligan R, Brolin T, Azar FM, Throckmorton TW: A retrospective comparative study of patient satisfaction following ambulatory outpatient and inpatient total shoulder arthroplasty. *Curr Orthop Prac* 2019;30:435-438.

51. Siddiqi A, White PB, Mistry JB, et al: Effect of bundled payments and health care reform as alternative payment models in total joint arthroplasty: A clinical review. *J Arthroplasty* 2017;32(8):2590-2597.

52. Maddox KE, Orav EJ, Zheng J, Epstein AM: Evaluation of Medicare's bundled payments initiative for medical conditions. *N Engl J Med* 2018;379:260-269.

53. Murphy WS, Siddiqi A, Cheng T, et al: 2018 John Charnley Award: Analysis of US hip replacement bundled payments – Physician-initiated episodes outperform hospital-initiated episodes. *Clin Orthop Relat Res* 2019;477(2):271-280.

54. Ellimoottil C, Ryan AM, Hou H, Dupree J, Hallstrom B, Miller DC: Medicare's new bundled payment for joint replacement may penalize hospitals that treat medically complex patients. *Health Aff (Millwood)* 2016;35(9):1651-1657.

55. Clement RC, Derman PB, Kheir MM, et al: Risk adjustment for Medicare total knee arthroplasty bundled payments. *Orthopedics* 2016;39(5):e911-e916.

56. Cairns MA, Moskal PT, Eskildsen SM, Ostrum RF, Clement RC: Are Medicare's "comprehensive care for joint replacement" bundled payments stratifying risk adequately? *J Arthroplasty* 2018;33(9):2722-2727.

57. Plate JF, Ryan SP, Black CS, et al: No changes in patient selection and value-based metrics for total hip arthroplasty after comprehensive care for joint replacement bundle implementation at a single center. *J Arthroplasty* 2019;34(8):1581-1584.

58. Dundon JM, Bosco J, Slover J, Yu S, Sayeed Y, Iorio R: Improvement in total joint replacement quality metrics: Year one versus year three of the bundled payments for care improvement initiative. *J Bone Joint Surg Am* 2016;98(23):1949-1953.

59. Ryan SP, Howell CB, Wellman SS, et al: Preoperative optimization checklists within the comprehensive care for joint replacement bundle have not decreased hospital returns for total knee arthroplasty. *J Arthroplasty* 2019;34(7 suppl):S108-S113.

60. Centers for Medicare & Medicaid Services: BPCI Advanced. Available at: https://innovation.cms.gov/innovation-models/bpci-advanced. Accessed July 20, 2020.

61. Yayac M, Schiller N, Austin MS, Courtney PM: 2020 John N. Insall Award: Removal of total knee arthroplasty from the inpatient-only list adversely affects bundled payment programmes. *Bone Joint J* 2020;102-B(6 supple A):19-23.

62. Theosmy E, Yayac M, Krueger CA, Courtney PM: Is the new outpatient prospective payment system classification for outpatient total knee arthroplasty appropriate? *J Arthroplasty* 2021:36(1):42-46.

63. Davis CM, Swenson ER, Lehman TM, Haas DA: Economic impact of outpatient Medicare total knee arthroplasty at a tertiary care academic medical center. *J Arthroplasty* 2020;35(6 suppl):S37-S41.

Orthopaedics as a Service Line

Ahmed Siddiqi, DO, MBA • Nicolas S. Piuzzi, MD
Ashley E. Chacko, MHA • Wael K. Barsoum, MD, FAAOS

INTRODUCTION

Orthopaedic surgery as a medical subspecialty has experienced significant progress over the past decade, contributing to the advancement of enabling surgical technologies and robotics, the propagation of ambulatory surgery centers, the evolution of the surgeon and vendor company relationship, and the upswing of gain-sharing models and surgeon co-management of growing orthopaedic businesses. As the demand of orthopaedics continues to rise, orthopaedic service lines are evolving and transforming delivery of patient care through standardized care pathways while curtailing cost. This is especially relevant during the current climate of healthcare reform that has shifted towards value-based care. Orthopaedic surgeons must be conscious of outcomes and resource utilization within their practice because failure to address clinical shortcomings may result in financial implications. This chapter focuses on the process of establishing and building a successful orthopaedic service line.

BACKGROUND

The concept of healthcare service lines strategies was introduced in the late 1980s in an effort to gain market share due to significant interhospital competition.[1] As the driving forces of health care advancement have progressed over time, interhospital competition has diminished with the introduction of specialty hospitals and ambulatory surgical centers.[2-4] Over the past decade, there has been a renewed focus on establishing streamlined service line management due to an increasing

Dr. Siddiqi or an immediate family member has stock or stock options held in AZSolutions, LLC, Monogram Orthopaedics, ROM Tech, and Stabl. Dr. Piuzzi or an immediate family member serves as a paid consultant to or is an employee of Stryker; has received research or institutional support from Osteal Therapeutics, Peptilogics, RegenLab, Signature Orthopaedics, and Zimmer; serves as a board member, owner, officer, or committee member of American Association of Hip and Knee Surgeons, ISCT, and Orthopaedic Research Society. Dr. Barsoum or an immediate family member has received royalties from Stryker; serves as a paid consultant to or is an employee of Cleveland Clinic and Healthcare Outcomes Performance Company (HOPCo); has stock or stock options held in Beyond Limits, Capsico Health, Custom Orthopaedic Solutions, Health XL, PeerWell, PT Genie, and Sight Medical; serves as a board member, owner, officer, or committee member of Florida Board of Medicine. Neither Ashley E. Chacko nor any immediate family member has received anything of value from or has stock or stock options held in a commercial company or institution related directly or indirectly to the subject of this chapter.

focus on value-based health care. Providing high-value care for patients has shifted to become the primary goal, with value defined as quality of care and outcomes relative to cost.[5] Because value is dependent on outcomes achieved, rather than volume of services rendered, there has been an ideologic paradigm shift within health care and orthopaedics, changing the focus from volume to value.[6]

Value improvement has shown to benefit patients, physicians, hospitals, and payers while further increasing health care economic sustainability.[5] Specialized service lines allow both hospital administrators and physicians to monitor outcomes objectively and allow resource allocation while delivering optimal patient care.[4,7,8] A notable trend has been reported in the establishment of orthopaedic service lines across large health systems nationally to achieve high quality care at lower expense.[4,7,9,10]

COMPONENTS OF AN ORTHOPAEDIC SERVICE LINE

An orthopaedic care transformation service line allows health care providers to adopt an integrated, streamlined patient care pathway, track relevant clinical and patient data, and allocate resource consumption efficiently. A streamlined care pathway through the establishment of a horizontal hierarchal system is critical, which allows simultaneous multidisciplinary patient management, especially those requiring subspecialty services.[4] Increased collaboration among clinicians can improve patient safety throughout the episode of care and generate better outcomes by using evidence-based practices and minimizing variations in care. However, physician alignment is one of the greatest challenges to a successful service line as multiple physicians and physician groups may have different ideas, goals, and priorities. Independent physician practices often have competing investments in ancillary services including ambulatory surgery centers, physical therapy, and imaging facilities that can further obscure a common vision with a hospital service line. Hospital administrators must be able to demonstrate to orthopaedic surgeons on staff at their facilities how a care transformation service line can directly benefit both physician and patient outcomes and further improve quality of care.

The value of orthopaedic service lines is embedded in the idea of value-based health care, which focuses on optimizing both clinical and economic success. Clinical success is measured through patient-reported outcome measures, complications, patient experience, and procedural survivorship.[11,12] Economic success is based on financial profitability for both hospitals and physicians alike, contribution margins, and overall market share.[4] A relatively new idea is that economic success is also based on saving the healthcare system and society money which can be passed along to patients through decreased premiums. It is critical for hospital administrators, payers, and surgeons to ascertain common goals before investing varying time, effort, and resources into establishing practices. The close working relationship with orthopaedic surgeons and vendor representatives can lead to the introduction of new, expensive products and technologies.[13] If hospital administrators and surgeons are not aligned in common principles and cost-containing strategies, the surgeon and hospital relationship can become strained if surgeons begin to view hospitals as inhibitors to progress.[13]

Identification of contributions of various personnel involved in the service line along with physician leaders among the health care providers enables greater alignment of goals and further allows clinicians to serve distinct leadership roles. Leaders from various specialties involved in orthopaedic patient care delivery, including anesthesiology, emergency medicine, internal medicine, physical therapy, and case management necessitate key involvement in service line implementation. The multidisciplinary integration and alignment encourages physician advocacy while maintaining transparency during program inception and through changes during development.[14] Different subcommittees are often necessary to focus on different aspects of optimizing orthopaedic care both clinically and financially. A close working relationship is important in establishing a successful service line.[13] Key stakeholders in and key elements of an orthopaedic service line are depicted in **Figures 1** and **2**, respectively.

HOW TO ALIGN ORTHOPAEDIC SURGEONS

Hospital merger and acquisitions (M&A) have substantially increased over the past decade, with healthcare systems aiming to create large corporations that optimize strategic and financial value.[15] The primary drivers of M&A include achieving economies of scale and decreasing cost while improving outcomes through increased volume.[15] Hospitals and physicians who perform procedures at hospitals that are newly acquired by larger health systems may often struggle with changes that transpire with M&A. Cost containment and streamlining patient care strategies can sometimes harbor resistance among clinicians and administrators. After M&A, it is especially critical to establish strong working relationships with

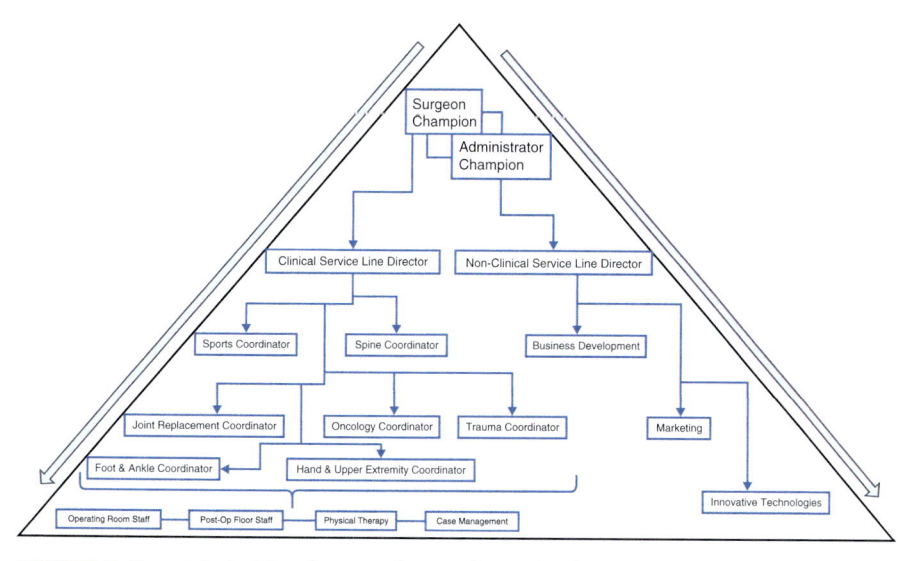

FIGURE 1 Key stakeholders in an orthopaedic service line with the primary focus on improving quality of care for patients.

Hip/Knee Osteoarthritis Care Pathways

Frequency of visits/touchpoints by treatment pathway

| Visits/touchpoints | Nonsurgical | | | | | | Surgical | |
| | Mild OA | | Mod OA | | Severe OA | | | |
	#	%	#	%	#	%	#	%
Prework	1	40%	1	40%	1	40%	1	40%
Initial Clinic Visit	1	100%	1	100%	1	100%	1	100%
Surgical Experience	0	0%	1	0%	0	0%	1	100%
Follow-up Visit	0.5	20%	1.5	70%	2.5	100%	2	100%
Home Rehab	7	25%	9	50%	15	75%	15	100%
Outpatient Rehab	0	0%	0	0%	0	0%	8	100%
Care Coordination	1	20%	2	25%	3	30%	2	30%
Smoking Cessation	4	10%	4	10%	4	10%	4	10%
Behavioral Health	1	20%	2	25%	3	30%	2	30%
Nutrition Counseling	1.5	40%	1.5	40%	1.5	40%	1.5	40%

*Mod = moderate, OA = osteoarthritis

FIGURE 2 Key elements of an orthopaedic service line.

surgeons to help align them with the health care system's service line mission statement and core values. By directing the focus toward optimizing patient care and improving outcomes, health care systems can show clinicians who are part of hospitals that are acquired that a teamwork approach is of utmost importance. Prior to implementing and expecting change within hospitals that have been merged with larger systems, it is critical for administrators to listen to surgeons' concerns and consider how a larger health system can help improve the surgeon and patient experience. Furthermore, creating gainsharing programs that financially reward high quality of patient care can also incentivize surgeons toward adoption of streamlined service line care pathways.

BUILDING A SERVICE LINE

Surgeon Champion

Building a service line starts with identifying a surgeon champion who will help drive programmatic change and leadership both macroscopically and microscopically within the healthcare organization. A few fundamental characteristics of a surgeon champion include an individual who places the program above individual needs and personal gains, someone who is motivated to optimize surgical volume and improve efficiency, an individual who is a team player with administrations, hospital staff, and other physicians, and a person who is supported by other orthopaedic surgeons to represent common interests and ideals. Identifying qualified surgeon champions is essential to improving patient outcomes, lowering complications and total cost of care, and enhancing overall patient and clinician experience and satisfaction.[16] A comprehensive list of surgeon champion characteristics is presented in **Table 1**.

TABLE 1 Surgeon Champion Characteristics and Goals

Energetic
Motivated to increase volume and improve clinical practice efficiency
Team player with administration and staff
Interested in controlling hospital costs
Supports the operational team and establishes a productive and positive operating room culture
Uses data and research to drive change

Administration Champion

Similar to identifying an executive surgeon champion, it is equally important to align with an administration champion who is able to understand a surgeon's perspective with regard to clinical, perioperative, and postoperative growth, and areas for improvement and optimization. Furthermore, administration leaders have to be willing to work creatively, have endurance to overcome frequent obstacles, and have the ability to invest time, money and appropriate personnel support to develop a service line. Ultimately, administration champions are responsible for ensuring return on investment through appropriate surgical volume with decreased expenditure in the correct site of care in conjunction with the surgeon.

Core Conflicts

Surgeons often have difficulty dividing their focus and attention between patient care and hospital management and administrative duties. Surgeons who are unable to allocate their time appropriately to meet clinical and administrative duties can often experience burnout. Burnout syndrome is marked with emotional exhaustion, depersonalization, and low job satisfaction and outcomes.[17] This is especially relevant as burnout rates among orthopaedic surgeons are substantially higher than those in the general population and many other medical subspecialties.[17] Surgeons also face a clash between goals and demands (providing value-based health care versus optimizing revenue but mitigating costs). Due to their innate nature, most surgeons may think that they possess the ability to personally fix all problems. It is important to realize that success in establishing a service line, and its longitudinal productivity, is an evolving process that requires constant learning, growth and potential for improvement by making and learning from mistakes. Unlike some orthopaedic complications that can often be rectified immediately in the short term, problems occurring during the business of running a service line may take longer to solve.

Nonclinical leaders may have difficulty seeing past costs to initiate a service line and through adoption of technologies that may require capital investment. Hospitals and surgery departments are often working with decreasing capital budgets that may make it difficult to satisfy surgeons who are seeking newer equipment or technologies that require substantial capital outlay. Administrators are also reliant on surgeon volume and an anticipated increase in volume to be able to demonstrate service line success. Therefore, common goal alignment with transparency is central to sustainability of an orthopaedic service line.

Culture Development

Service line development and commitment from all stakeholders revolves around establishing a culture of trust.[16] An important aspect of building trust is clearly articulating common goals that provide all staff members and physicians a clear direction and sense of purpose. Transparency can be further optimized by making all data accessible to staff so there is no confusion on how decisions and changes are implemented. Identifying tasks that can be improved upon easily during the first year of service line inception is prudent to further help instill trust among all participants. After fostering an environment of trust, data (accessible to staff) should be used to pursue and outline strategic priorities focusing on growth, positive contribution margins, operational excellence, and decreasing variation in expenditure management.[16]

OPEN COMMUNICATION

Orthopaedic service line success is dependent on the creation of a forum for meaningful dialogue between stakeholders and clinicians devoted to the process.[4,13] Interactions between administrators and orthopaedic surgeons may be erratic and contentious, usually occurring in response to obstacles and issues rather than proactive discussions. Therefore, establishing open communication is a challenging yet fundamental task for service line viability. The development of an orthopaedic steering committee is generally a method health systems use to cultivate an environment for the exchange of ideas and concerns. Decisions made during committee meetings should be implemented in a timely manner to further establish trust and rapport among stakeholders. Involvement of majority and/or all stakeholders, including administrators and clinicians, may not only help address trepidation but also improve compliance.[4,9] Because administrative and business training is often lacking during medical education, physicians may aspire to obtain business and financial education to help minimize vulnerability. Similarly, hospital administrators should educate themselves clinically on trends, emerging technologies, and procedural value related to orthopaedics.[6,13] Open communication and multidisciplinary care continue to be the focus of an effective service line, especially as legislative reform has driven health care from being volume and margin driven to being value driven based on quality and performance.[4]

LEADERSHIP STRUCTURE OF A SERVICE LINE

An ideal orthopaedic service line requires a leadership structure that includes parallel clinical and nonclinical personnel. A surgeon champion and administration champion are at the top and in charge of the constituents who report to them. A clinical (registered nurse, nurse practitioner, certified physician assistant) and

Value-Based Health Care in Orthopaedics

administrator service line director are both required to comprehensively understand both the clinical and business aspects. The service line should be further
subdivided into subspecialities to address the needs of subspeciality surgeons to
further optimize and streamline patient care. The subspeciality leaders should
have direct communication with operating room personnel along with staff members involved in postoperative care including floor leadership, physical therapy,
and case management (**Figure 3**).

COSTS AND CONTRIBUTION MARGIN

When implementing a new program, hospitals often track revenue from services
provided with associated expenditures to determine profits or loss. In orthopaedic
service lines, financial leaders evaluate and monitor hospital surgical caseloads,
discharge volume, and discharge dispositions, which represents most "sales"
attributed to orthopaedic procedures.[4] Financial leaders often compare orthopaedic "sales" relative to all direct and indirect expenses, which helps outline
the overall financial effect of an orthopaedic service line to the hospital (**Table 2**).
Contribution margins are the primary markers that are tracked to determine
profitability.[4,18]

If direct costs and/or expenses are unable to be covered, clinical and nonclinical leaders have to investigate areas of inefficiencies and consider efforts for
improvement without affecting patient quality of care.[4,18] Financial metrics that
assess time-driven and activity-driven costs are necessary in identifying factors
contributing to resource wastage and money loss. The challenge for most service
line administrators and directors during financial loss, however, is often managing
physician practices that drive the use of resources during patient care. Physicians
may be accustomed to using more expensive modalities, instruments, and technologies that lead to improved patient outcomes. It is important for health systems to

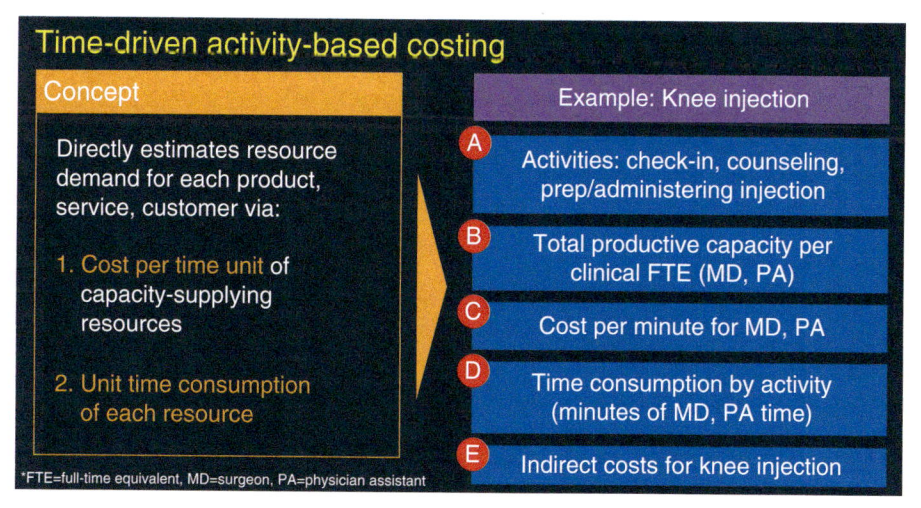

FIGURE 3 Ideal leadership structure of an orthopaedic service line. FTE = full-time
equivalent

TABLE 2 The Costs and Contribution Margin of an Orthopaedic Service Line

Cost Principles	Definition	Example
Direct costs	Cost of surgical care directly provided to patients; may be fixed or variable	Cost of implants used in surgical procedure
Indirect costs	Expenses associated with services that are often seen as overhead; may be fixed or variable	Facility expenses, laundry, and electrical costs
Fixed costs	Incrementally fixed within every episode of providing care	Cost of a specific knee implant regardless of patient
Variable costs	Incrementally changes with respect to various episodes of providing care	Duration of operating room use and associated cost, salary of operating room nurse, and anesthetic agents
Contribution margin	Most frequently cited markers of profitability for a service line; there are two types: 1. Variable contribution margin: net revenue (all the revenue the hospital receives for patient care), the variable direct cost for patients 2. Direct contribution margin: net revenue (variable direct cost + fixed direct cost)	—

Reproduced with permission from Sayeed Z, El-Othmani MM, Anoushiravani AA, Chambers MC, Saleh KJ: Planning, building, and maintaining a successful musculoskeletal service line. *Orthop Clin North Am* 2016;47(4):681-688.

have surgeons engaged in service line development and management to be able to make informed decisions that are fiscally responsible without adverse effect on patients outcomes.[18]

HOW TO MEASURE COST

Although there has been tremendous improvement in measuring and delivering higher quality of care, understanding how to quantify the costs associated with improved outcomes remains challenging. Traditional cost accounting methods use relative value units (RVU) to estimate indirect and direct costs.[19] However, traditional cost calculations are arbitrary and do not highlight the major intangible drivers of cost and are dependent on fixed costs.[19] Time-drive activity-based costing (TDABC) has garnered increased attention in health care as a cost estimation method that more accurately identifies drivers of cost by allocating indirect costs to activities performed by capacity-supplying resources, including clinical/

nonclinical staff and equipment.[19] TDABC cost calculations are based on two primary parameters: per minute cost for each resource involved and the average time required for each resource.[19] Personnel cost is calculated using salary and benefit data divided by the actual time worked, whereas utilization times are recorded either through direct observation or by interviewing personnel involved in the episode of care. Understanding and accounting for labor costs is critical; this factor is often overlooked and a major determinant in all episodes of care. Applying TDABC is a collaborative effort that requires both clinical and nonclinical knowledge and clear pathways identifying all steps in the involved care delivery pathways (**Figures 4** and **5**). Although the infrastructure to establish TDABC is more involved, with focus on the indirect costs, it allows for a more accurate representation of expenditures associated with any episode of care that can substantially improve care pathways, profitability, and influence pricing strategies.[19,20]

HIGH-TOUCH MUSCULOSKELETAL PATIENT CARE

Delivery of orthopaedic patient care requires a unique combination of resources regarding personnel, facility capabilities, patient amenities, and widespread staff education (nursing, physical therapy, case management). Administrators and directors managing orthopaedic service lines often inadvertently focus primarily on cost containment and cost reduction strategies while sometimes

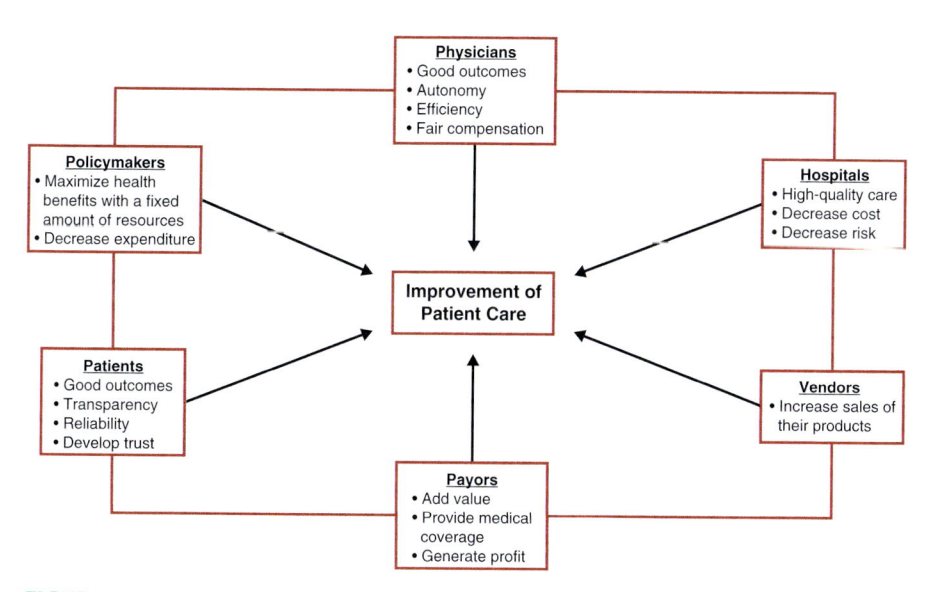

FIGURE 4 Process map of lower extremity osteoarthritis care pathway (including patient visits) by disease severity and treatment approach (surgical versus nonsurgical). (Data from Keswani A, Sheikholeslami N, Bozic KJ: Value-based healthcare: Applying time-driven activity-based costing in orthopaedics. *Clin Orthop Relat Res* 2018;476[12]:2318-2321.)

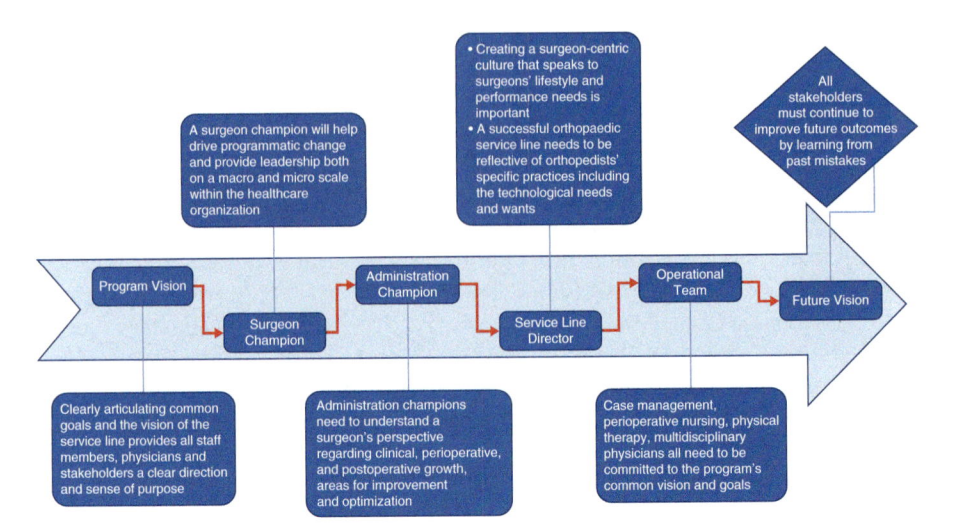

FIGURE 5 Example of time-drive activity-based costing (TDABC) of a knee injection procedure. The left side describes the components of TDABC. The right side outlines all the steps that are used to calculate estimated cost. (Data from Keswani A, Sheikholeslami N, Bozic KJ: Value-based healthcare: Applying time-driven activity-based costing in orthopaedics. *Clin Orthop Relat Res* 2018;476[12]:2318-2321.)

neglecting the necessary resources to provide a special patient experience.[13] Because orthopaedic care is predominantly elective for quality-of-life improvement, patients often select their physicians. Perioperatively, the care provided often transforms a medically stable individual into a sick patient for the short term. Because transient patient disability is often anticipated postoperatively from orthopaedic surgeries, approaching patient care with a high-touch model by proactively addressing patient concerns by preventing any potential pitfalls and obstacles will improve the patient experience. This approach to patient care can help distinguish orthopaedic service lines from its competitors and help bolster its clinical reputation in the community, which can ultimately drive procedural volume.

MUSCULOSKELETAL POPULATION HEALTH

As health care transitions from volume-based to value-based care, alternative payment models have been created to incorporate quality and cost into the reimbursement process. The fee-for-service (FFS) reimbursement model is the traditional and most commonly used health care model, whereby providers charge based on individual services (including diagnostic and therapeutic) rendered. FFS is a variable system, unless explicitly capped, because providers can increase their profits (indefinitely) by providing more services. Although FFS facilitates access to care, it places little to no value on coordinating care across activities, providers, or settings, which results in a fragmented healthcare system that makes it a challenge for patients and providers to navigate.

The value-based care reimbursement model has been growing in popularity in recent years as patients seek out simpler and higher quality health care services. There are several alternative reimbursement models available in the value-based system. These include pay-for-performance, shared savings, bundled payments, and capitation. The main objective in pay-for-performance models is to improve quality of care; however, there is little evidence of significant, uniform, or sustained improvements for select quality indicators. There is also increased risk of miscoding and upcoding under this model. The shared savings model takes the percentage of net savings and distributes it among providers through bonuses. Last, in a capitated model, clinicians are prospectively paid a sum of money per enrolled patient to provide all the care needed by the enrolled patient.[18]

With a population health model such as capitation, clinicians can participate in the savings and continued growth of capitated payments, providing strong incentives for the coordination of care and maximizing efficiency. In partial capitation, a monthly fee is paid to the clinician for a defined set of health care services for a particular population. Although the clinician bears full risk for the capitated clinical services, any services that are not covered are typically reimbursed on a FFS basis. Conversely, in a full capitation model, the provider network assumes 100% financial risk for the covered population. Reimbursement is determined on a per-member, per-month basis.[19]

Capitation can occur both at a clinician and system level. At the clinician level, for example, general practitioners can receive capitation payments for each patient enrolled in their respective program. At a system level, population-based funding models use information on physician practices and hospital and postacute care, along with demographic and socioeconomic data, to project the health care needs and expenditures for a region's population. System-level capitation allows networks to benefit from driving down medical costs relative to the expected cost. Clinicians have financial incentives to lower utilization and deliver care focused on health prevention and promotion. The longer the capitation period, the more likely clinicians will make use of health prevention and promotion treatments.[19]

The fully capitated model is ideal in orthopaedics because it controls costs while monitoring and managing risk. It aligns all stakeholders, patients, clinicians, payers, and health systems in a data-driven, evidence-based ecosystem that provides surgeons with clinical and surgical care pathways and promotes high-quality outcomes. A population-based approach of global, capitated care has the potential to allow the management of the full scope of medical economics related to musculoskeletal care while engaging providers in continued improvement, cost containment, and higher value.[20]

SUMMARY

It is important for physicians to become engaged in service line management in order to represent their value to the health system when negotiating for resources. Furthermore, the establishment of service lines with key stakeholders fosters a patient-centric multidisciplinary approach in an effort to optimize patient quality of care, productivity, and growth. Establishment of a successful orthopaedic service line begins with a clear program vision with transparent priorities. Identifying qualified surgeon and administration champions is important to forge a strong physician-hospital relationship toward a common goal. A service line director is critical in creating a surgeon-centric culture to optimize productivity and procedural volume and growth long term. A streamlined service line necessitates a large multifaceted team committed to aligning themselves with the common vision and having an individual sense of purpose for contribution. Finally, ultimate service line success relies on the stakeholder's motivation and commitment for continued improvement, especially learning from past missteps.

REFERENCES

1. Gee EP: Divide and compete. A new look at service lines. *Healthc Financ Manage* 2004;58(3):60-65.

2. Parker VA, Charns MP, Young GJ: Clinical service lines in integrated delivery systems: An initial framework and exploration. *J Healthc Manag* 2001;46(4):261-275.

3. Patterson C: Orthopaedic service lines – Revisited. *Orthop Nurs* 2008;27(1):12-20.

4. Sayeed Z, El-Othmani MM, Anoushiravani AA, Chambers MC, Saleh KJ: Planning, building, and maintaining a successful musculoskeletal service line. *Orthop Clin North Am* 2016;47(4):681-688.

5. Porter ME: What is value in health care? *N Engl J Med* 2010;363(26):2477-2481.

6. Novikov D, Cizmic Z, Feng JE, Iorio R, Meftah M: The historical development of value-based care: How we got here. *J Bone Joint Surg Am* 2018;100(22):e144.

7. Kwon B, Tromanhauser SG, Banco RJ: The spine service line: Optimizing patient-centered spine care. *Spine (Phila Pa 1976)* 2007;32(11 suppl):S44-S48.

8. Turnipseed WD, Lund DP, Sollenberger D: Product line development: A strategy for clinical success in academic centers. *Ann Surg* 2007;246(4):585-590.

9. Dundon JM, Bosco J, Slover J, Yu S, Sayeed Y, Iorio R: Improvement in total joint replacement quality metrics: Year one versus year three of the bundled payments for care improvement initiative. *J Bone Joint Surg Am* 2016;98(23):1949-1953.

10. Dummit LA, Kahvecioglu D, Marrufo G, et al: Association between hospital participation in a medicare bundled payment initiative and payments and quality outcomes for lower extremity joint replacement episodes. *J Am Med Surg* 2016;316(12):1267-1278.

11. Gray CF, Prieto HA, Deen JT, Parvataneni HK: Bundled payment "creep": Institutional redesign for primary arthroplasty positively affects revision arthroplasty. *J Arthroplasty* 2019;34(2):206-210.

12. Canovas F, Dagneaux L: Quality of life after total knee arthroplasty. *Orthop Traumatol Surg Res* 2018;104(1 suppl):S41-S46.

13. Lang S, Powers K: Strategies for achieving orthopedic service line success. *Healthc Financ Manage* 2013;67(12):96-100, 102.

14. Horwitz DS: Orthopaedic surgeon-hospital alignment at Geisinger health system. *Clin Orthop Relat Res* 2013;471(6):1846-1853.

15. Hospital Mergers and Acquisitions. Deloitte US. Available at: https://www2.deloitte.com/us/en/pages/life-sciences-and-health-care/articles/hospital-mergers-and-acquisitions.html. Accessed August 16, 2021.

16. Masson G: *How Hackensack Meridian Health's Robotic Surgery Service Line Achieved Lower Costs, Increased Surgeon Satisfaction.* Becker's Health IT, 2020. Available at: https://www.beckershospitalreview.com/digital-transformation/how-hackensack-meridian-health-s-robotic-surgery-service-line-achieved-lower-costs-increased-surgeon-satisfaction.html. Accessed November 30, 2020.

17. Daniels AH, DePasse JM, Kamal RN: Orthopaedic surgeon burnout: Diagnosis, treatment, and prevention. *J Am Acad Orthop Surg* 2016;24(4):213-219.

18. Olson SA, Mather RC: Understanding how orthopaedic surgery practices generate value for healthcare systems. *Clin Orthop Relat Res* 2013;471(6):1801-1808.

19. Keswani A, Sheikholeslami N, Bozic KJ: Value-based healthcare: Applying time-driven activity-based costing in orthopaedics. *Clin Orthop Relat Res* 2018;476(12):2318-2321.

20. Chen A, Sabharwal S, Akhtar K, Makaram N, Gupte CM: Time-driven activity based costing of total knee replacement surgery at a London teaching hospital. *Knee* 2015;22(6):640-645.

17 Role of Advanced Practice Providers in Orthopaedic Care

Ryan Desgrange, DMSc, MPAS, PA-C
Stephanie Muh, MD, FAAOS

INTRODUCTION

The addition of advanced practice providers (APPs), including physician assistants (PA) and nurse practitioners (NP) within an orthopaedic setting, has proved to be invaluable in not only providing safe and reliable care, but also in driving efficiency and profitability within a practice or hospital setting. Time and research have shown that APPs are a cost-effective solution to enhancing the patient care experience and in offering an affordable solution in both an established and an expanding orthopaedic practice. Although commonly grouped together at times for administrative purposes, PAs and NPs have their own respective differences regarding education, training, scope of practice, and salary. The goal of this chapter is to provide the orthopaedic clinician or administrator with the background and information about these two professions in order to decide how to best use the APPs for their specific goals.

Within the orthopaedic practice, APPs have traditionally been used to provide inpatient hospital care, outpatient clinic care, operating room first assist, emergency room consultations, and community outreach and education, as well as possible call coverage. The needs of the specific orthopaedic practice need to be taken into consideration when deciding how to best use an APP. Although sometimes grouped into APPs with PAs and NPs, certified athletic trainers may be a useful adjunct to an orthopaedic practice to offload clinical and administrative burdens of the physician. They can be used to assist with wound management, completing office paperwork, providing patient education, fielding patient care questions, and many other tasks that are helpful to an orthopaedic practice. The focus of this chapter will be the use of PAs and NPs within the orthopaedic setting.

Dr. Muh or an immediate family member serves as a paid consultant to or is an employee of Arthrex, Inc., DePuy, a Johnson & Johnson Company, and Exactech, Inc.; has received research or institutional support from Exactech, Inc. and Smith & Nephew; and serves as a board member, owner, officer, or committee member of American Academy of Orthopaedic Surgeons, American Orthopaedic Association, and American Shoulder and Elbow Surgeons. Neither Dr. Desgrange nor any immediate family member has received anything of value from or has stock or stock options held in a commercial company or institution related directly or indirectly to the subject of this chapter.

PHYSICIAN ASSISTANTS

PAs and NPs are being increasingly integrated in orthopaedic systems of care due to the exponentially increasing service demand by the aging population.[1] According to the 2023 U.S. News Best Jobs rankings, the PA profession ranks fourth overall behind nurse practitioner, software developer, and dentist.[2] PAs are educated in a manner similar to their physician colleagues with regard to the medical model of learning, where the focus is more on the pathologic and biologic components of patient health[3] (**Table 1**). The profession began in the mid-1960s as a response to a shortage of primary care physicians. Through the Duke University Medical Center, Dr. Eugene Stead Jr chose four Navy Hospital Corpsmen who had extensive medical field training to be among the first individuals to be a part of the first graduating PA program in the United States. The PA curriculum was based on the "fast-track" training of doctors during World War II.[4]

The PA profession is a master's level degree, with most programs lasting 26 months. Recently, hybrid tracks have allowed PAs to pursue an online learning component rather than the traditional in-person didactic route. There are currently 268 Accreditation Review Commission on Education for the Physician Assistant approved PA programs.[5] PAs during their training complete more than 2,000 hours of clinical rotations (surgical rotation is a mandatory item). Upon successful program completion, the candidate may sit for the Physician Assistant National Certifying Exam administered by the National Commission on Certification of Physician Assistants.

Maintenance of certification is achieved by successful completion of 100 continuing medical education credits every 2 years along with passing the recertification every 10 years.[6] Over the past few years, PA programs also have started to offer a doctorate level degree that can be completed in 1 year, typically while continuing to practice as a PA.[7] It is an attractive emerging trend for those wanting to transition into education, administration, and leadership.[8] PAs may also apply to various orthopaedic fellowship or residency programs in the United States to further develop their education and improve marketability for future job opportunities in orthopaedics. Most of these programs last 12 months and provide exposure to all orthopaedic subspecialties, and often include a stipend, health insurance, textbooks, meal allowance, vacation, and a certificate of completion in some programs.[9]

PAs can also obtain specialty certification (one of seven specialties) in terms of an Orthopaedic Surgery CAQ (certificate of additional qualifications) by accumulation of at least 4,000 hours of experience in orthopaedics, knowledge/skill attestation by a physician or lead PA, and successful completion of the National Commission on Certification of Physician Assistants - approved specialty examination.[10] The specialty certification has been seen as a way to show competency in the specialty, justify increased pay, and expand one's knowledge base. All PAs are required to obtain a state licensure to practice medicine; some states also require a controlled substance license to prescribe opioid medications. A collaborative or practice agreement is required for scope of practice and supervision of the PA

TABLE 1 Physician Assistant/Nurse Practitioner Comparison

	Physician Assistant	Nurse Practitioner
Required background before program eligibility	Bachelor's degree with program-specific prerequisites in conjunction with generally more than 2,000 direct patient contact hours	Bachelor of science in nursing with state licensure as a registered nurse
Degree upon graduation	Master of Science as a physician assistant. Doctorate level available at some campus and online locations	Master of Science in nursing with specialty concentration focus. Doctorate level available (encouraged by American Association of Colleges of Nursing)
Program details	At least 1,000 didactic hours and a minimum 2,000 clinical hours over 24 to 36 months depending on the program	At least 500 didactic hours and 500 clinical hours over 15 to 24 months depending on the program
Accreditation	Accreditation Review Commission on Education for the Physician Assistant	Accreditation Commission for Education in Nursing Commission on Collegiate Nursing Education
Licensure	Master's degree as PA with national certification	Registered nurse licensure as well as master's or doctorate level nurse practitioner degree with national certification
Certification	Successful completion of the Physician Assistant National Certifying examination through the National Commission on Certification of Physician Assistants	Specialty certification from: American Academy of Nurse Practitioners American Nurses Credentialing Center
Recertification	100 hours of continuing medical education (CME) every 2 years with recertifying exam every 10 years by passing the Physician Assistant National Recertification Exam	Must be completed within 5 years every cycle with option clinical practice hours (at least 1,000) and minimum 100 continuing education hours (American Academy of Nurse Practitioners Certification Board) or sit for specialty concentration exam
Practice restrictions	Practice medicine with a practice agreement with participating physician	Depending on state regulations, nurse practitioners in almost half the states possess full practice authority. Most often work with a supervising physician

(Continued)

TABLE 1 Physician Assistant/Nurse Practitioner Comparison (Continued)

	Physician Assistant	Nurse Practitioner
Additional specialty designation	Certificate of added qualifications (CAQ) in orthopaedic surgery recertifying every 10 years with concurrent physician assistant licensure and at least 125 continuing medical education credits in specialty during 10-year cycle	Orthopaedic nurse practitioner (ONP-C) recertifying every 5 years with concurrent nurse practitioner licensure

with a reporting physician assigned in accordance with state law or at the practice level.[11] PAs can write prescriptions in all 50 states, but Kentucky does not allow PAs to prescribe controlled substances.[12]

According to the US Bureau of Labor Statistics 2021, the median annual salary of a PA was $121,530 per year (**Table 2**), with an expected growth of 28% between the years 2021 to 2031.[13] Historically, PAs in surgical specialties such as orthopaedics

TABLE 2 Physician Assistant/Nurse Practitioner Salary Demographics

	Physician Assistant	Nurse Practitioner
Overall median base salary (orthopaedic specialty)	$112,000	$113,000
Median base salary per US region (nonspecialty)		
Region 1 (CT, MA, ME, NH, RI, VT)	$110,000	$115,000
Region 2 (NY, NJ)	$113,000	$123,000
Region 3 (DE, MD, PA, VA, WV, DC)	$103,205	$114,000
Region 4 (KY, NC, SC, TN)	$101,888	$110,000
Region 5 (IL, IN, MI, MN, OH, WI)	$107,000	$110,000
Region 6 (AR, LA, OK, TX)	$105,000	$118,000
Region 7 (IA, KS, MS, NE)	$102,500	$110,000
Region 8 (CO, MO, ND, SD, UT, WY)	$109,750	$113,000
Region 9 (AZ, CA, HI, NM, NV)	$117,500	$133,000
Region 10 (AK, ID, OR, WA)	$117,500	$125,000
Region 11 (AL, FL, GA, MS)	$102,750	$110,000

have a higher salary in comparison with other nonsurgical specialties. The 2020 American Academy of Physician Assistants salary review showed that the base salary of an orthopaedic surgery PA in the 50th percentile was $120,000, with an average bonus of $7,750.[14] The 2022 Physician Assistants in Orthopaedic Surgery salary survey of 1,159 of its members demonstrated that mean annual base salary was $128,585 with a mean total compensation (including bonus, office/hospital call, and other resources) of $144,282, with slight variations based on geographic location.[15]

NURSE PRACTITIONERS

The first NP program was created in 1965 at the University of Colorado by Drs. Loretta Ford and Henry Silver as a response to the physician shortage across the United States. Initially a certificate program, the NP program became a master's level degree in the early 1970s, and most NPs worked with the pediatric population. As time advanced, NPs moved into adult and other specialty areas. In 2004 the American Association of Colleges of Nursing published an article on the position of a doctorate (DNP) level education.[16] There are DNP programs currently in 50 states and it is widely considered to be the preferred degree for individuals pursuing the NP profession.[17] There are approximately 400 academic institutions with NP programs in the United States. Programs have both in-person and online-only options to allow students the ability to maintain a full-time job and complete the program.[18]

NPs must complete at least 500 direct patient care clinical hours of practice in areas such as pediatric, adult, or geriatric medicine in order to successfully complete their degree in conjunction with their didactic hours (at least 500 hours as NP, and higher at DNP level).[19] Their education is rooted in the patient-centered model approach, which focuses on disease prevention and health education.[3] Recertification as an NP is typically every 5 years, but these laws can vary due to continuing medical education requirements and recertification intervals.[12] According to the American Academy of Nurse Practitioners, NPs must submit a minimum 1,000 clinical work hours working as an NP, as well as a minimum of 75 contact hours of continuing education in their respective specialty area of focus.[20] Laws for NPs vary from state to state, as almost half of practitioners can practice independently without oversight of a physician.

Similar to their PA colleagues, NPs also have access to multiple residencies and fellowships across the United States that span 1 to 2 years of orthopaedic concentration. These advanced learning opportunities are often offered to both PA and NP professions as many specialties consider the professions interchangeable. Although not required to assist in the operating room setting (varies per practice policy), NPs can obtain (if not previously) a Registered Nurse First Assistant certification to further expand their familiarity and skillset in the surgical setting. NPs also may obtain an orthopaedic specialty delegation (Orthopaedic Nurse Practitioner) by obtaining 2,000 or more hours of practice as an NP in conjunction with the successful passing of the exam by the Orthopaedic Nurses Certification Board.[21]

NPs do enjoy full prescriptive authority, with the inclusion of controlled substances in the United States.[12] According to the US Bureau of Labor Statistics 2021, an NP's median annual salary was $123,780 per year with an expected growth of 40% between the years 2021 to 2031.[22] Although sources are much more scarce on NPs in orthopaedics, one resource points to a 2020 average base salary equating to $100,035 with an average bonus of $4,943.[23] It has been in the experience of the authors that PA and NP salaries are very comparable in large healthcare systems, given that both professions are used similarly and interchangeably. According to the 2023 U.S. News Best Jobs rankings, the NP profession ranks second overall.[2]

OPERATING ROOM UTILIZATION

APPs are critical to help enhance a surgeon's efficiency and throughput in the operating room. This is especially useful when "room-to-room" opportunities exist as this allows the surgeon to efficiently move from one operating room to another once the critical portions of the case are complete. The APP plays a critical role in all three phases of care. In the preoperative holding area, the APP can perform the history and physical examination, patient education, and any orders necessary. In the operating room, APPs can prepare a surgical case by ensuring all instruments and equipment for the case are present and that the patient is properly prepped and draped prior to the surgeon entering the room. Finally, APPs can finish closing the wound and complete transfer of the patient to the recovery room while the surgeon moves to a different operating room for better efficiency.

As discussed previously, PAs are required to do a surgical rotation as part of their clinical training. This is not a requirement of NPs, and the ability to use them as a first assistant can be dependent on state and facility restrictions. Although there are residencies and fellowships to develop PA surgical skills (sterile technique, prepping/draping, wound closure, etc), there is no certification that can be obtained as a PA. In contrast, NPs have the ability as a registered nurse to obtain a Registered Nurse First Assistant certificate separate from their bachelor's and master's level degrees. This allows for billing of Medicare and Medicaid for their services as well.[24]

Measuring APP productivity in regard to relative value units and profitability has always been difficult to calculate.[25] There are many unbilled added benefits of a PA or NP that do not have a direct monetary value, or that are somehow hidden within the boundaries of a global billing package. As health care reimbursement switches to an increasingly consumer-focused and value-based care focus, PAs and NPs can be seen as essential in optimizing patient satisfaction and clinical outcomes while maintaining efficiency and quality.[1] An evaluation of the Medicare breakdown fee schedule used in the global surgical packages include the preoperative, intraoperative, and postoperative phase of care and is credited as 10%, 69%, and 21%, respectively (cms.gov). Approximately 31% of this surgical package could be attributed to the work of the midlevel practitioner (MLP) performing the duties previously described while allowing the surgeon to use their time in a second operating room or on other clinical responsibilities.

For example, the Medicare reimbursement physician fee for a total knee arthroplasty (CPT 27447) is \$1,413.[26] Taking 31% of the direct physician fee for the preoperative/postoperative workup performed by the APP would equate to \$438.03 generated by the APP. The potential first assist reimbursement bills approximately 13.6% of the surgeon's fee. Additionally, if the MLP sees 200 surgical patients for their preoperative and postoperative care yearly this would approximate \$87,606 annually. Taking into account the patient visits seen by the APP instead of the physician, this would allow 200 additional revenue-generating patient visits for the practice. Clearly indirect revenue generation should be considered in the orthopaedic practice as direct measurement of only CPT codes for revenue does not provide the additional important contributions of an APP.

These hidden contributions of APPs are usually not reflected as direct revenue items in bundled payments and Medicare's "incident to" billing.[27] In "incident to" billing, the APP professional services are attributed to a physician (billed under the physician's name and National Provider Identifier [NPI]) with whom the APP works alongside. Medicare guidelines instruct on the eligibility for this type of billing, but nonetheless, it does not account for the value that a PA or NP brings into a practice if looking strictly at relative value units. This same understanding can be seen as demonstrated in the global surgical package, whereas some of the preoperative, postoperative, and intraoperative work performed by APPs is lost in the billing under the surgeon. Therefore, it is important that the physician understands the indirect productivity provided by the APP when determining their utilization in the surgical setting.

CLINIC UTILIZATION

Three basic clinic models are utilized within the orthopaedic setting with APPs (**Table 3**). Each of these models has advantages and disadvantages, and a better understanding of these models will allow the orthopaedic practice to choose the best model to meet their needs. The first model is an independent clinic, where the PA or NP practices in a clinic setting independent of the physician's input and the encounter is billed under the APP's NPI. This model is generally considered the most financially productive for the utilization of an APP. This model allows for greater patient access to the orthopaedic practice as the APP evaluates and treats patients autonomously.

This model is especially helpful for those nonrevenue-generating encounters (postoperative global billing) for which the APP can decompress the physician's clinic schedule in order to allow for revenue-generating new patient access. The independent model also allows for patients to see the APP as a suitable adjunct to the physician for orthopaedic needs in times of physician absence (vacation, illness, surgical procedures) as well as allowing for a capable clinician to see new patients and urgent add-ons. As expected, this model requires the most amount of time to train and mentor a PA or NP to feel comfortable as well as having the knowledge base to safely function at this level.

The second model, the shared clinic model, allows the APP to evaluate a patient and formulates a plan that is then staffed and reviewed by the physician.

TABLE 3 Physician Assistant/Nurse Practitioner Clinical Models

	Independent	Split	Shared
Description	Clinic setting where advanced practice provider (APP) independently evaluates and treats their own scheduled patients	Clinic setting where the APP and physician share a clinic schedule and split the patient volume with or without involvement of the physician in the APP evaluation and treatment of their patients	Physician and APP share a clinic schedule where the APP will have all of their patients in some capacity seen by the physician with treatment plan guided by the physician
Advantages	Endorses independent thinking on behalf of the APP Allows potentially for more comfort evaluating new patients in physician absence Financially more cost effective than the other models Allows APP to practice at top of scope Offloads nonbillable or global period patient encounters	Endorses independent thinking on behalf of the APP, but allows for ease of direct contact with physician for patient evaluation Can show a "team" approach to patient care Can allow top of scope practice when independently formulating assessment and plan Increases patient clinic volume for the physician Allows for APP to perform procedures and freeing up physician Removes potential burden for clinical tasks such as peer review, charting, prescription ordering, patient education	Excellent for new APP training and competency evaluation Can show a team approach to patient care Increases patient clinic volume for the physician Allows for APP to perform procedures and freeing up physician Removes potential burden for clinical tasks such as peer review, charting, prescription ordering, patient education
Disadvantages	Can be difficult for new APP to function at independent level Potential to decrease clinic relative value units of the physician Decreased insurance reimbursement compared to physicians in some cases May require more clinical staff and space to support	Potential to inhibit independent thinking and growth of midlevel practitioner (MLP) by staffing patients with physician Can compete with physician relative value unit obtainment Potential for decreased patient insurance reimbursement Potential for added resources and staffing	May prove difficult for clinic coverage in physician's absence due to normal process of evaluation and management dictated by the physician Potential for added resources and staffing Financially the least cost-effective clinical model utilizing MLP and physician combined time on each patient

This helps create a sense of a team-based approach to patient care, and is especially helpful for new graduates or hires into the practice setting. This allows for the potential of increasing patient access in the clinic with the addition of another provider working on the same schedule, but is the most financially detrimental taking into consideration the time spent with two providers evaluating and treating the same patient. In some instances, the APP acts as a scribe in offloading patient charting and orders that would otherwise require the surgeon's time. The APP could be best used offloading the physician's nonrevenue-generating encounters such as preoperative history and physical examinations and postoperative follow-ups, allowing the physician to have access for new patient appointments or schedule surgical cases during the APP clinic time.[25]

The last option is a split model in which the PA/NP shares the same patient schedule as a physician but has the ability to independently see patients from the schedule with or without the input of the physician. In the opinion of the authors, if there are constraints of support staff and space as well as the need for additional training/support of the APP, this model may be the most advantageous when compared with the shared model. This team-based approach allows the APP to evaluate and treat a patient without the need for physician oversight, but allows for intervention should a patient request to be seen by the physician or additional expertise is needed. If the patient is discussed or seen by the physician, then billing can be done under the physician's NPI if guidelines are met appropriately; otherwise, pending the type of insurance, the billing would be charged under the APP NPI. Once again, this model is particularly helpful if the physician becomes unavailable due to schedule conflicts such as add-on surgeries, unexpected illness, or other physician obligations.

The physician must consider the advantages and disadvantages of each clinic model and determine the right fit for their practice. As noted earlier in the independent clinic model, the APP practices without direct physician interaction. Financially, the traditional way to look at this is to generalize the reimbursement of APPs at 85% billing using the Medicare model (commercial/private payers may reimburse at 100%). The contribution margin is higher when a PA or NP sees a patient in the clinic setting for a visit rather than their physician counterpart. APPs cost approximately one-half to one-third that of a physician in terms of salary (generalized from Medical Group Management Association data).

If an orthopaedic physician's annual salary of approximately $300,000 is broken down to an hourly rate of $144.23, in contrast to that of an MLP using an average example salary of $111,000, this equates to $53.37 per hour. If Medicare reimburses 100% for an evaluation and management visit for a physician at $100, and $85 for an MLP at 85% there is a loss of $44.23 (100-144.23) using the physician to evaluate the patient versus the positive profit margin of $31.63 (85-53.37). Assuming a clinic day of 8 hours (1 hour cumulative break) with both clinicians seeing four patients per hour (28 patients per day) the MLP would make a positive contribution margin of $1953.04 compared to the physician at $1646.16 even at the 85% of Medicare.

This demonstrates the importance of utilizing the APP in more of an independent nature in the clinic setting to allow the physician to focus more on administrative, surgical, or physician-only tasks. The ability of APPs to read and interpret imaging studies is another important component in the ambulatory clinic setting. Downstream revenue can also be looked at briefly by referral services provided by PA/NP care of the patient for therapy, durable medical equipment, and other specialty services. There is an increase in the development of orthopaedic walk-in clinics staffed by PAs and NPs (autonomously or with physician oversight) and can be an indispensable component to help drive new patients into the practice, but also help contribute to future surgical cases. Pending the oversight and experience of the APPs, they can provide services such as imaging, splinting/casting, suturing, injections/aspirations, and fracture reductions, as well as ordering of therapy, advanced imaging, and durable medical equipment that are additional billable services.

A more recent consideration for the utilization of APPs in the orthopaedic practice includes the evolution of telemedicine in orthopaedics. Telemedicine is a more modern option in the ambulatory setting that can take advantage of the experience of an APP to see patients in the global billing period or where the patient is unable to physically meet the provider. Finally, it should be noted that in some ambulatory settings the use of athletic trainers has been helpful by providing services such as history and physicals, patient education, durable medical equipment fitting and assisting with diagnostic form completion that would otherwise be tasked with the physician or other support staff.[28] Optimizing and choosing the right APP can maximize one's practice by utilizing the care provider at the top of their scope of practice.

INPATIENT HOSPITAL UTILIZATION

Inpatient PA and NP productivity has long been a difficult area to account for billable services. It requires an emphasis by the orthopaedic practice to understand the nonbillable services provided that help with safety and efficiency in regard to the value of APP. Most commonly in academic teaching institutions APPs provide care for patients admitted to the hospital for postoperative care and disposition. The clinician assists in home and inpatient medication reconciliation, progress notes, rounding, dressing changes, physical therapy and specialty consultations, and discharging patients from the hospital. Many times, there is a specified orthopaedic APP inpatient service that allows for consistency in the care and management of the patient per the physician's protocols. This process allows for ease in training new APPs, vacation/illness coverage, as well as potentially limiting the potential in delay in discharges.

In many institutions with an orthopaedic residency, the resident may be used in a manner similar to APPs in regard to inpatient care, often working in collaboration with PAs and NPs. It has been the experience of the authors that the APP-resident interaction can be mutually beneficial in not only providing efficient care to the patients they serve, but also with clinicians understanding one another's role in health care delivery. PAs and NPs can help serve as educators regarding protocols and service specific needs to incoming orthopaedic interns and residents, and serve as the permanent team member on services with rotating residents. Many APPs take on the role of educator and precept PA and NP students, which serves as a way to educate future clinicians, and allow for assistance with floor procedures and chart reviews. It also serves a way for potential future employment of the student by way of work ethic and knowledge base during the rotation.

Finally, APPs can function as consultants in the emergency department and on the inpatient floors. Their roles can be as simple as the assessment of the patient and any required imaging with discussion of the supervising physician, to the APP formulating a plan and executing based on experience level. A PA or NP pending hospital privileging and scope of practice can perform procedures such as joint or fracture reductions, aspiration, injections, bedside digital amputation revisions, splinting or casting, and skeletal traction application. These procedural competencies would allow training for future staff and residents, as well as give the APP a component of educational oversight that may prove to be a job satisfier. Regardless of how the provider would fit the needs of an inpatient service, it is favorable for the physician to advocate for top-of-scope practice for the APP in order to fully maximize the clinician's potential.

SUMMARY

APPs play a critical role in a successful orthopaedic practice. This chapter introduces the role of the PA and NP and a variety of options an orthopaedic practice can implement in the use of APPs effectively. It is critical that the practice understands the differences and capabilities between the APPs as well as the direct and indirect productivity provided by the APP when determining the best utilization in the orthopaedic practice.

REFERENCES

1. Manning BT, Bohl DD, Redondo ML, et al: Midlevel providers in orthopaedic surgery: The patient's perspective. *Iowa Orthop J* 2019;39(1):211-216.

2. U.S. News Reveals the 2023 Best Jobs. Available at: https://money.usnews.com/careers/articles/u-s-news-ranks-the-best-jobs. Accessed May 29, 2023.

3. Staff Writers. Nurse practitioner vs. Physician assistant. 2020. Available at: Nursepractitionerschools.com website: https://www.nursepractitionerschools.com/faq/np-vs-physician-assistant/. Accessed November 20, 2020.

4. History of the AAPA. Available at: https://www.aapa.org/about/history/. Accessed November 20, 2020.

5. Accredited Programs. Available at: http://www.arc-pa.org/accreditation/accredited-programs/ Accessed November 19, 2020.

6. Becoming a PA. Available at: https://www.aapa.org/career-central/become-a-pa/. Accessed November 19, 2020.

7. Carder P: About the DMSc Program. Available at: https://www.lynchburg.edu/graduate/doctor-of-medical-science/faqs/. Accessed November 19, 2020.

8. Stephens S: *Physician Assistants Weigh Benefits of Professional Doctorates*. Health eCareers. Available at: https://www.healthecareers.com/article/physician-assistants-weigh-benefits-of-professional-doctorates. Accessed November 19, 2020.

9. Arrowhead Orthopaedics - ARMC Orthopaedic Surgery PA Fellowship - APPAP, 2013. Available at: https://appap.org/appap-programs/arrowhead-orthopaedics-armc-orthopaedic-surgery-pa-fellowship/. Accessed November 20, 2020.

10. Orthopaedic Surgery CAQ. Available at: https://www.nccpa.net/orthopaedicsurgery. Accessed November 20, 2020.

11. Byrnes JF Jr: Physician assistants: An overview, in Cernaianu AC, DelRossi AJ, Spence RK, eds: *Critical Issues in Surgery.* Springer, 1995, pp 177-181.

12. Current Evidence and Controversies: Advanced Practice Providers in Healthcare. Available at: https://www.ajmc.com/view/current-evidence-and-controversies-advanced-practice-providers-in-healthcare. Accessed November 20, 2020.

13. Physician Assistants. Available at: www.bls.gov/ooh/healthcare/physician-assistants.htm. U.S. Bureau of Labor Statistics. Accessed May 29, 2023.

14. AAPA Salary Report 2023. Available at: https://www.aapa.org/research/salary-report/. Accessed May 29, 2023.

15. PAOS Practice/Salary Survey Findings 2022. Available at: https://cdn.ymaws.com/paos.org/resource/resmgr/files/surveys/paos_2022_survey_report.pdf. Accessed May 29, 2023.

16. AACN Position Statement on the Practice Doctorate in Nursing. Available at: https://www.aacnnursing.org/news-data/position-statements-white-papers/practice-doctorate-in-nursing. Accessed November 20, 2020.

17. AACN Fact Sheet-DNP. Available at: https://www.aacnnursing.org/news-data/fact-sheets/dnp-fact-sheet#:~:text=DNP%20programs%20are%20now%20available,plus%20the%20District%20of%20Columbia. Accessed November 20, 2020.

18. Planning your nurse practitioner (NP) education. Available at: https://www.aanp.org/student-resources/planning-your-np-education. Accessed November 20, 2020.

19. Clinical practice experiences FAQs. Available at: https://www.aacnnursing.org/CCNE-Accreditation/Resources/FAQs/Clinical-Practice. Accessed November 20, 2020.

20. Frequently Asked Questions AANPCB recertification application and CE. Available at: https://www.aanpcert.org/faq-ce. Accessed November 20, 2020.

21. How to become orthopedic nurse practitioner (ONP), 2020. Available at: https://nursinglicensemap.com/advanced-practice-nursing/nurse-practitioner/orthopaedic-nurse-practitioner-onp/. Accessed November 20, 2020.

22. Nurse anesthetists, nurse midwives, and nurse practitioners. Available at: https://www.bls.gov/ooh/healthcare/nurse-anesthetists-nurse-midwives-and-nurse-practitioners.htm. Accessed May 29, 2023.

23. Orthopedic nurse practitioner salary. Available at: www.payscale.com/research/US/Job=Orthopedic_Nurse_Practitioner/Salary. Accessed November 19, 2020.

24. APRN RNFA Program for Nurse Practitioners. Available at: https://www.rnfa.org/aprn-rnfa/. Accessed November 20, 2020.

25. American Academy of Physician Assistants: Reimbursement. Available at: https://www.aapa.org/topic/advocacy/reimbursement/page/7/. Accessed November 20, 2020.

26. Procedure Price Lookup for Outpatient Services. Available at: https://www.medicare.gov/procedure-price-lookup/cost/27447. Accessed November 20, 2020.

27. American Academy of Physician Assistants: Quantifying PA productivity can be challenging. Available at: https://www.aapa.org/news-central/2020/05/quantifying-pa-productivity-can-be-challenging/. Accessed November 20, 2020.

28. National Athletic Trainers Association: Physician Practice, 2015. Available at: https://www.nata.org/sites/default/files/outpatient-rehab-clinic-faq.pdf. Accessed November 20, 2020.

Predictive Modeling, Machine Learning, and Artificial Intelligence

Bryan C. Luu, MD • Heather S. Haeberle, MD
Prem N. Ramkumar, MD, MBA

INTRODUCTION

Artificial intelligence (AI) represents the fourth industrial revolution and the next frontier in medicine, poised to transform the field of orthopaedics and sports medicine. However, widespread understanding of the fundamental principles and adoption of applications remains nascent. Recent research efforts into implementation of AI in the field of orthopaedic surgery and sports medicine have demonstrated great promise in predicting future athlete injury risk, interpreting advanced imaging, evaluating patient-reported outcomes, reporting value-based metrics, and augmenting the patient experience. AI has the capability of automating redundant tasks, allowing physicians to spend more time with patients. The technology should be viewed as a physician's aid, a tool that can better augment a physician's capabilities rather than replace their responsibilities. Additionally, it is important that physicians not consider this explosive area of research outside of their scope of practice. The future practice of orthopaedic surgery necessitates surgeons to gain a sufficient familiarity with AI and machine learning (ML) concepts, seizing the opportunity to wield a powerful tool and to take a participatory role in its responsible deployment.

AI AND ML

What is AI?

The application of AI in the field of medicine has been widely forecasted since the term was first coined by John McCarthy more than 60 years ago.[1] In 1955, McCarthy originally envisioned AI as "the science and engineering of making intelligent

Dr. Haeberle or an immediate family member serves as a board member, owner, officer, or committee member of American Academy of Orthopaedic Surgeons. Dr. Ramkumar or an immediate family member has received royalties from Globus Medical; serves as a paid consultant to or is an employee of Globus Medical and Stryker; has stock or stock options held in ConforMIS, Johnson & Johnson, and Overture; has received nonincome support (such as equipment or services), commercially derived honoraria, or other non–research-related funding (such as paid travel) from Stryker; and serves as a board member, owner, officer, or committee member of American Association of Hip and Knee Surgeons. Neither Dr. Luu nor any immediate family member has received anything of value from or has stock or stock options held in a commercial company or institution related directly or indirectly to the subject of this chapter.

machines." He predicted that these machines would be capable of performing feats previously thought to be exclusively in the domain of human intelligence, such as abstract thought, advanced problem-solving, and iterative self-improvement. At that time, this extremely innovative concept sparked much discussion over potential applications of such a technology and the implications such an innovation would have on the worldwide economy. In 1976, Jerrold S. Maxmen, a professor of psychiatry at Columbia University, predicted that AI would bring about the "post-physician era" by the 21st century,[2] describing the change as "possible, inevitable, and desirable".[3] Although AI has not replaced the role of physicians, this technology has already profoundly affected other industries. Some examples of the utilization of AI can be seen in the development of autonomous self-driving cars, online purchase recommendations, targeted advertisements, and high-frequency stock trading. Although the end user is generally insulated from seeing its direct employment, AI has already been established and fundamentally ingrained within many facets of today's society. However, the employment of AI in medicine has lagged behind that of other industries.[4,5] Despite initial excitement over the possibilities of AI in the medical field, practical applications of AI have only recently begun to materialize.

Topol[6] outlined several large-scale factors that are likely playing a role in the recent acceleration of AI implementation in health care. The first factor is economic: it is becoming progressively apparent that health care in the United States is a failing business model. Rapidly increasing expenditures are paradoxically paired with deteriorating key outcomes and decreasing reimbursements for health care providers. Despite having the highest health care expenditure per capita among developed countries, the United States consistently ranks poorly in key quality metrics such as average life expectancy, maternal and infant mortality, and health equity.[7,8] Innovation in the form of AI offers exciting potential in both improving health care outcomes and reducing inefficiencies that currently plague modern medicine globally. The second factor is the generation of patient data at an unprecedent large scale. From high-resolution medical imaging, continuously evolving electronic medical records, genome sequencing, and numerous diagnostic testing capabilities, each patient encounter produces a considerable number of discrete points of information, generating big data that cannot be effectively analyzed with human processing or standard statistical methods. One study of electronic medical records found that a single patient's health record was associated with an average of approximately 32,000 data elements.[9] In an age of information overload, a physician is tasked with integrating this overwhelming amount of data and synthesizing a clinical decision, a seemingly impossible task for a physician already given "insufficient time, insufficient context, and insufficient presence," as described by Topol.[6] Judicious employment of AI and its predictive abilities may provide a solution to these problems of economic sustainability and overwhelming data.

What is ML and its Relationship to AI?

ML is a subset of AI that involves the use of computational algorithms that can analyze large data sets in order to classify, predict, or gain useful inference.[6,10] In its most simplistic form, ML models are given inputs and outputs of training sets of real-world data to analyze and make connections from using various methods of pattern recognition.[11] The models are then tasked with creating predictions given inputs from a testing set, and its predictions are compared with actual known outcomes in order to quantify the accuracy of the algorithm. These algorithms exhibit the same experiential learning associated with human intelligence, having the capacity to continually assess and improve the quality of its analyses given an adequate amount of data inputs, with the potential to continue learning after implementation as new data are available.[11-13]

Deep learning can be thought of as an additional subset of ML (**Figure 1**). Made possible with increasingly powerful computational processing capabilities, deep learning models are more sophisticated algorithms that require less human supervision for development. Also known as deep neural networks, these models can mimic the structure and function of the biologic neuronal brain. Unlike traditional ML algorithms, which generally require human expertise and the predetermined transformation of raw data into a suitable format, deep learning models are a form of representation learning.[14] They work autonomously, allowing the system to discover alternative representations with differing levels of abstractions (**Figure 2**). The neural network begins with an input tier that receives the raw data. The network then progresses to a number of hidden tiers that each respond to different features of the input.[15] Through this process of developing multiple hidden layers, the model continues to develop more and more abstract representations of the

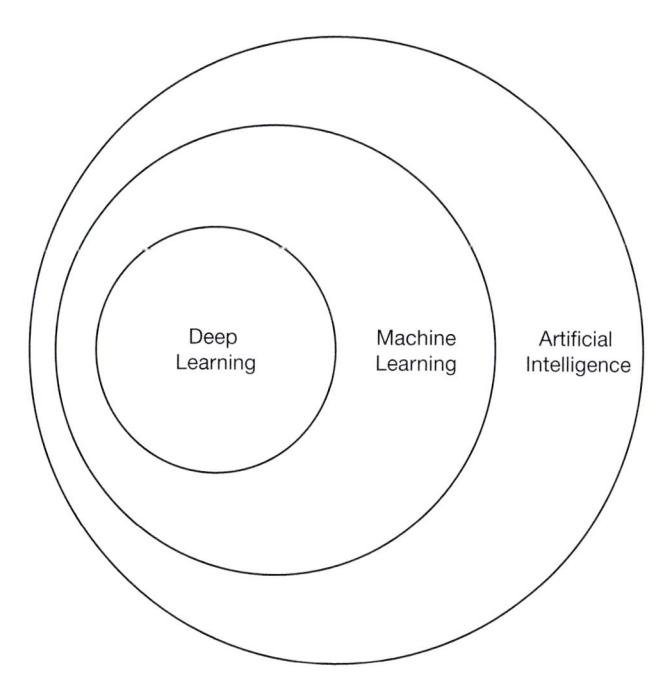

FIGURE 1 Diagram demonstrated the relationship between artificial intelligence (AI), machine learning (ML), and deep learning. (Courtesy of Prem N. Ramkumar, MD.)

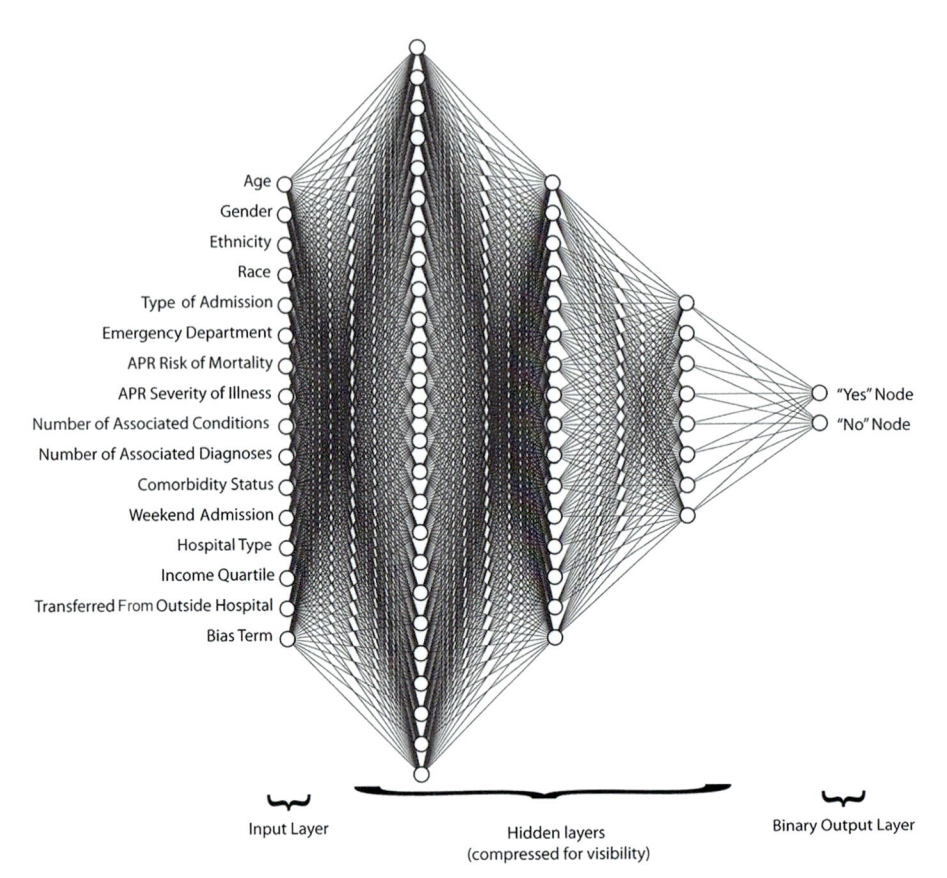

FIGURE 2 Diagram representing an artificial neural network model, demonstrating inputs, hidden layers, and binary outputs ("yes" or "no"), used to predict value-based outcomes (cost, length of stay) following primary total hip or knee arthroplasty. APR = All Patient Refined. (Reproduced with permission from Ramkumar PN, Karnuta JM, Navarro SM, et al: Preoperative prediction of value metrics and a patient-specific payment model for primary total hip arthroplasty: Development and validation of a deep learning model. *J Arthroplasty* 2019;34[10]:2228-2234.e1.)

data. Similar to the way the human brain functions, the machine is able to make "neuronal" connections from "dendrites" on multiple hierarchical data levels.[12] Eventually, the model learns to appreciate a concept on multiple layers and dimensions, building on itself to create a web of interconnected relationships.[11]

ML in Orthopaedic Surgery: Current Uses

In the field of orthopaedics, ML technology is still somewhat new, with limited studies detailing potential uses. ML can be used in orthopaedics for the identification of fractures from plain radiographic images, the identification of orthopaedic implants for hardware removal and/or modular revision,[16-21] the prediction of postoperative opioid use following total hip arthroplasty (THA),[20] and the evaluation of remote patient monitoring systems.[22] Some of these topics are reviewed in greater detail later in this chapter. Although the maturity of AI in the field of orthopaedics has lagged behind fields such as radiology, dermatology, and ophthalmology, research interest in ML in orthopaedics has increased rapidly in the past 2 decades.

In 2018, Cabitza et al[23] conducted a systematic review and reported massive growth in the number of studies detailing ML strategies applied to the field of orthopaedics in the years immediately preceding. Most papers focused on the areas of osteoarthritis (OA) detection and prediction, bone and cartilage imaging, and spine pathology detection. Evaluating the development of ML in the field of orthopaedics in the manner of traditional health technologies, the application of ML is still limited to phase 2 studies. It is vitally important for orthopaedic surgeons to gain a fundamental appreciation for ML and the paradigm shift it represents, not just in orthopaedic surgery, but in the practice of medicine as a whole.

ML IN THE ORTHOPAEDIC LITERATURE

In this section, the use of ML techniques in the execution of value-based health care in the field of orthopaedics is reviewed as it relates to (1) remote patient monitoring, (2) postoperative outcomes and cost, (3) injury prediction, (4) imaging and gait analysis, and (5) implant design.

Remote Patient Monitoring

Remote patient monitoring systems are an avenue to increasing the value of care, applied either in the preoperative and postoperative period. Although many companies have developed software to monitor step counts and activity level, the application of ML allows patients and health care providers to track their participation in home exercise programs and general activity levels. The surgical team can therefore track rehabilitation and intervene with calls or additional office visits if postoperative milestones are not being met. Although patients and practitioners have embraced digital technology (eg, glucose monitors), wearable fitness devices are a relatively untapped resource for patients and physicians to access personal analytics that can contribute to preventive care, postoperative care, or aid in the management of a chronic disease. This new technology understandably raises questions concerning the effect on users' health and well-being: the margin of error may be high when patients without medical training attempt to interpret the data from these devices. With appropriate frameworks in place, wearable devices that are integrated into health care systems could improve postoperative care.

In the context of research, these wearable technologies present an opportunity to collect data that can further support the goals outlined previously: collecting more data on patients' activity level before and after surgery to stratify risk levels of future patients based on their specific demographics, comorbidities, and injury or disease.[24] Of course, these wearable fitness devices may, as with other technologic gadget trends, drift out of popular favor. Furthermore, concerns about privacy and security of personal data are valid as users do not "own" the data that they create when wearing these devices. However, given their current popularity, the adoption of these technologies has potential.

Remote patient monitoring systems have been proven to be effective for patients undergoing primary total knee arthroplasty (TKA) for OA. In one cohort study of 25 patients,[22] patients who underwent this procedure downloaded a mobile application onto their personal iPhones and recorded preoperative mobility and patient-reported outcome measures, beginning 2 to 4 weeks before surgery. A knee sleeve was paired with the patient's iPhone via Bluetooth and the application notified the patient to complete weekly exercises. The knee sleeve and phone collected data on mobility (daily step count), a weekly range of motion checks, weekly patient-reported outcomes, daily home exercise program compliance, and self-reported daily opioid consumption. Some of these data points required active engagement by the patient/user and others were collected passively through the smartphone's native sensors. For this group, this system was found to be reliable, low maintenance and well received during the process of recovery from TKA.[22] Although this small cohort may not represent a broadly generalizable experience, the experience guides an ongoing effort to reduce cost and physician resources required to efficiently distinguish a patient who is thriving after surgery from one who needs additional intervention. It may be a feasible option to engage patients, communicate procedural value, and survey patients postoperatively. More studies are required to evaluate the clinical significance of the intervention and its effect on population health.

Currently, capturing patient data relies on administrators, mail, and faxed or phoned questionnaires, which may be inefficient and costly in comparison with the promise of wearable technology. For these reasons, wearable technology may also be an efficient alternative in collecting postoperative outcomes to improve both patient care and research endeavors.

Postoperative Outcomes and Cost

ML has been shown to be useful in utilizing patient-specific factors to predict postoperative outcomes. This feature can be applied to further improve payment models by bringing greater, more nuanced specificity to tiered reimbursement.[25] The Comprehensive Care for Joint Replacement model for bundled payments and quality measures was established to improve value and incentivize high-quality care at lower costs. However, hospitals that have demonstrated savings with bundled payments are more likely to be large, high volume, and associated with postacute care facilities.[26] Although bundling care has been shown to improve outcomes (readmissions decreased from 5% to between 1.6% and 2.7% and patients are more likely to be discharged home), bundling care does not account for the specific factors each patient possesses.[27] Patient-level factors are essential in predicting the likely actual cost and outcome of a procedure.[28,29] These specificities may shape or determine the course of treatment. A single reimbursement fee for a single procedure may therefore fall short, failing to acknowledge or incorporate patient-level factors that influence cost. A comprehensive model that can identify patient-specific factors that influence cost may be able to help determine more appropriate reimbursements and reduce the phenomenon of "cherry-picking" (selecting patients with fewer health risks) or "lemon-dropping" (avoiding selection of patients who would require more resources).[30,31]

For example, ML has been applied to predict the necessity of prolonged opioid prescription after an operation. In 2019, Karhade et al[20] developed ML algorithms for the preoperative prediction of prolonged opioid use after THA. Using data from 5,507 patients, five algorithms were developed, singling out risk factors for prolonged addiction such as age, duration of exposure, preoperative hemoglobin levels, and preoperative medications. This application of ML can be used to improve preoperative screening and prediction of patients at risk for prolonged postoperative opioid use. Understanding the risk factors associated with prolonged opioid use is a valuable application of ML technology because early identification in high-risk cases presents an opportunity for intervention. Additionally, the algorithm's predictive power presents an opportunity to more accurately estimate the true cost of a procedure, a cost estimate that includes the likelihood of prolonged opioid prescription or dependence, in addition to the direct costs of the procedure.[20]

In this manner, ML technologies can be applied to determine patients' likelihood of increased resource utilization; in this study, investigators predicted prescription utilization, but others have examined length of stay and inpatient charges. These specific outcomes help characterize a case's predicted complexity based on the patient's specific factors. Identifying and understanding the complexity of a case creates an opportunity to more accurately understand value. Although value has been understood as the relative benefit of the outcome to the cost, value is not standardized, as individuals may require different resources, bring different goals, and achieve different outcomes.

Beyond identifying risk factors for increased cost, risk stratification for the purpose of improving cost may be a useful tool to improve equity. In 2018, Navarro et al[32] used a bayesian model to forecast length of stay and cost, using factors such as age, race, sex, and comorbidity scores. A proposed risk-based patient-specific payment model was created based on the output. As patient complexity increased, cost add-ons then increased in tiers of 3%, 10%, and 15% for moderate, major, and extreme mortality risks, respectively. This proposition has the potential to encourage cost sharing, reduce patient selection, and reinforce patient access by reimbursing in proportion to complexity. The ability to predict a specific patients' outcomes and resource utilization based on their preoperative variables has important implications in increasing the efficiency of payment models to improve population health. Currently, risk is not distributed equally between payers and the treating team: surgeons are not incentivized to take on a large proportion of patients with increased comorbidities or case complexity. However, using ML to predict complexity offers an opportunity to fairly reward surgeons and institutions that take on greater risk. In the context of an aging population with increased comorbidities, a flat bundle reimbursement fee for patients with varying risk fails to match value with reimbursement.

Similarly, a 2019 study by Ramkumar et al[33] developed and validated an artificial neural network that was able to use patient-specific factors and outcomes to "learn" and predict length of stay, inpatient charge, and discharge disposition in unfamiliar patients undergoing TKA. Furthermore, this predictive model was applied in order to propose a risk-based, patient-specific payment model. The neural network was created using 175,042 TKAs and had an area under the curve of 0.748 for length of stay, 0.828 for charges, and 0.761 for discharge disposition. The model "learns" iteratively from training groups until it is able to predict value-based patient outcomes. This predictive capability has promise in application to patient-specific payment models and tiering reimbursement based on case complexity in which patients may be preoperatively assigned to a tier based on their risk factors, with a reimbursement commensurate with their stratified risk.

With the advancement of data aggregation and deep learning algorithms, the field of orthopaedics is on the cusp of a transformation. The adoption of ML in orthopaedics has the power to improve patient care by estimating complexity of cases and supporting progress toward patient-specific payment models that are more capable of incorporating specificities of each case.[12]

Injury Prediction

Professional sports are a billion-dollar industry that depends on the maintenance of player health as premium asset commodities. This involves many expenses including dieticians, trainers, physicians, and physical therapists, all with the goal of maximizing player performance and availability. As such, injury prevention is a focal point in optimizing player health. For the 2014 to 2015 National Basketball Association season, missed games due to injury accounted for a loss of $344 million in player salaries.[34] For the 2019 to 2020 season, the National Football League spent an estimated $521 million on injured players.[35] With the breadth of statistics and player metrics surrounding professional sports, ML may provide a competitive advantage franchises seek as they search for an ideal tool to aid with injury prevention and prediction.

In 2018, the Department of Orthopaedic Surgery at the Cleveland Clinic established the Machine Learning Arthroplasty Laboratory, with the goal of exploring practical implementation of AI techniques in the practice of orthopaedics, specifically in arthroplasty and sports medicine.[22,33,36-38] Most recently, this group applied ML techniques to predict next-season injury risk for both National Hockey League and Major League Baseball players.[39,40] For National Hockey League players, Karnuta et al[39] compiled yearly injury data as well as player-specific metrics such as age, 85 different performance metrics, and injury history. Multiple ML algorithms were trained and compared in performance for predicting next-season injury. This study demonstrated that the best performing algorithm (XGBoost) predicted next-season injury with an accuracy of 94.6% (SD = 0.5%), outperforming logistic regression and demonstrating good to excellent reliability. For Major League Baseball players, data encompassed 1,931 position players and 1,245 pitchers, as well as player age, performance, and injury history. Of the 84 algorithms tested, the best performing algorithm (top three ensemble) demonstrated an accuracy of

70% (SD = 2%) at predicting next-season injury. The model outperformed logistic regression and demonstrated fair reliability. In both studies, ML techniques were superior to logistic regression at predicting future player injury. Further studies may look into obtaining official professional league databases, which contain metrics unavailable to the public as well as more granular injury data that could improve the predictive power of these algorithms.

Imaging and Gait Analysis

ML has important applications in diagnosis, using both imaging and gait analysis. It has been used to automatically detect OA using imaging patterns and movement patterns, a feature that has potential for efficient and objective automated diagnosis.[28]

For example, preprogrammed mathematical algorithms and measurements have been shown to accurately diagnose arthritis on a radiograph. Urish and Reznik[41] described the use of medical imaging data in a technique that analyzes pixels in a radiograph to recognize pertinent structures and specific features to create a pattern. When presented with an unknown image, the algorithm was shown to "decide" if it was consistent with a known model for OA, or if it did not match. This algorithm may be used in both clinical applications and research applications to confirm the presence of OA. Furthermore, it could be expanded to predict which patients have more advanced pathology or would benefit most from surgical intervention. With an algorithm capable of processing images, a health system may be able to more efficiently triage a patient to the appropriate care provider, whether it be a specialist arthroplasty surgeon, sports medicine surgeon, or a nonsurgeon physician. These clinical decisions can be made using data rather than reliance on nonclinical schedulers. Additionally, they provide the benefit of increasing efficiency.

ML has utility in detecting knee OA using gait analysis. A computer system developed by Kotti et al[42] takes as input body kinetics and produces as output an estimate of the likelihood of the presence of knee OA. In addition, it identifies the discriminating parameters and set of rules that led to the decision. This explanation mimics "interpretation," and increases the value of the diagnosis. In the study, locomotion data from 47 patients with OA and 47 patients without OA were collected as patients walked on a walkway with force plates with piezoelectric force sensors. These sensors created output with the following parameters: vertical, anterior-posterior, and mediolateral ground reaction forces such as mean value, push-off time, and slope. With three steps or less, a reliable clinical measure could be extracted that would, in a rule-based approach, allow an appropriate analysis regarding the patient's likelihood of having OA, with an accuracy of 72.6%. Again, this automatic detection of knee OA provides a unique opportunity to create objective, sensitive diagnostic tools that can increase efficiency and quality of care delivered to patients.

In 2020, Ramkumar et al[43] applied a ML model to discern, for patients undergoing arthroscopic correction of femoroacetabular impingement syndrome, which preoperative radiographic indices from preoperative CT scans of the hip predicted significant changes in 1- and 2-year patient-reported outcome measures (PROMs).

These indices included the modified Harris Hip Score (mHHS), the Hip Outcome Score Activities of Daily Living Subscale (HOS-ADL) and Sport Specific Subscale (HOS-SS) as well as the international hip outcome tool (iHOT-33). Separate random forest models, trained on a database of 1,735 patients with femoroacetabular impingement syndrome, were created for each of the four outcome measures. The study found that no specific radiographic index or combination of indices was found to be predictive of improvement in any of the four PROMs at either 1- or 2-year follow-up in the setting of strict surgical indications. **Figure 3** illustrates a workflow diagram of how the ML algorithm interprets the relationship between radiographic hip indices and PROMs.

Implant Design

Optimization of implants and devices can increase the value that they provide both to the patient, and the value of investments made by developers. Currently, implant design is not as efficient as possible due to constraints in testing fit.

Kozic et al[44] present a method to assess specific anatomic and morphologic criteria that transcend shape variability in a population in order to optimize orthopaedic implant design. Although implants are mostly designed and tested through fitting on cadaver bones, which provide only a limited sample that does not represent the entire variability of the patient population, this technology provides an alternative. The framework allows an implant design to be virtually fit to samples drawn from a statistical model, determining which range of the population is most appropriate for a particular implant. Certain patterns of bone variability are more important for implant fitting, and this method allows for improvement of implant design such that a maximum target population can have a benefit.

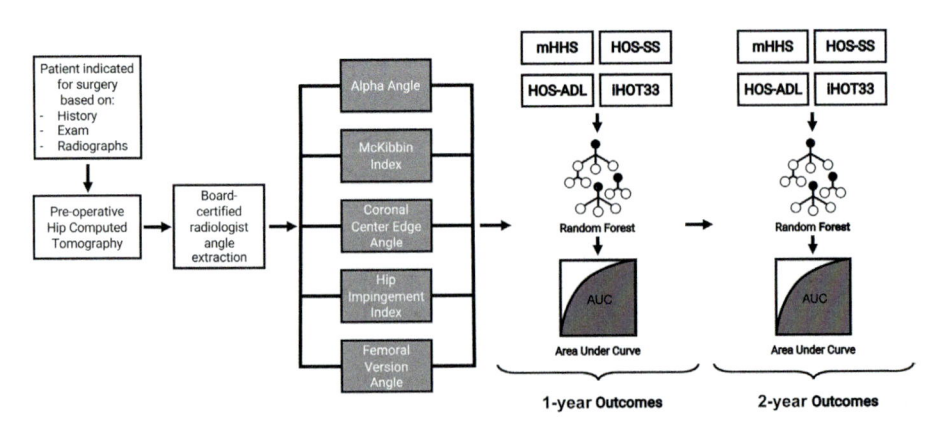

FIGURE 3 Schematic of the constructed machine learning models assessing for the relationship between critical radiographic indices and patient-reported outcome measures at 1 and 2 years. (Reproduced with permission from Ramkumar PN, Karnuta JM, Haeberle HS, et al: Radiographic indices are not predictive of clinical outcome among 1,735 patients indicated for hip arthroscopy: A machine learning analysis. *Am J Sports Med* 2020;48[12]:2910-2918.)

This study demonstrated the optimization of implant design, utilizing their proposed design and virtual validation method, of a proximal human tibia used for internal fracture fixation. Overall, implant design can benefit from these methods to improve fit for the patient, designer, and physician.

ML AND ORTHOPAEDIC PRACTICES

The day-to-day use of ML in an independent orthopaedic practice is not yet widely utilized. However, individual orthopaedic services across the United States have pioneered the use of ML technology in recent years and may serve as examples of what future deployment will look like. In 2019, Goltz et al[45] released a 90-day readmission risk calculator following primary unilateral THA and TKA. Using patient data from 10,155 primary unilateral THAs and TKAs performed at a single institution, a multivariable regression model was created to "adequately predict" the likelihood of 90-day readmission, based on preoperative parameters, duration of surgery, postoperative laboratory results (hemoglobin and blood urea nitrogen level), and nine comorbidities. This tool is available online for any provider to use and serves as an example of how applied statistical techniques, in conjunction with large amounts of available patient data, can be harnessed to provide benefit in patient care. Although many may not consider such regression models as "machine learning," it may be useful to consider ML as a natural extension of statistical techniques that have been used in the profession of health care for decades. Other online applications are similarly available, ranging from predicting risk of increased length of stay after joint arthroplasty to predicting inpatient payments.[20,46,47] It is likely that the use of such applications and online tools, powered by ML algorithms, will become more ubiquitous in the future, as well as paid private consulting services.

In 2018, the Cleveland Clinic's Orthopaedic and Rheumatology Institute established the Machine Learning Arthroplasty Laboratory (MLAL), with the goal of exploring practical implementation of ML techniques in the practice of orthopaedic medicine.[36,37] This program lays the groundwork for the future design and application of ML to musculoskeletal medicine. The team has developed and validated several ML models in several areas of research interest, all with the ultimate focus of providing patient-specific, value-based care.[22,33,36,38] The team has recently developed an image classifier to read preoperative radiographs and identify arthroplasty implant class and manufacturer before revision. Such a tool would be valuable to any arthroplasty surgeon, avoiding the increase in costs associated with delays in care, as well as misidentifications leading to lack of appropriate equipment available during the procedure.[12] Another area of study for the group has been the establishment of value-based payment models for THA and TKA.[32,38] Although the development of these theoretical payment models may not serve any utility for a single orthopaedic practice, these studies represent an initial foray exploring the use of ML in better informing reimbursement. As this research develops, lower extremity arthroplasty surgeons may be able to leverage these data for fair arbitration among hospitals, insurance carriers, and the Centers for Medicare & Medicaid Services.

LIMITATIONS

There are several limitations to ML and AI that have hindered widespread use. Arguments against include concerns over potential overreliance on so-called black box models, the subsequent deskilling of physicians and other health care providers, and the displacement of physician jobs. This fear of seemingly nontransparent ML algorithms directly underscores the need for interdisciplinary collaboration between ML engineers/developers and medical providers to improve understanding of ML tools.[48] It is also important to note that, for practicing physicians, there are likely several aspects of medicine that are not clearly understood or remain unexplained. For example, many physicians may not know the specific biologic mechanisms of actions of every drug they prescribe, especially if the mechanism has not proven to be clinically salient. Although a future physician may never need to fully develop and validate an ML algorithm, one would greatly benefit from having enough working knowledge to adapt such algorithms into their clinical workflow and systemic infrastructure with the ultimate goal of improving patient care.

There are additional ethical considerations that must be addressed in the future, such as issues relating to data sharing and patient privacy. Another concern is the introduction of uncertainty and accountability when a physician's desired course of action differs from what is recommended by an expert system ML tool. In medicine, making good decisions is an integral aspect of the profession, whether in regard to making an accurate diagnosis, an appropriate treatment plan, or laboratory interpretation.[49] It may be understandably frustrating for a physician to have their decision undermined, a phenomenon already experienced by doctors in the age of widely available online medical resources.[50,51] Additionally, ML may cloud clinical decision making or make physicians wary of deviating from definitive, seemingly infallible ML algorithms. However, gold standards of treatment and decision-making algorithms have existed in medicine for decades and only serve to improve patient care and the promotion of evidence-based medicine.[52]

SUMMARY

The general reaction toward AI and ML in medicine is mixed, with many in the field expressing apprehension over the disruptive nature of the technology and the effect it will have on the practice of medicine.

Despite its potential limitations, ML has demonstrated its ability to revolutionize the technology industry and is poised to transform medicine, particularly orthopaedics. ML has the capability of automating redundant tasks, allowing physicians to spend more time with patients. The technology should be viewed as a physician's aid and a tool that can augment a physician's capabilities rather than replace their responsibilities. Additionally, it is important that physicians not consider this explosive area of research outside of their scope of practice. The future practice of orthopaedic surgery necessitates surgeons to gain sufficient familiarity with AI and ML concepts, seizing the opportunity to wield a powerful tool and to take a participatory role in its responsible deployment.

REFERENCES

1. McCarthy J, Minsky ML, Rochester N, Shannon CE: A proposal for the Dartmouth summer research project on artificial intelligence. *AI Mag* 1955;27(4):12-14.

2. Maxmen JS: *The Post-Physician Era: Medicine in the Twenty-First Century.* John Wiley & Sons, 1976. pp 1-35.

3. Maxmen JS: *Long-Term Trends in Health Care: The Post-Physician Era Reconsidered.* Springer, 1987, pp 109-115.

4. Beam AL, Kohane IS: Big data and machine learning in health care. *J Am Med Assoc* 2018;319(13):1317-1318.

5. Poduval M, Ghose A, Manchanda S, Bagaria V, Sinha A: Artificial intelligence and machine learning: A new disruptive force in orthopaedics. *Indian J Orthop* 2020;54(2):109-122.

6. Topol EJ: High-performance medicine: The convergence of human and artificial intelligence. *Nat Med* 2019;25(1):44-56.

7. Papanicolas I, Woskie LR, Jha AK: Health care spending in the United States and other high-income countries. *J Am Med Assoc* 2018;319(10):1024-1039.

8. Macdorman MF, Declercq E, Cabral H, Morton C: Recent increases in the U.S. maternal mortality rate: Disentangling trends from measurement issues. *Obstet Gynecol* 2016;128(3):447-455.

9. Milinovich A, Kattan MW: Extracting and utilizing electronic health data from Epic for research. *Ann Transl Med* 2018;6(3):42.

10. Naylor CD: On the prospects for a (Deep) learning health care system. *J Am Med Assoc* 2018;320(11):1099-1100.

11. Haeberle HS, Helm JM, Navarro SM, et al: Artificial intelligence and machine learning in lower extremity arthroplasty: A review. *J Arthroplasty* 2019;34(10):2201-2203.

12. Helm JM, Swiergosz AM, Haeberle HS, et al: Machine learning and artificial intelligence: Definitions, applications, and future directions. *Curr Rev Musculoskelet Med* 2020;13(1):69-76.

13. Myers TG, Ramkumar PN, Ricciardi BF, Urish KL, Kipper J, Ketonis C: Artificial intelligence and orthopaedics: An introduction for clinicians. *J Bone Joint Surg Am* 2020;102(9):830-840.

14. Esteva A, Robicquet A, Ramsundar B, et al: A guide to deep learning in healthcare. *Nat Med* 2019;25(1):24-29.

15. Mintz Y, Brodie R: Introduction to artificial intelligence in medicine. *Minim Invasive Ther Allied Technol* 2019;28(2):73-81.

16. Adams M, Chen W, Holcdorf D, McCusker MW, Howe PDL, Gaillard F: Computer vs human: Deep learning versus perceptual training for the detection of neck of femur fractures. *J Med Imaging Radiat Oncol* 2019;63(1):27-32.

17. Lindsey R, Daluiski A, Chopra S, et al: Deep neural network improves fracture detection by clinicians. *Proc Natl Acad Sci U S A* 2018;115(45):11591-11596.

18. Gan K, Xu D, Lin Y, et al: Artificial intelligence detection of distal radius fractures: A comparison between the convolutional neural network and professional assessments. *Acta Orthop* 2019;90(4):394-400.

19. Kang YJ, Yoo JI, Cha YH, Park CH, Kim JT: Machine learning–based identification of hip arthroplasty designs. J Orthop Translat 2019;21:13-17.

20. Karhade AV, Schwab JH, Bedair HS: Development of machine learning algorithms for prediction of sustained postoperative opioid prescriptions after total hip arthroplasty. *J Arthroplasty* 2019;34(10):2272-2277.e1.

21. Zhang J, Dushaj K, Rasquinha VJ, Scuderi GR, Hepinstall MS: Monitoring surgical incision sites in orthopedic patients using an online physician-patient messaging platform. *J Arthroplasty* 2019;34(9):1897-1900.

22. Ramkumar PN, Haeberle HS, Ramanathan D, et al: Remote patient monitoring using mobile health for total knee arthroplasty: Validation of a wearable and machine learning–based surveillance platform. *J Arthroplasty* 2019;34(10):2253-2259.

23. Cabitza F, Locoro A, Banfi G: Machine learning in orthopedics: A literature review. *Front Bioeng Biotechnol* 2018;6:75.

24. Piwek L, Ellis DA, Andrews S, Joinson A: The rise of consumer health wearables: Promises and barriers. *PLoS Med* 2016;13(2):e1001953.

25. Ramkumar PN, Karnuta JM, Navarro SM, et al: Preoperative prediction of value metrics and a patient-specific payment model for primary total hip arthroplasty: Development and validation of a deep learning model. *J Arthroplasty* 2019;34(10):2228-2234.e1.

26. Navathe AS, Liao JM, Shah Y, et al: Characteristics of hospitals earning savings in the first year of mandatory bundled payment for hip and knee surgery. *J Am Med Assoc* 2018;319(9):930-932.

27. Mouille B, Higuera C, Woicehovich L, Deadwiler M: How to succeed in bundled payments for total joint replacement. *NEJM Catal* 2016;10:370.

28. Rondon AJ, Tan TL, Greenky MR, et al: Who goes to inpatient rehabilitation or skilled nursing facilities unexpectedly following total knee arthroplasty? *J Arthroplasty* 2018;33(5):1348-1351.e1.

29. Courtney PM, Bohl DD, Lau EC, Ong KL, Jacobs JJ, Della Valle CJ: Risk adjustment is necessary in medicare bundled payment models for total hip and knee arthroplasty. *J Arthroplasty* 2018;33(8):2368-2375.

30. Clement RC, Derman PB, Kheir MM, et al: Risk adjustment for medicare total knee arthroplasty bundled payments. *Orthopedics* 2016;39(5):e911-e916.

31. Humbyrd CJ: The ethics of bundled payments in total joint replacement: "Cherry picking" and "lemon dropping." *J Clin Ethics* 2018;29(1):62-68.

32. Navarro SM, Wang EY, Haeberle HS, et al: Machine learning and primary total knee arthroplasty: Patient forecasting for a patient-specific payment model. *J Arthroplasty* 2018;33(12):3617-3623.

33. Ramkumar PN, Karnuta JM, Navarro SM, et al: Deep learning preoperatively predicts value metrics for primary total knee arthroplasty: Development and validation of an artificial neural network model. *J Arthroplasty* 2019;34(10):2220-2227.e1.

34. Lewis M: It's a hard-knock life: Game load, fatigue, and injury risk in the national basketball association. *J Athl Train* 2018;53(5):503-509.

35. Injuries Cost NFL Teams Over $500 Million In 2019. https://news.hss.edu/injuries-cost-nfl-teams-over-500-million-in-2019/. Accessed June 28, 2020.

36. Ramkumar PN, Haeberle HS, Bloomfield MR, et al: Artificial intelligence and arthroplasty at a single institution: Real-world applications of machine learning to big data, value-based care, mobile health, and remote patient monitoring. *J Arthroplasty* 2019;34(10):2204-2209.

37. Artificial Intelligence and Machine Learning Across the Care Continuum in Lower Extremity Arthroplasty – Consult QD. https://consultqd.clevelandclinic.org/artificial-intelligence-and-machine-learning-across-the-care-continuum-in-lower-extremity-arthroplasty/. Accessed May 14, 2020.

38. Ramkumar PN, Navarro SM, Haeberle HS, et al: Development and validation of a machine learning algorithm after primary total hip arthroplasty: Applications to length of stay and payment models. *J Arthroplasty* 2019;34(4):632-637.

39. Karnuta J, Luu B, Haeberle H, et al: Machine learning outperforms regression analysis to predict next season mlb player injury: Epidemiology and validation of 13,982 player-years from performance and injury profile trends between 2000-17. *Orthop J Sport Med* 2020;8(11):2325967120963046.

40. Luu B, Wright A, Haeberle H, et al: Machine learning outperforms logistic regression analysis to predict next-season NHL player injury: An analysis of 2322 players from 2007 to 2017. *Orthop J Sport Med* 2020;8(9):2325967120953404.

41. Urish K, Reznik A: How would a computer diagnose arthritis on a radiograph? *AAOS Now* 2018;2018:32-33.

42. Kotti M, Duffell LD, Faisal AA, McGregor AH: Detecting knee osteoarthritis and its discriminating parameters using random forests. *Med Eng Phys* 2017;43:19-29.

43. Ramkumar PN, Karnuta JM, Haeberle HS, et al: Radiographic indices are not predictive of clinical outcomes among 1735 patients indicated for hip arthroscopic surgery: A machine learning analysis. *Am J Sports Med* 2020;48(12)2910-2918.

44. Kozic N, Weber S, Büchler P, et al: Optimisation of orthopaedic implant design using statistical shape space analysis based on level sets. *Med Image Anal* 2010;14(3):265-275.

45. Goltz DE, Ryan SP, Hopkins TJ, et al: A novel risk calculator predicts 90-day readmission following total joint arthroplasty. *J Bone Joint Surg Am* 2019;101(6):547-556.

46. Manning DW, Edelstein AI, Alvi HM: Risk prediction tools for hip and knee arthroplasty. *J Am Acad Orthop Surg* 2016;24(1):19-27.

47. Karnuta JM, Golubovsky JL, Haeberle HS, et al: Can a machine learning model accurately predict patient resource utilization following lumbar spinal fusion? *Spine J* 2020;20(3):329-336.

48. Ting DSW, Pasquale LR, Peng L, et al: Artificial intelligence and deep learning in ophthalmology. *Br J Ophthalmol* 2019;103(2):167-175.

49. Grote T, Berens P: On the ethics of algorithmic decision-making in healthcare. *J Med Ethics* 2020;46(3):205-211.

50. Semigran HL, Linder JA, Gidengil C, Mehrotra A: Evaluation of symptom checkers for self diagnosis and triage: Audit study. *BMJ* 2015;351:h3480.

51. Wyatt JC: Fifty million people use computerised self triage. *BMJ* 2015;351:h3727.

52. Podgorelec V, Kokol P, Stiglic B, Rozman I: Decision trees: An overview and their use in medicine. *J Med Syst* 2002;26(5):445-463.

Lessons From Abroad: Cases of Innovative, High-Value Musculoskeletal Care

Olivia Manickas-Hill, BA • Eugenia Lin, MD
Toby Colegate-Stone, MA (Oxon), MBBS, MRCS, MSc, FRCS (Tr and Orth) • Prakash Jayakumar, MD, PhD

INTRODUCTION

The fundamental principles of value-based care and high-value care for the orthopaedic patient can be observed in various global settings. This chapter provides an overview of six national health care systems and the current initiatives and challenges around the provision of high-quality care.

CURRENT ISSUES WITH US HEALTH CARE

Health care spending in the United States is much higher than in other high-income countries.[1] As a share of the economy, the United States spends more than 17% of gross domestic product (GDP) on health care.[2] This is nearly twice as much as the average for members of the Organisation for Economic Co-operation and Development (OECD): the United States spent $10,207 per capita in 2017 and out-of-pocket costs were above average at $1,122 per capita. However, this higher spending does not result in better population health outcomes. The United States has the lowest life expectancy and highest suicide rate, chronic disease burden, and obesity rate of any other OECD country. In addition, rates of preventable hospitalizations and deaths are among the highest across high-income countries. In addition to higher costs and poorer outcomes, the US health care system is characterized by inequalities in access to care and insurance coverage. Poor health outcomes are exacerbated by societal inequalities that affect social determinants of health, such as access to healthy food, housing, or financial security.[1-3]

None of the following authors or any immediate family member has received anything of value from or has stock or stock options held in a commercial company or institution related directly or indirectly to the subject of this chapter: Olivia Manickas-Hill, Dr. Lin, Dr. Colegate-Stone, and Dr. Jayakumar.

CURRENT GLOBAL ISSUES WITH HEALTH CARE

Although the United States faces some tough challenges, health care costs in many nations across the globe are also rising rapidly, due in part to demographic changes such as aging populations and increasing rates of obesity.[4-6] These demographic shifts have led to increased use of health care services[7,8] and subsequent inefficiencies in treatment pathways. Many health systems now experience the systemic consequences of inappropriate use of tests and procedures, waste of resources, inequity, inequality, and variation in care.[9,10] To treat a more health-burdened patient population, many nations are focusing on improving the quality of care delivered, based not only on objective clinical and process-level metrics but also on outcomes that are important to the patient.[11-14] Initiatives being implemented and lessons learned are described as the six countries discussed herein variably adopt the principles of value-based health care implementation in delivering high-value musculoskeletal care. These principles are (1) understand shared health needs of patients; (2) design solutions to improve health outcomes; (3) integrate learning teams; (4) measure health outcomes and costs; and (5) expand partnerships.

THE EFFECT OF MUSCULOSKELETAL HEALTH AND ORTHOPAEDIC CARE

As health care expenditures increase across the globe, it has been imperative to contain spending while simultaneously improving the quality of care.[11-14] Musculoskeletal conditions are common and providing health care for these conditions represents a significant portion of current and projected spending increases.[12] This is fueled by an increase in population age, obesity rates, and the use of costly surgical interventions.[12,15-17] In the United States alone, the estimated cost of musculoskeletal expenditures was $237 billion.[18] The high-cost, high-volume nature of musculoskeletal conditions and interventions, as well as inefficiencies in current management pathways provide substantial opportunity for improvement and a call for orthopaedic value-based health care initiatives.[16,17]

Several factors have led to experimentation in value-based orthopaedic care. Surgical interventions are common treatment options for many musculoskeletal conditions, are high in volume with discrete and easily definable pathways and workflows, and, for appropriate candidates, can yield excellent clinical and patient outcomes.[12,15-17,19] Orthopaedic care that is volume-driven and procedure-focused, rather than based on value, condition, or outcomes, at times does not require a 360° whole-person approach. Many traditional care pathways remain focused on delivering high volumes rather than evidence-based best practices designed around the biopsychosocial needs of the patient, some of which can be highly effective, low-cost, nonsurgical strategies.[12,20-24] The lack of attention to the holistic needs of patients, whether or not they proceed with surgical treatment, may result in suboptimal outcomes. This opportunity for improvement has launched a variety of value-oriented initiatives globally that are variably driven to improve patient outcomes[17,25] and costs.[15,26,27] Some of these efforts also focus on utilization and limiting the use of inappropriate interventions, promoting strategies to prevent unnecessary hospitalization, and methods to accelerate the development of standardized patient-centered care pathways over the full cycle of care.

The navigation of value-based health care reform is naturally receptive to the surrounding health care ecosystem and patient population. The following section includes a sample of international health care systems and initiatives that seek to implement value-based care in the treatment of musculoskeletal conditions. Lessons learned may help move US orthopaedic practices toward value-based health care.

THE UNITED KINGDOM: PATHWAY REDESIGN TOWARD HIGH-VALUE, INTEGRATED, MULTIDISCIPLINARY CARE
The United Kingdom National Health Service

Most United Kingdom (UK) residents access health care through the National Health Service (NHS), a publicly funded universal health care system.[28] Enrollment is automatic for UK residents who also have the option to enroll in private insurance plans for access to a private health care network. Health care accounts for a significant portion of government spending. In 2016, 9.8% of the UK's GDP was spent on health care, with an average of $3,943 spent per capita in 2017. Average out-of-pocket health care spending was $629 in 2017 and the NHS recorded a deficit of $6.1 billion US (£4.3 billion) in 2020. In addition to increasing debt, the NHS also faces a growing shortage of primary and specialty care physicians. This financial pressure has been associated with a deterioration in some aspects of care quality, such as patient wait times. Recent cost-containing strategies include halting staff pay raises, promoting the use of generic drugs, and reducing payments to hospitals. In 2016, NHS Improvement launched a program to promote more efficient use of staff, equipment, and facilities that was projected to save up to $7.1 billion (£5.0 billion) over the subsequent 4 years.

Primary care is typically delivered by general practitioners (GPs) who are the first point of contact for patients seeking care. GPs are tasked with coordinating care as part of their NHS contract, and direct patients to community-based or hospital-based specialists when appropriate. Most specialists are salaried employees of NHS hospitals who are compensated based on nationally determined rates. Specialists may also have private practices alongside their NHS practice. Providers must register with the Care Quality Commission, the national body that monitors performance. A National Quality and Outcomes Framework provides practices with financial incentives to improve quality when the practices meet certain benchmarks for compliance with best-practice standards and maintenance of patient disease registries. A series of legislative measures have promoted improved integration of care between hospital-based and community-based health services. In 2016, the NHS formed voluntary integrated care systems modeled on Accountable Care Organizations in the United States. The Getting It Right First Time program was also introduced in 2016 as a national initiative designed to improve medical care within the NHS by reducing unwarranted variations.

Pathway Redesign in Primary Hip Osteoarthritis Care: King's College Hospital, London, England

Local initiatives directed at improving outcomes relative to cost have been implemented outside broader government mandates focused on enhancing the quality of care. Physician-researchers operating within the King's College Hospital NHS Trust pursued value-based health care solutions for patients with primary hip osteoarthritis (OA).[29] Primary hip OA is a common condition (affecting 10.9% of adults in the United Kingdom older than 45 years) with high rates of surgical utilization (the rate of hip replacements in adults older than 45 years in the United Kingdom is between 0.1% and 0.4%), presenting significant costs to the health system and demonstrating variable patient outcomes.[30]

A retrospective assessment of 50 patients (20 men, 30 women) compared two surgical care models for total hip arthroplasty to identify elements that could advance the delivery of high-value care.[29] One model was a traditional hip OA pathway and the other an integrated multidisciplinary care pathway. In the traditional pathway model, patients were referred directly to an orthopaedic hip surgeon. These referrals were made at various points along the pathologic continuum in patients with hip OA care and came from multiple sources. In the second model, patients were treated within a multidisciplinary team integrated practice unit (**Figure 1**). This pathway began with patient triage involving extended-scope physiotherapists and consultations from orthopaedic surgeons before proceeding with multidisciplinary team care prior to surgery and postoperative physiotherapy. Patients were operated on by the same surgeons at the same orthopaedic elective surgical center with preoperative workups being conducted by the same teams. The primary differences between the two models were in the preoperative phase, specifically, the initial triage, prehabilitation, and overall care coordination by the multidisciplinary team in the preoperative and perioperative phases.

Value was assessed by a combination of patient-reported outcome measures (PROMs) and economic outcomes. PROMs included the Oxford Hip Score (OHS), European Quality of Life Index -5L (EQ-5D-5L), and European Quality of Life Index – Visual Analog Scale (EQ-VAS), all PROMs set by NHS England for the assessment of hip OA following total hip arthroplasty. Economic evaluation was conducted using Patient Level Information Costing System methodology and verified using the electronic patient record. Per-patient margin was calculated by subtracting the cost per individual patient from the reimbursement set by NHS England tariffs for the procedure. There was no difference in the preoperative to postoperative PROM changes between model 1 and model 2. Overall improvements in EQ-5D-5L, EQ-VAS, and Oxford Hip Score in both models exceeded the national expected average, and improvements were noted in pain, function, and psychological domains. Notably, there were disproportionate delays in postoperative physiotherapy for patients in model 1 through the lack of care coordination. Model 2 had lower costs than model 1. In combining the patient-reported outcomes and economic results, model 2 was deemed to provide the optimal approach through delivering improved patient outcomes relative to cost.

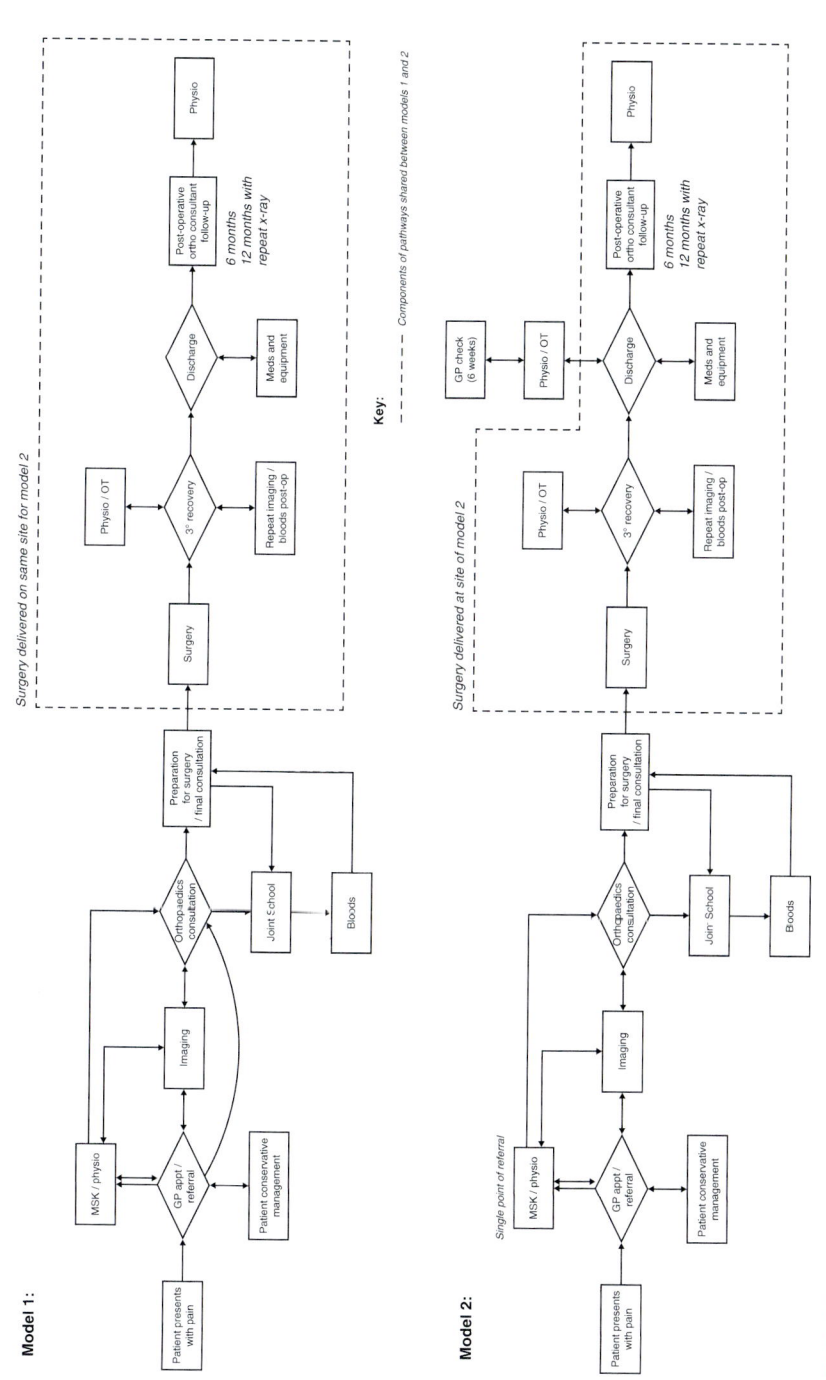

FIGURE 1 Integrated care pathway for hip osteoarthritis, Kings College London. GP = general practitioner, MSK = musculo-skeletal, OT = occupational therapist. (Reproduced with permission from Tikkanen R, Abrams MK: U.S. Health Care from a Global Perspective, 2019: Higher Spending, Worse Outcomes? The Commonwealth Fund, 2020. Available at: https://www.commonwealthfund.org/publications/issue-briefs/2020/jan/us-health-care-global-perspective-2019. Accessed May 8, 2023.)

Integrated Practice Unit-Driven Surgical Care for Rotator Cuff Tear: King's College Hospital, London, England

Surgeon-scientists at the King's College Hospital NHS Trust also conducted a prospective study of patients undergoing treatment for rotator cuff tears to measure the outcomes and costs of surgical repair over each phase of the full care pathway.[31] Surgical repair of rotator cuff tears continues to be a fairly common elective procedure in orthopaedic surgery (more than 300,000 surgeries are performed to repair torn rotator cuffs in the United States annually), and variations in costs and outcomes offer an opportunity for improvement.

A cohort of 20 patients (12 men, 8 women) undergoing surgical repair of symptomatic full-thickness rotator cuff tears was treated using a standardized integrated care pathway that was designed using value-based care principles (**Figure 2**). Assessment of the quality of clinical outcomes was achieved using a validated set of PROMs. Economic evaluation was accomplished through detailed mapping of the costs of each component of the care pathway and establishment of a baseline cost of care, followed by a comparison of this established baseline with individual patient costs. Outcomes were assessed using PROMs including the Oxford Shoulder Score (OSS), EQ-5D-5L, and EQ-VAS. Cost per patient was calculated using Patient Level Information Costing System methodology and verified using the electronic patient record. Per-patient margin was calculated by subtracting the cost per individual patient from the reimbursement set by NHS England tariffs for the procedure.

Patients reported improvements in postoperative EQ-5D-5L, EQ-VAS, and Oxford Shoulder Score. The average standard care pathway resulted in a lower cost than reimbursement, and consistently generated a positive profit margin.

ROTATOR CUFF TEAR PATHWAY

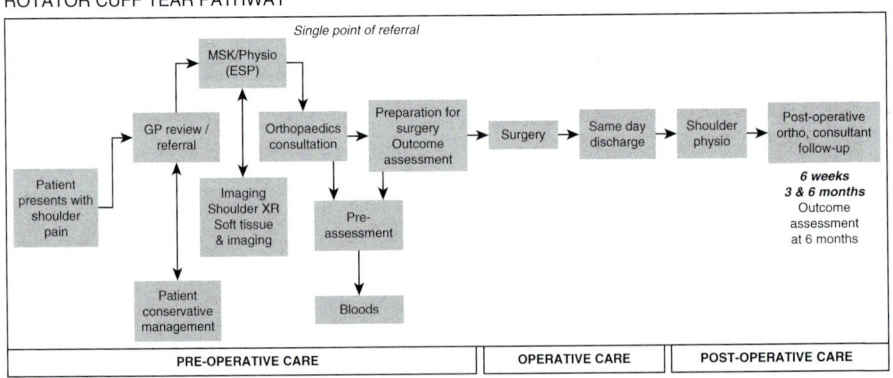

FIGURE 2 Integrated care pathway for rotator cuff tears, Kings College, London. (Reproduced with permission from Holzer-Fleming C, Tavakkolizadeh A, Sinha J, Casey J, Moxham J, Colegate-Stone TJ: Value-based healthcare analysis of shoulder surgery for patients with symptomatic rotator cuff tears – Calculating the impact of arthroscopic cuff repair. *Shoulder Elbow* 2022;14[suppl 1]:59-70.)

This standardized pathway for surgical repair of rotator cuff tears demonstrated increased value in both the improved clinical outcomes and the positive profit margins. Positive economic and clinical outcomes in these procedure-focused models of care for hip OA and rotator cuff tear highlight opportunities for innovative pathway redesign oriented around the principles of value. They demonstrate how rethinking pathways of care through relatively cost-effective care redesign can achieve value within a broader national health system.

However, the study researchers of the King's College Hospital NHS Trust underlined the time-consuming nature of data capture, even among the relatively small cohort, as a significant barrier to their approach. Low prioritization of data collection by frontline workers perceiving collection as optional rather than integral to a new approach also highlights the need for culture change and potential for linking data collection, and specifically patient-reported outcomes, more closely to routine performance evaluation and financial remuneration. These researchers also stressed that the methodology used to calculate value requires substantial buy-in from business managers and hospital administration in gaining access and control of cost information systems. This component highlighted the need for an effective, consistent, and communicative clinician-administrator relationship. Caution was expressed that any disconnect between clinicians and costing information system managers could make an already time-consuming process more arduous and less effective. These hip OA and rotator cuff care delivery models demonstrate that intentional care pathway design can result in savings for high-volume, high-cost orthopaedic conditions without sacrificing patient outcomes. A standardized value calculation could enhance implementation but would require a universal consensus on an approach to outcomes and cost measurement to remain meaningful, replicable, and comparable. Significant upfront investment is required for setup followed by consistent and coordinated efforts to maintain longitudinal PROMs collection and billing data acquisition and analysis. These pilot programs aim to be scaled across the orthopaedic practice.

SWEDEN: LEVERAGING BUNDLED PAYMENTS FOR PROCESS AND QUALITY IMPROVEMENT IN ORTHOPAEDICS

The Swedish Healthcare System

Legal residents of Sweden are entitled to health care under its universal, publicly funded health system, and 6% of Swedish residents are covered by additional supplementary insurance, which is typically purchased by employers to avoid waitlists for elective treatments and provide a greater choice of private ambulatory care specialists.[32] Less than 1% of health expenditures are associated with private health insurance. Health care expenditures amounted to 10.9% of the GDP in 2016 and an average of $5,264 was spent per capita in 2017. Out-of-pocket health care spending averaged $791 per capita in 2017. Costs containment strategies have included the institution of value-based pricing, subsidization of drugs, setting budget and volume caps, and capitation formulas. Recent policies have encouraged active patient participation in the health care process through shared decision-making and sought to reduce wait times for procedures.

Primary care accounts for 16% of Swedish physicians and 17% of all health care expenditures, with GPs or district nurses being the typical entry point for health care. The most common form of practice is team-based primary care, consisting of four to five GPs, nurses, midwives, physiotherapists (PTs), and psychologists. Provider fees are set by region and payment is based on quality targets, such as those related to patient satisfaction, care coordination, and compliance with clinical best-practice guidelines. Specialists are usually salaried employees working at university and regional hospitals or private clinics. Public and private physicians are typically compensated based on regionally defined levels, and publicly employed physicians may also work in private settings. Quality is monitored at the regional level and evaluated based on achievement of national and regional performance targets. Patient safety in surgical specialties is monitored based on indicators such as infection, injury, and complications. Care coordination and the shift of inpatient care to outpatient and primary care settings have been the focus of policies since the 1990s.

Orthochoice Bundled Payment for Total Joint Replacement for Hip and Knee OA, Stockholm, Sweden

In 2008, Sweden's health care expenditures accounted for 9.2% of its GDP.[33-35] Wait times for nonemergency treatments were long, and the wait list for orthopaedic procedures at times exceeded 2 years. In response to concerns of increasing costs and growing wait times for joint replacement surgeries, Sweden launched OrthoChoice in 2009, a bundled payment program for total hip and total knee replacements based in Stockholm County. The program was launched across all major hospitals and three private specialized centers. As one of the earliest examples of bundled payment systems in Sweden, OrthoChoice reimbursed health care providers based on outcomes and close monitoring of quality and care delivery. The scheme covered the patient's preoperative visit, diagnostic tests, surgery, implant, postoperative care, and follow-up visits with clinicians maintaining responsibility for nonacute complications up to 5 years postoperatively. Low-risk patients were expected to be discharged directly home after the procedure, with the potential for eliminating many of the expenses accrued by overnight stays or transfer to rehabilitation facilities. Care quality was measured based on patient-reported pain and quality of life. Evaluation was based on a combination of patient-reported outcomes, complication rates, wait time, costs, and savings per procedure. Clinicians qualified for a payment of a total of 3.2% of the €6,300 fee, an amount that is withheld and paid retroactively only if the clinician meets a predefined set of outcome goals.

Initial results demonstrated a positive effect on outcomes and costs in the Orthochoice program).[36] By 2011, substantial savings were achieved along with decreases in wait time (rate of patients waiting 90 days or more for their joint replacement surgery) despite a simultaneous increase in procedural volume, and without adversely affecting patient and clinical outcomes. Specifically, there was an overall decrease in complication rates (a reduction by almost 40% over 2 years since the program's introduction) and revision surgery rates (by approximately 20%) compared with control groups using traditional reimbursement plans. The overall per-patient costs were reduced by 17% primarily through lower payments to providers.[34] Changes in patient-reported pain and quality of life remained unaffected by cost-saving measures.

In addition, Orthochoice also signaled opportunities for improvement. Patient selection criteria for this program were based on the American Society of Anesthesiologists (ASA) classification and included only patients from the lowest risk categories (ie, ASA 1 and 2). Selecting individuals with lower risk and comorbidity profiles (or "cherry-picking") can naturally skew outcomes as individuals may be less likely to experience costly complications or readmissions. Definition of selection criteria that account for sociodemographic and personal characteristics as well as clinical factors, episode triggers, alongside robust risk adjustment are important elements of value-based care delivery models including bundled payment arrangements. These components should be incorporated into service lines and care pathways tailored to meet the needs of patients. For instance, engaging patients early in the pathway, managing their expectations, and empowering them with appropriate education and skills through effective communication can lead to postoperative discharge home rather than a rehabilitation facility. This not only reduces costs but enables patients to recover safely and effectively in familiar settings.

The program has added more recent trends, including an increase in the volume of surgeries at specialized orthopaedic centers while decreasing the number performed at hospitals, providing a general range of specialty services. In addition, new private operators have also been developed that have engaged in less complicated procedures whereas acute hospitals provide care for the more complex procedures.[37]

Building on the OrthoChoice experience, Stockholm County proceeded to implement further advanced bundled episode payment arrangements, including a spinal care bundle in 2013 that encompasses the full cycle of care, incorporates risk- and outcome-adjusted payments, and requires providers to cover the costs of complications up to 2 years after treatment.[37] These initiatives have also played a part in the development of SVEUS, a Swedish value-based health care knowledge development and sharing project that has guided other counties to introduce additional quality-related payment programs. The OrthoChoice program effectively showed how the delivery of a package of services for a well-defined, high-volume, high-cost procedure through a specialized network of designated providers and hospitals can result in substantial savings and positive outcomes. Implementation and assessment of the fidelity and feasibility of such pilot programs provide an opportunity to observe, learn, develop, and expand such models at scale.

DENMARK: IMPLEMENTING EVIDENCE-BASED 360° WHOLE-PERSON CARE FOR OA

The Danish Healthcare System

Denmark has a universal healthcare system originating from the Danish sickness funds of the late 19th century.[38] The current health program has been in operation since 1973. Danish residents are automatically enrolled in one of two insurance options. Group 1 (chosen by 98%) operates with GPs as gatekeepers to specialist care for which patients require a referral. Group 2 (chosen by the remaining 2%) allows patients to access specialists directly and without a referral, though patients are subject to copayments. Forty-two percent of Danish residents choose to purchase voluntary health insurance that covers certain copayments and services not covered by the national health system. They may also choose to purchase supplementary insurance that increases access to private providers and elective procedures; 30% of Danes are enrolled in supplementary insurance. The average out-of-pocket health care spending per capita was $690 in 2017. In 2016, a 10.4% share of Denmark's GDP was spent on health care (with an average of $5,025 spent per capita in 2017), of which 84% was spent on the public sector. To manage health care costs, the national government has set budgets and sanctions for regions and municipalities that incorporate a surplus. National guidelines and promotion of generic pharmaceuticals are also used to control health care expenditures.

Most GPs are self-employed, comprising 22% of doctors. Compensation is accounted for by fee-for-service (FFS; 70% of income) and capitation (30% of income), paid by the regions using nationally determined rates. Specialist care is delivered at ambulatory clinics operated by hospitals or private facilities and is reimbursed through a combination of FFS paid by the region, out-of-pocket paid by individual patients, and private insurance.

The Danish Health Authority has developed multiple standard treatment pathways to improve consistency in care quality, with a particular focus on chronic disease prevention and follow-up. However, there are no national economic incentives bound by quality. Recent national initiatives have concentrated on shifting care from the hospital to primary care and care in the community. Government guidelines for the allocation of regional funding tied financial incentives to lower rates of hospitalization per capita, reduction of in-hospital treatment for chronic conditions (reducing unnecessary readmissions) and increase in the use of telemedicine.

Good Life with OsteoArthritis in Denmark (GLA:D), Southern Denmark

In response to the slow uptake of evidence-based clinical guidelines for OA management, the University of Southern Denmark launched the Good Life with OsteoArthritis in Denmark (GLA:D) initiative in 2013.[39] The aim of the program was to increase the application of evidence-based guidelines in clinical practices to improve outcomes for patients with hip and knee OA.

GLA:D was administered by PTs trained in delivering guideline-adherent OA care. The PTs led patients through an 8-week course consisting of 2 weeks of educational sessions designed to increase the patient's understanding of OA and its treatment options, and 6 weeks of biweekly supervised neuromuscular exercise sessions

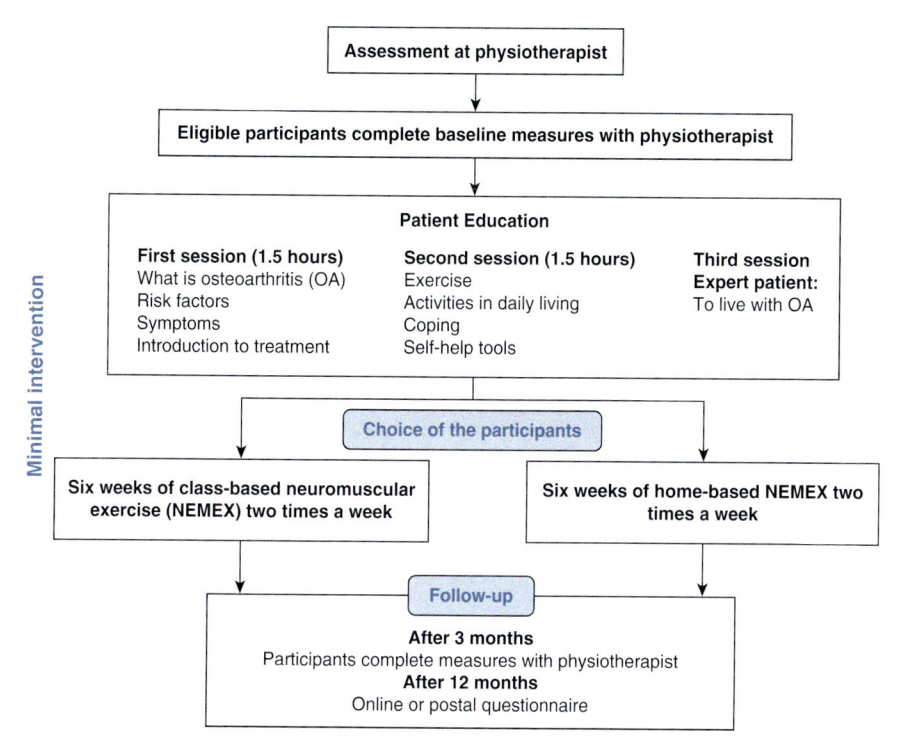

FIGURE 3 Flow diagram for the good life with osteoarthritis in Denmark. (Reproduced with permission from Skou ST, Roos EM: Good Life with osteoArthritis in Denmark (GLA:D™): Evidence-based education and supervised neuromuscular exercise delivered by certified physiotherapists nationwide. *BMC Musculoskelet Disord* 2017;18[1]:72.)

(**Figure 3**). Patients were also encouraged to participate in a supplemental group exercise program under PT supervision; those who opted out were given the option of completing the exercises at home. Patients were encouraged to continue to exercise with a PT in their community or on their own after the program ended.

Outcomes were measured through objective PT-assessed tests and PROMs. Objective physical activity-related outcomes included the 40-m fast-paced walk test and the 30-second chair-stand test. PROMs assessed symptom intensity, activity tolerance, and quality of life. Analgesic intake was also assessed. Data were collected at baseline, 3 months, and 12 months, and stored in a national electronic GLA:D registry.

Between 2013 and 2015, 9,825 patients with hip and/or knee OA registered baseline GLA:D data. Of these patients, most completed the program and attended the 3-month and 1-year follow-ups. Significant improvements in pain intensity were reported at 3 and 12 months, even among patients who had not undergone total joint arthroplasty. There was a reduction in the number of patients taking analgesics for both knee and hip OA. Patients experienced improvements in objective measures of functionality (the 30-second chair-stand test and 40-m fast-paced walk test) at 3 and 12 months, and changes were similar for patients who had undergone total joint arthroplasty as well as those receiving nonsurgical treatment only. PROM results indicated improvements in activity tolerance, quality of life, and reduction in time off work for sickness at both follow-up time points.

Many patients eventually underwent surgery and healthier patients (those with lower comorbidity indices) unsurprisingly tended to have fewer complications and undergo less intensive postoperative care with improved outcomes and lower costs compared to those with multiple comorbidities.[3,9,14] The improvements in general health and quality of life have implications for other chronic diseases. More comprehensive models of OA care potentially reduce the health care costs associated with the management of concurrent high-cost medical conditions such as diabetes and obesity.

The GLA:D program demonstrated that whole-person treatment of OA could help improve patient outcomes and manage costs. The initiative also highlighted the feasibility of designing large-scale care models using evidence-based clinical guidelines for a full range of nonsurgical and surgical treatment strategies for OA. The program has continued to improve over time since its inception with increasing interoperability of the database, increased consistency in longitudinal outcomes collection with patient and clinician involvement to enhance the data collection platform.

NEW ZEALAND: EXPANDING MUSCULOSKELETAL TEAMS AT THE POINT OF CARE

New Zealand's Healthcare System

New Zealand operates a universal health system;[40] however, 33% of New Zealanders purchase private insurance, which covers elective surgeries and faster access to certain other treatments. In 2017, 9% of New Zealand's GDP was spent on health, 78.7% of which was accounted for by public spending. The per-capita cost of health care came to an average of $3,742 in 2017, with an average of $508 spent out of pocket. Costs are contained through setting budgets and requiring district health boards to design proposals that fit within these budgets. The national government subsidizes certain drugs and charges patients the full cost if they opt to use an unsubsidized drug.

GPs are reimbursed through a mix of capitation by primary health organizations at government-determined rates, patient copayments, and payments from the Accident Compensation Corporation. They act as gatekeepers to specialist care and comprise approximately 40% of physicians in New Zealand. Most specialists are salaried employees of district health boards who work in public hospitals. They may also work in private hospitals or run private clinics, where they are paid via FFS systems. District health boards monitor quality of care, based on achieving preset health care performance targets, wait times, and mental health outcomes. Quality measures focus mainly on district trends rather than individual physician performance. Partnerships between district health boards and primary health organizations are working on improving health system integration to varying levels of success. Several districts have launched initiatives to shift health care away from the hospital toward the home, particularly for chronic conditions.

Orthopaedic Musculoskeletal Physiotherapy Clinic, Auckland, New Zealand

The Orthopaedic Musculoskeletal Physiotherapy Clinic (OMPC)[41] was launched in 2018 in response to long wait times experienced by patients referred to orthopaedic services as part of the Auckland District Health Board Greenbelt Project. The Auckland District Health Board serves approximately 545,640 people (per 2018 to 2019 estimate) and includes three major public hospitals with multiple clinics. Escalating referrals for surgical consultations without administering evidence-based nonsurgical strategies exacerbated the long wait times.

In the OMPC model, a senior musculoskeletal PT assesses patients with knee and shoulder pain who have been triaged as unlikely to require surgery (termed priority D patients). These therapists determine which patients would likely benefit from nonsurgical treatment strategies, providing reassurances to the patient about their condition and ongoing referrals to physical therapy and other services as needed. An audit assessing OMPC released in November 2019 involving 49 half-day clinics assessed patient wait times, cost-effectiveness, and patient satisfaction. The cost of a comprehensive musculoskeletal assessment performed by a PT accredited by the Auckland District Health Board was substantially lower (by approximately one-third) compared with that performed by an orthopaedic surgeon. Wait times to see a PT or orthopaedic surgeon were also significantly reduced from 120 to 40 days following the institution of the program. Patient satisfaction ratings were high, with no recorded complaints and few patient requests for assessment by a surgeon instead of a PT.

Long wait times for musculoskeletal assessment can have a detrimental effect on a patient's quality of life while also placing a substantial burden on society. PT-guided triage of patients based on various factors including suitability for surgery may lead not only to more appropriate referral trends but also the right care for the right patient at the right time. PTs embedded in an orthopaedic setting providing this type of service reduced wait times for surgical candidates by an orthopaedic surgeon while also expediting access to effective nonsurgical care, which could delay or avert surgery altogether. The OMPC model demonstrated how substantial savings could be made without a major overhaul of an orthopaedic practice.

ARGENTINA: EVIDENCE-BASED MANAGEMENT OF PERSISTENT MUSCULOSKELETAL PAIN

Argentina's Healthcare System

Argentina operates a decentralized, segmented healthcare system divided into three main sectors: a public sector, a union-run social security sector, and a private sector.[42] The social security sector is Argentina's largest health care sector, covering 60% of Argentinians, followed by 36% relying solely on public health insurance, and slightly more than 13% covered by private insurance. Public health funds are distributed from the national level to the provincial and local levels. Funding is not contingent on any national criteria, so the national Ministry of Health has little sway over provincial health care spending and limited ability to enforce efficiency or quality standards.

The Social Security sector includes approximately 300 different coverage programs. The Obras Sociales Nacionales (OSNs) account for 40% of health expenditures and are largely managed by trade unions and consist of numerous sick funds that cover workers within the same labor activity as well as their family members. Funding comes from compulsory payroll contributions from employees. The Obra Social Provincial includes public workers in each province. Many of the elderly and disabled are covered by the Programa de Asistencia Medica Integral, a national fund for retirees. In practice, many Social Security funds purchase health services in private clinics and hospitals, as they are too small to provide the services themselves. The Social Security sector struggles with high administrative costs, fragmentation, and instability in risk pools that make coverage of high-cost events challenging. There are also significant differences between different OSNs in terms of benefits and coverage.

Slightly more than 13% of Argentinians are covered by private insurance, which accounts for 30% of health expenditures. Two-thirds of those privately insured are covered by OSNs, which contract supplementary private plans, and one-third enroll in private insurance on an individual basis. There is also a significant socioeconomic disparity in insurance coverage: most of the poorest fifth of the population has no insurance coverage, whereas only 10% of the wealthiest one-fifth of the population do not have health insurance.

In 2015, Argentina spent 10.2% of its GDP on health care, with one of the highest health expenditures in Latin America. Private insurance was equal to or lower than that in similar Latin American countries. In contrast, private health expenditures accounted for 30%, 39%, and 57% of all health spending in Uruguay, Chile, and Brazil, respectively. Competition with neighboring countries has been a significant driver of health care reforms in Argentina. Notably, neighboring countries of Chile and Uruguay spend similar amounts on health care but offer more dynamic health programming to address health outcomes.[43,44] Proposed reforms variably focus on public, Social Security, or private sectors, but no widespread efforts have been implemented to date. Due in part to economic pressures, there is comparatively little financial support from the government or academic medical institutions for large-scale innovation in health care.

FLENI Interdisciplinary Outpatient Pain Rehabilitation Program

Persistently painful musculoskeletal disorders are a major burden in Argentina. The FLENI interdisciplinary outpatient pain rehabilitation program (IOPRP) was instituted in 2006 and involved a comprehensive 16-session pain management program.[45] The FLENI IOPRP targeted treatments for persistently painful conditions such as low back pain and neck pain with a goal of improving self-efficacy in pain management, reducing medication use, improving psychosocial well-being and sleeping patterns, and helping patients to gain independence and return to normal daily activities. The program was driven by a multidisciplinary health care team including physicians, psychologists, nurses, PTs, occupational therapists, and nutritionists. Patients completed two 5-hour sessions every week for 8 weeks as individuals, in group settings, or at home. Many treatments focused on coaching patients in self-management of pain. Behavioral therapies such as cognitive behavioral therapy and therapies focused on pain coping strategies were introduced alongside relaxation techniques, lifestyle coaching, physical exercise, and sleep hygiene.

Outcomes were measured through questionnaires administered at baseline, 3 months, and 1 year, including quality of life (SF36, HAQ [Health Assessment Questionnaire]), insomnia (Insomnia Severity Index [ISI]), pain intensity (VAS), mental health (Beck Depression Inventory [BDI]), physical therapy (Oswestry Disability Index [ODI], low back pain disability Roland Morris test [RMT], Back Performance Scale [BPS], body mass index, and Global Impression of Change (GIC).

Patients demonstrated improvements in outcomes that were sustained at 3 months and 1 year after completion of the program, although robust longer-term follow-up was challenging considering most patients completed the program within 2 months. Overall PROMs improved, including measures of quality of life, insomnia, pain intensity, and symptoms of depression. Patients reported a reduction in prescription medication use and improvement in physical function. Satisfaction rates and patient feedback for the overall program were largely positive.

These results were sustained over the 8 years that the intervention was assessed. A key component of the program's success was patient commitment to the relatively high intensity of interventions over a sustained period of time, and commitment from providers to supporting patients in maintaining these practices in daily life. Group-based treatments structured around best practices allowed patients to receive high-quality care for persistent pain while increasing the program's patient capacity (and cost-effectiveness) and contributed to the program's long-term sustainability. Despite a relatively fragmented health care system with constrained resources, the FLENI IOPRP demonstrated the potential for positive outcomes and patient experiences through the implementation of a musculoskeletal care program compliant with best-practice guidelines.

NORWAY: UPSTREAM CARE INTEGRATION FOR HIGH-VALUE TREATMENT OF OA

Norway's Healthcare System

Although Norwegians are automatically enrolled in the country's universal health care system,[46] 10% purchase private insurance, which provides quicker access to certain services and a greater choice of private providers. Health care expenditures accounted for 10.5% of Norway's 2016 GDP, of which 85% was spent by public sources. The average health care spending in 2017 was $6,064 per capita and $860 in out-of-pocket payments. Pharmaceuticals and medical devices are a major focus of Norway's cost-containing strategies, and the government has undertaken several price-reduction schemes such as subsidization and the establishment of a common procurement trust to negotiate discounts on supplies and drugs. Clinical guidelines and patient out-of-pocket payments are also used to contain costs and reduce the utilization of low-value procedures. GPs comprise 26% of Norwegian physicians, who serve as gatekeepers to specialty care. Most are self-employed; 35% are paid by Norway's municipalities, 35% on a FFS basis by the national government, and 30% receive out-of-pocket payments. Hospital specialists are mostly salaried employees, or in private practices, where they have the option of working under contract with the National Health Service.

Quality of care is monitored by the National Board of Health Supervision. Systems for governance and accountability continue to evolve. In 2017, the board refocused regulation from "internal control for health services" to "leadership and quality improvement in the health services," which required hospitals to initiate quality and safety improvement activities while measuring performance quality. Patient pathways and bundles have been developed using national evidence-based guidelines for conditions such as stroke and cancer, with expansion into other conditions. Norway maintains a robust system of national clinical and health registries. Since 2013, Norway has been experimenting with quality-based reimbursement, although such programs are still in development.

SAMhandling for Bedre Artrosebehandling I Kommunehelsetjenesten Model

In response to the underutilization of evidence-based treatment guidelines for the management of OA, a Norwegian research team designed an integrated care model based on best-practice guidelines for OA patients[46] (**Figure 4**). The SAMhandling for Bedre Artrosebehandling I kommunehelsetjenesten (SAMBA) program was launched in 2015 and aimed to improve the treatment of patients with hip and knee OA, mainly in the primary care setting. The program assessed the effectiveness of an integrated management program on PROMs and clinically relevant markers in patients with hip and knee OA.

The SAMBA model included group-based OA education led by PTs, an 8- to 12-week individualized exercise program, an optional nutritional program, and preprogram and postprogram debriefings with GPs. PTs completed a standardized workshop-based education program before treating SAMBA patients, and both GPs and PTs regularly participated in workshops with updates to current treatment recommendations. Workshops included presentations by orthopaedic surgeons about the importance of employing nonsurgical treatments first and when to consider referral to orthopaedic consultation. PROMs were administered at baseline, 3, 6, 9, and 12 months. The study also included a control phase consisting of usual patient care by GPs and PTs who were unaware of the SAMBA model. These patients received PT but did not attend the OA education program nor did they participate in individualized exercise programs.

Surveys also included questions to determine whether guideline-adherent care had been administered. Self-reported referral data to PTs, MRI, or orthopaedic surgery were also collected, along with patient satisfaction, exercise frequency and intensity, and body mass index. The experimental group reported high satisfaction with care and improved levels of physical activity. They also reported higher rates of referral to PTs and lower rates of referral to orthopaedic surgeons, a trend that led to an overall lowering of costs.

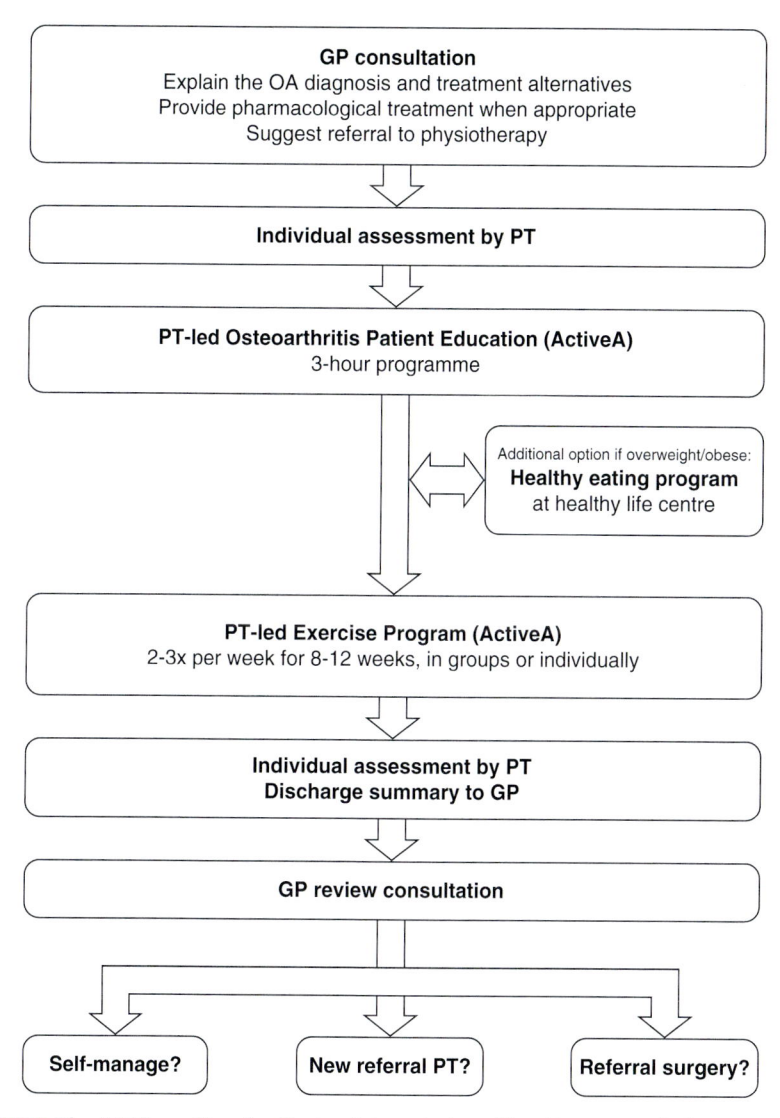

FIGURE 4 The SAMhandling for Bedre Artrosebehandling I kommunehelsetjenesten model for integrated osteoarthritis care. (Reproduced with permission from Østerås N, Moseng T, van Bodegom-Vos L, et al: Implementing a structured model for osteoarthritis care in primary healthcare: A stepped-wedge cluster-randomised trial. *PLoS Med* 2019;16[10]:e1002949.)

Overutilization or inappropriate utilization of health care services for hip and knee OA in Norway has led to high spending on low-impact interventions such as MRI to assess this condition. The SAMBA model demonstrates that it is possible to implement high-quality, evidence-based care while improving affordability and accessibility of care through group-based interventions led by teams of GPs and musculoskeletal therapists. Educating and supporting GPs and PTs in the use of structured, evidence-based care models may improve guideline-adherent treatment of patients with hip or knee OA earlier in the care continuum. Facilitating early secondary prevention strategies can reduce the burden of disease and potentially reduce direct and indirect OA-related costs. Utilizing group-based care in the right settings can be highly effective in terms of outcomes and costs. Consistent and reliable data collection and provider engagement were key to the program's success and ongoing improvement.

SUMMARY

Although value-based care has not been adopted at a national scale in any country, there are several examples of initiatives driving a more value-oriented approach to improving outcomes that matter to patients relative to cost.

In the United Kingdom, the implementation of integrated practice unit-based, multidisciplinary team care for total hip arthroplasty and rotator cuff tear repair created an optimal integrated set of services redesigned in a standardized and coordinated care pathway. In Sweden's OrthoChoice program, a procedure-focused bundled care package delivered at specialized units over a set period of time facilitated improved patient outcomes, reduced costs, and the ability to regain control of long waits for surgery. In Denmark, an evidence-based 360° whole-person program of care resulted in improved patient outcomes stimulating implementation at scale. In New Zealand, extending the scope of practitioners enabled orthopaedic surgeons and PTs to work at the top of their license and reduce patient wait times without disrupting patient satisfaction or the flow of the orthopaedic practice. In Argentina, taking a holistic, symptom-level approach to address persistently painful musculoskeletal conditions yielded sustained improvements in patient outcomes ranging from pain and disability to psychosocial distress. In Norway, the SAMBA program focused on shifting care and delivering value upstream, which facilitated a successful population-based approach to OA care.

Although the programs described in this chapter operate in a variety of different health care settings and take differing procedure- or condition-focused approaches to delivering high-value musculoskeletal care, they have some common underlying threads. Many of the programs demonstrate that it is critical to incorporate evidence-based nonsurgical strategies when designing pathways to deliver high-value musculoskeletal care. Such strategies include lifestyle management, behavioral therapies such as cognitive behavioral therapy, physical therapy, exercise and self-management, and coaching of coping strategies. Most programs place a strong focus on data and outcomes that benefit patients (eg, patient-reported outcome measurements), while also concentrating on the actual costs of care.

These examples also demonstrate that both small-scale and large-scale efforts (requiring varying degrees of structural, functional, normative, interpersonal, and process integration), to achieve value-based health care require a commitment for change, along with the right level of resources upfront. Effective initiatives were implemented when those designing value-oriented programs truly understood the key problems facing health systems while identifying gaps in existing care pathways.

The potential is great for value-based models of care to overcome several of the issues faced by different countries around delivering high-quality orthopaedic care. These global lessons may be valuable for US health systems and orthopaedic practices as they look to transition toward delivering high-value musculoskeletal care.

REFERENCES

1. Papanicolas I, Woskie LR, Jha AK: Health care spending in the United States and other high-income countries. *J Am Med Assoc* 2018;319(10):1024-1039.

2. Tikkanen R, Abrams MK: U.S. Health Care from a Global Perspective, 2019: Higher Spending, Worse Outcomes? The Commonwealth Fund, 2020. Available at: https://www.commonwealthfund.org/publications/issue-briefs/2020/jan/us-health-care-global-perspective-2019. Accessed May 8, 2023.

3. Tikkanen R, Osborn R, Mossialos E, et al: International Health Care Systems Profiles. The Commonwealth Fund, 2020. Available at: https://www.commonwealthfund.org/international-health-policy-center/countries/united-states. Accessed May 8, 2023.

4. Global Health and Aging: National Institute on Aging, National Institutes of Health, World Health Organization, 2011. Available at: https://www.nia.nih.gov/sites/default/files/2017-06/global_health_aging.pdf. Accessed May 12, 2023.

5. Global Spending on Health: A World in Transition. World Health Organization, 2019. Available at: https://www.who.int/publications/i/item/WHO-HIS-HGF-HFWorkingPaper-19.4. Accessed May 15,2023.

6. Thorpe KE, Florence CS, Howard DH, Joski P: The impact of obesity on rising medical spending. *Health Aff (Millwood)* 2004;23(6).

7. Promoting Healthy Ageing: Background report for the 2019 Japanese G20 Presidency. Organisation for Economic Co-operation and Development, 2019. Available at: https://www.oecd.org/g20/topics/global-health/G20-report-promoting-healthy-ageing.pdf. Accessed May 8, 2023.

8. Tremmel M, Gerdtham UG, Nilsson PM, Saha S: Economic burden of obesity: A systematic literature review. *Int J Environ Res Public Health* 2017;14(4):435.

9. National Academies of Sciences, Engineering, and Medicine; Health and Medicine Division; Board on Health Care Services; Committee on Health Care Utilization and Adults with Disabilities: Factors that affect health care utilization, in *Health-Care Utilization as a Proxy in Disability Determination*. National Academies Press, 2018.

10. Pizer SD, Prentice JC: What are the consequences of waiting for health care in the veteran population? *J Gen Intern Med* 2011;26(suppl 2):676-682.

11. Øvretveit J, Zubkoff L, Nelson EC, Frampton S, Knudsen JL, Zimlichman E: Using patient-reported outcome measurement to improve patient care. *Int J Qual Health Care* 2017;29(6):874-879.

12. Speerin R, Needs C, Chua J, et al: Implementing models of care for musculoskeletal conditions in health systems to support value-based care. *Best Pract Res Clin Rheumatol* 2020;34(5):101548.

13. Mensah Abrampah N, Syed SB, Hirschhorn LR, et al: Quality improvement and emerging global health priorities. *Int J Qual Health Care* 2018;30(suppl 1):5-9.

14. Syed SB, Leatherman S, Mensah-Abrampah N, Neilson M, Kelley E: Improving the quality of health care across the health system. *Bull World Health Organ* 2018;96(12):799.

15. Keswani A, Koenig KM, Bozic KJ: Value-based healthcare: Part 1 – Designing and implementing integrated practice units for the management of musculoskeletal disease. *Clin Orthop Relat Res* 2016;474(10):2100-2103.

16. Lentz TA, Goode AP, Thigpen CA, George SZ: Value-based care for musculoskeletal pain: Are physical therapists ready to deliver? *Phys Ther* 2020;100(4):621-632.

17. Annaswamy TM, Kasitinon D, Royston A: Value-based care and musculoskeletal rehabilitation. *Curr Phys Med Rehabil Rep* 2018;6(1)49-54.

18. Medical Services Expenditures by Disease: Diseases of the Musculoskeletal System and Connective Tissue, Blended Account Basis. Federal Reserve Bank of St. Louis, 2020. Available at: https://fred.stlouisfed.org/series/DIMSCTEXPBLEND. Accessed May 9, 2023.

19. Babatunde OO, Jordan JL, Van der Windt DA, Hill JC, Foster NE, Protheroe J: Effective treatment options for musculoskeletal pain in primary care: A systematic overview of current evidence. *PLoS One* 2017;12(6):e0178621.

20. Daigle ME, Weinstein AM, Katz JN, Losina E: The cost-effectiveness of total joint arthroplasty: A systematic review of published literature. *Best Pract Res Clin Rheumatol* 2012;26(5):649-658.

21. Basedow M, Esterman A: Assessing appropriateness of osteoarthritis care using quality indicators: A systematic review. *J Eval Clin Pract* 2015;21(5):782-789.

22. Gademan MG, Hofstede SN, Vliet Vlieland TP, Nelissen RG, Marang-van de Mheen PJ: Indication criteria for total hip or knee arthroplasty in osteoarthritis: A state-of-the-science overview. *BMC Musculoskelet Disord* 2016;17(1):463.

23. Dakin H, Gray A, Fitzpatrick R, Maclennan G, Murray D, KAT Trial Group: Rationing of total knee replacement: A cost-effectiveness analysis on a large trial data set. *BMJ Open* 2012;2(1):e000332.

24. Lin I, Wiles L, Waller R, et al: What does best practice care for musculoskeletal pain look like? Eleven consistent recommendations from high-quality clinical practice guidelines: Systematic review. *Br J Sports Med* 2020;54(2):79-86.

25. Allen KD, Oddone EZ, Coffman CJ, et al: Telephone-based self-management of osteoarthritis: A randomized trial. *Ann Intern Med* 2010;153(9):570-579.

26. Teisberg E, Wallace S, O'Hara S: Defining and implementing value-based health care: A strategic framework. *Acad Med* 2020;95(5):682-685.

27. Vail T: *Achieving Super-Outcomes Without Super-Costs: Reducing Orthopedic Surgery Costs and Improving Care in Managed Care Environment*. AJMC, 2020. Available at: https://www.ajmc.com/view/achieving-superoutcomes-without-supercosts-reducing-orthopedic-surgery-costs-and-improving-care-in-managed-care-environment. Accessed May 9, 2023.

28. Tikkanen R, Osborn R, Mossialos E, et al: International Health Care System Profiles: The Commonwealth Fund, 2020. Available at: https://www.commonwealthfund.org/international-health-policy-center/countries/england. Accessed May 9, 2023.

29. Gabriel L, Casey J, Gee M, et al: Value-based healthcare analysis of joint replacement surgery for patients with primary hip osteoarthritis. *BMJ Open Qual* 2019;8(2):e000549.

30. Prevalence of osteoarthritis in England and local authorities. Public Health England. Arthritis Research UK, Available at: https://www.versusarthritis.org/media/13374/birmingham-oa-1.pdf. Accessed May 9, 2023.

31. Holzer-Fleming C, Tavakkolizadeh A, Sinha J, Casey J, Moxham J, Colegate-Stone TJ: Value-based healthcare analysis of shoulder surgery for patients with symptomatic rotator cuff tears – Calculating the impact of arthroscopic cuff repair. *Shoulder Elbow* 2022;14(1 suppl):59-70.

32. Tikkanen R, Osorn R, Mossialos E, et al: International Health Care System Profiles. The Commonwealth Fund, 2020. Available at: https://www.commonwealthfund.org/international-health-policy-center/countries/sweden. Accessed on May 9, 2023.

33. Porter ME, Marks CM, Landman ZC: *OrthoChoice: Bundled Payments in the County of Stockholm (A)*. Harvard Business School, 2015. Available at: https://www.hbs.edu/faculty/Pages/item.aspx?num=47439. Accessed May 9, 2023.

34. Porter ME, Marks CM, Landman ZC: *OrthoChoice: Bundled Payments in the County of Stockholm (B)*. Harvard Business School, 2015. Available at: https://www.hbs.edu/faculty/Pages/item.aspx?num=47450. Accessed May 9, 2023.

35. Manickas-Hill O, Feeley T, Bozic KJ: A review of bundled payments in total joint replacement. *JBJS Rev* 2019;7(11):e1.

36. The Economist Intelligence Unit: Value based health care in Sweden – Reaching the next level. Available at: https://impact.economist.com/perspectives/sites/default/files/value-basedhealthcareinswedenreachingthenextlevel_infographic.pdf. Accessed May 5, 2023.

37. Pross C, Geissler A, Busse R: Measuring, reporting, and rewarding quality of care in 5 nations: 5 policy levers to enhance hospital quality accountability. *Milbank Q* 2017;95(1):136-183.

38. Tikkanen R, Osorn R, Mossialos E, et al: International Health Care System Profiles. The Commonwealth Fund, 2020. Available at: https://www.commonwealthfund.org/international-health-policy-center/countries/denmark. Accessed May 9, 2023.

39. Skou ST, Roos EM: Good Life with osteoarthritis in Denmark (GLA:D™): Evidence-based education and supervised neuromuscular exercise delivered by certified physiotherapists nationwide. *BMC Musculoskelet Disord* 2017;18(1):72.

40. Tikkanen R, Osorn R, Mossialos E, et al: International Health Care System Profiles. The Commonwealth Fund, 2020. Available at: https://www.commonwealthfund.org/international-health-policy-center/countries/new-zealand. Accessed May 9, 2023.

41. Donaldson B: *One Year Audit of the Orthopaedic Musculoskeletal Physiotherapy Clinic (OMPC)*, 2019. Available at: https://vimeo.com/378403351.

42. Rubinstein A, Zerbino MC, Cejas C, López A: Making universal health care effective in Argentina: A blueprint for reform. *Health Syst Reform* 2018;4(3):203-213.

43. Gilardino RE, Valanzasca P, Rifkin SB: Has Latin America achieved universal health coverage yet? Lessons from four countries. *Arch Public Health* 2022;80(1):38.

44. Oliver HC: In the wake of structural adjustment programs: Exploring the relationship between domestic policies and health outcomes in Argentina and Uruguay. *Can J Public Health* 2006;97(3):217-221.

45. Tikkanen R, Osborn R, Mossialos E, et al: International Health Care System Profiles. The Commonwealth Fund, 2020. Available at: https://www.commonwealthfund.org/international-health-policy-center/countries/norway. Accessed May 9, 2023.

46. Østerås N, Moseng T, van Bodegom-Vos L, et al: Implementing a structured model for osteoarthritis care in primary healthcare: A stepped-wedge cluster-randomised trial. *PLoS Med* 2019;16(10):e1002949.

Comparative Effectiveness Research: Applications to Orthopaedics and Sports Medicine

Prem N. Ramkumar, MD, MBA • Spencer W. Sullivan, BS
Benedict U. Nwachukwu, MD, MBA

INTRODUCTION

The orthopaedic and sports medicine literature has embraced comparative effective research (CER), which focuses on evidence-based research to improve patient health. This chapter explores the various ways in which CER has been used and reviews its history and arrival as it relates to orthopaedic surgery and sports medicine.

BACKGROUND

CER was first established on June 30, 2009 with the introduction of the American Recovery and Reinvestment Act of 2009.[1,2] This stimulus bill, alongside the passing of the 2010 Patient Protection and Affordable Care Act, enacted a shift in American health care, focusing on evidence-based research to improve patient health. CER represents the synthesis of available evidence and commitment to the generation of new research that identifies the value of interventions through the lens of outcomes and cost. This evidence is then used to guide decision-making in the most effective methods of prevention, diagnosis, and treatment of specific ailments, injuries, and diseases. Thus, CER was established to improve value in the United States across all major fields of medicine.[2,3] With a budget of $1.1 billion, Congress allocated $400 million to the National Institutes of Health, $300 million the Agency for Healthcare Research and Quality and $400 million the Department of Health

Dr. Ramkumar or an immediate family member has received royalties from Globus Medical; serves as a paid consultant to or is an employee of Globus Medical and Stryker; has stock or stock options held in ConforMIS, Johnson & Johnson, and Overture; has received nonincome support (such as equipment or services), commercially derived honoraria, or other non–research-related funding (such as paid travel) from Stryker; and serves as a board member, owner, officer, or committee member of American Association of Hip and Knee Surgeons. Dr. Nwachukwu or an immediate family member serves as a paid consultant to or is an employee of Figur8 and has stock or stock options held in BICMD. Neither Spencer W. Sullivan nor any immediate family member has received anything of value from or has stock or stock options held in a commercial company or institution related directly or indirectly to the subject of this chapter.

and Human Services to promote and support the implementation of CER projects in the United States. To begin this endeavor, the Institute of Medicine and Congress recommended specific priorities to create and sustain a robust CER strategy moving forward. These priorities were aimed at addressing health care delivery systems and disparities, as well as cardiovascular disease, psychiatric conditions, neurologic disorders, and individuals with functional limitations and disabilities.[4]

To promote the continued support of CER, the Patient-Centered Outcomes Research Institute was enacted under the Affordable Care Act in 2010. This federally funded, nonprofit organization aimed to support the ideals of CER and guide governing bodies in making informed decisions regarding health care issues and health policy.[3,5] Prompted by the mission of executing national health care research, Patient-Centered Outcomes Research Institute board members and stakeholders identified the following priorities to categorize their funding agenda: person-centered outcomes, health disparities, health care systems, communication and dissemination, and methodologic research.[6] Since its inception, a total of $3.6 billion was allocated for CER-related activities during the 2010 to 2019 fiscal years. Under this funding agenda, 1,987 research awards, 379 research infrastructure awards, 103 engagement awards, and 60 dissemination and implementation awards have been granted for both ongoing and completed projects.[7]

OBSERVATIONAL ANALYSES: REGISTRY AND ELECTRONIC MEDICAL RECORD DATA

It is common knowledge that experimental clinical research, namely the randomized controlled trial (RCT), is the gold standard for assessing the value of an alternative medical intervention. The increased validity and low bias associated with RCTs provide high causal evidence to the value of an intervention.[8] However, the RCI has become increasingly impractical at both the patient and population level.[8] The emergence of CER has prompted renewed interest within observational research methods in assessing the value of various medical interventions. Anglemeyer et al[9] reported that health outcomes (risk, odds and hazard ratios) using observational methods were comparable to those from RCTs. As such, the value of clinical registries and electronic medical records has skyrocketed because of their capacity to store large volumes of data capable of fueling observational study designs.[10-12]

Similar to the hospital electronic medical record, clinical registries contain important data for longitudinal research capable of comparing various orthopaedic interventions. Lake et al[13] described the role of CER in spine surgery, specifically highlighting the need to determine the optimal treatment paradigm for common degenerative spinal disorders through the Swedish Spine Registry and the Registry of the Scoliosis Research Society.[13] Spine surgery professional organizations are not the only orthopaedic subspecialty taking a recent interest in procedural-based and diagnosis-based registries. For example, the Hospital for Special Surgery conducts a number of registries to collect and analyze patient-reported health outcomes, including their total joint replacement registry.[14] Funded through grant support by the Agency for Healthcare Research and Quality, more than 10,000 patients have been enrolled in this registry since 2007.[15] The Cleveland

Clinic Health System developed a scientifically valid, cost-effective, and scalable prospective registry, called the Outcomes Management and Evaluation system, that collects demographic data, general health patient-reported outcome measures (PROMs), joint-specific PROMs, and disease severity at the time of surgery for all elective hip, knee, and shoulder procedures across seven different hospitals within the system.[16] Of the eligible 15,610 patients, 97.4% of patients completed PROMs and 99.9% of surgeons provided the necessary patient details of disease severity; at 1 year, the patient follow-up rate was 72.5%.[16] Currently, more than 50,000 patients are prospectively enrolled in this registry. Other institutional registries have been established around the world to best explore outcomes for various interventions, including St. Vincent's Melbourne Arthroplasty Outcomes Registry. To date, this registry reports more than 13,000 arthroplasties in more than 10,000 patients, with follow-up extending to 20 years after surgical intervention.[17] From this registry alone, more than 46 observational studies have been published using this registry's data.[17] Though registry data are imperfect and less exact than the RCT, high-quality data with appropriate statistical analysis can yield similarly meaningful discoveries.[18] Therefore, both the electronic medical record and clinical registry remain critical in CER for orthopaedics and sports medicine.

PATIENT-REPORTED OUTCOME MEASURES

In order to compare surgical effectiveness in elective orthopaedic surgery, the advent of PROMs embodies the recent shift to patient-centered care and provides the quantitative springboard to allow comparison. PROMs have come to represent the greatest commitment to CER in orthopaedic research through the administration of survey instruments that capture patient perspectives and experiences following a procedure. Often encompassing subjective measures of symptoms, functional status, health perception, health-related quality of life, and satisfaction,[19] **Table 1** details various PROMs used among sports medicine surgeons: anterior cruciate ligament (ACL) reconstruction,[20,21] hip arthroscopy,[22-24] and rotator cuff repair and shoulder stabilization.[25] Nwachukwu et al[26] systematically reviewed 12 cost effectiveness analyses in the sports medicine literature and found the available evidence is limited to select procedures, primarily ACL reconstruction and rotator cuff repair.

Similar to clinical trials, PROMs can be statistically analyzed to determine the effectiveness of a given orthopaedic procedure. Beyond the characteristics of the musculoskeletal disease, PROMs can capture overall health status, including physical, mental, and emotional health. The most common global health measure administered in orthopaedics is the Short Form-36, which contains the Physical Component Summary Score and a Mental Component Summary Score to measure health-related QOL.[27] The advent of PROMs serves to elucidate the previously nebulous relationship between mental and physical health to identify ideal surgical candidates and provide reasonable prognoses for at-risk populations. As an example, Ramkumar et al[28] applied machine learning to PROMs collected in an institutional cartilage registry to establish that patients who preoperatively report poor mental health, catastrophize pain symptoms, compensate with higher

TABLE 1 Common Patient-Reported Outcomes in Sports Medicine Procedures

Patient-Reported Outcome Measure	Short Name	Joint	Function	Symptoms	Pain	Activity Level	Quality of Life
International Knee Documentation Committee Subjective Knee Form	IKDC	Knee	X	X	X	—	—
Lysholm Knee Scoring Scale	Lysholm	Knee	X	X	—	—	—
Tegner Activity Scale	Tegner	Knee	—	—	—	X	—
Knee Injury and Osteoarthritis Outcome Score	KOOS	Knee	X	X	X	—	X
Marx Activity Scale	Marx	Knee	—	—	—	X	—
Western Ontario and McMaster Universities Arthritis Index	WOMAC	Knee	X	X	X	—	—
Copenhagen Hip and Groin Score	HAGOS	Hip	X	X	X	X	X
Hip Disability and Osteoarthritis Outcome Score	HOOS	Hip	X	X	X	—	X
Hip Outcome Score	HOS	Hip	X	X	X	—	X
International Hip Outcome Tool	iHOT	Hip	X	X	X	—	X
Modified Harris Hip Score	mHHS	Hip	X	—	X	—	—
Oxford Hip Score	OHS	Hip	X	—	X	—	X
Nonarthritic Hip Scale	NAHS	Hip	X	X	X	—	—

TABLE 1	Common Patient-Reported Outcomes in Sports Medicine Procedures (Continued)						
Patient-Reported Outcome Measure	Short Name	Joint	Function	Symptoms	Pain	Activity Level	Quality of Life
Lower Extremity Functional Scale	LEFS	Hip	X	—	—	—	—
Rowe Score for Instability	Rowe	Shoulder	X	X	—	—	—
Western Ontario Shoulder Instability Index	WOSI	Shoulder	X	X	X	—	X
Constant-Murley Score	CMS	Shoulder	X	X	X	—	—
Visual Analog Scale for Pain	VAS	Shoulder	—	—	X	—	—
American Shoulder and Elbow Surgeons Shoulder Score	ASES	Shoulder	X	—	X	X	—
University of California, Los Angeles Shoulder Rating	UCLA	Shoulder	X	X	X	—	—

physical health and knee function, and exhibit lower activity demands are at risk for failing to reach clinically meaningful outcomes after osteochondral allograft of the knee.

CUSTOMIZED OUTCOME REPORTING

Although many studies report successful interventions using PROMs, completion and follow-up rates are lacking due to survey length and burden.[29-31] In response, the National Institutes of Health has introduced the Patient-Reported Outcomes Measurement Information System (PROMIS) to help relieve question burden and standardize outcome collection in CER. Using item response theory and computer-adaptive testing (CAT) to identify a specific set of questions tailored to the patient, PROMIS is considered efficient, flexible, and precise.[32-35] **Table 2** details PROMIS instruments and their specific health domain.

TABLE 2 Common PROMIS Instruments in the Orthopaedic Literature

Patient-Reported Outcome Measure	Function	Symptoms	Pain	Activity Level	Quality of Life
PROMIS physical function	X	—	—	—	—
PROMIS mobility	X	—	—	—	—
PROMIS upper extremity	X	—	—	—	—
PROMIS pain Interference	—	—	X	—	X
PROMIS fatigue	—	X	—	—	—
PROMIS depression	—	—	—	—	X
PROMIS anxiety	—	—	—	—	X
PROMIS social satisfaction	—	—	—	—	X

PROMIS has seemed to pave the way for CAT and item response theory within orthopaedic CER and has been validated across a number of surgical procedures and joints. In the spine literature, PROMIS has demonstrated moderate to strong correlations with legacy spine-specific PROMs with less administrative burden for the patient.[36,37] Within knee arthroscopy, PROMIS instruments were found to be clinically useful with high responsiveness both preoperatively and postoperatively.[38,39] Similar findings have been replicated in the ACL reconstruction multiligament knee injury populations.[40,41] Within the periacetabular osteotomy literature, strong correlations have been found between PROMIS and legacy hip-specific PROMs.[29,42] Again, PROMIS has demonstrated moderate to excellent reproducibility for shoulder-specific legacy PROMs among patients who underwent rotator cuff repair, stabilization, and other shoulder procedures.[43,44] PROMIS has generated successful outcome assessment and represents a well-established pillar of orthopaedic CER.

There exist customized outcome reporting systems outside of PROMIS that reconcile the lower responsiveness, floor and ceiling effects of certain joint-specific PROMs, and inconsistent correlations with legacy instruments.[45,46] As an example, the American Shoulder and Elbow Surgeons Shoulder Score led the way by applying computer adaptive testing for shoulder conditions that better capture pain and function.[47] Similar investigations have applied computer adaptive testing to legacy outcomes for total hip and knee arthroplasty.[48,49] Customized outcome reporting represents a leaner approach to better understanding and comparing the numerator of the value equation across orthopaedic interventions.

CLINICALLY MEANINGFUL OUTCOMES

Over the past decade, PROMs have been well reported in the orthopaedic literature, initially emphasizing statistically significance. However, statistical significance does not confer clinical meaning capable of guiding informed decision making.[19] In an attempt to bridge research instruments (ie, PROMs) with real-world clinical significance, the following metrics have arrived at the forefront of CER: the minimal clinically important difference (MCID), substantial clinical benefit (SCB), and the patient acceptable symptom state (PASS).[50]

MCID is defined as the smallest outcome improvement that a patient considers meaningful following a given intervention.[51-53] PASS increases the threshold and is considered an intermediate outcome between MCID and SCB that is also acceptable to the patient.[54-56] The PASS has been defined as a dichotomous value between a patient considering themselves either "well" or "unwell" following an intervention.[55] Within sports medicine procedures specifically, PASS has been identified for a number of hip,[55,57] shoulder,[58,59] and knee-specific[60-62] legacy PROMs, including a number of PROMIS instruments.[63,64] SCB is the ideal clinically significant outcome defined as an improvement the patient considers clinically considerable.[53,65] Both measures have been highlighted recently in the sports medicine literature. For osteochondral allograft transplants in the setting of knee cartilage injury, Wang et al[66] identified the MCID and SCB for the International Knee Documentation Committee and Knee Outcome Survey Activities of Daily Living Scale as 17 ± 3.9 and 10 ± 3.7, respectively.[66] Similarly, Nwachukwu et al and Martin et al identified the MCID and SCB in both primary and revision hip arthroscopy, establishing critical pain thresholds and expected convalescence time following hip arthroscopy.[67-70] In a 2019 systematic review, MCID was used to report that patients achieved maximal subjective improvement 1 year after ACL reconstruction.[71] The MCID has additionally been used in identifying predictors of achieving the MCID and return to play 2 years after ACL reconstruction.[72] In rotator cuff repair, a recent study analyzed the MCID and SCB alongside PASS at 1-year follow-up for the visual analog scale for pain, American Shoulder and Elbow Surgeons score, University of California, Los Angeles score, and Single Answer Numeric Evaluation for function scores.[58] However, there is a paucity of MCID and SCB data for shoulder-specific legacy patient-reported outcomes in sports medicine, warranting further research to define the MCID and SCB.[73] Through identifying critical thresholds isolating the MCID and SCB for PROMs, high-level CER can be accomplished by answering questions that go beyond statistical significance to discover clinical meaning surrounding orthopaedic interventions.

SHARED DECISION-MAKING MODELS

CER seeks to provide evidence supporting the relative value of alternative courses of action, which involves estimates of the likelihood of desirable and undesirable outcomes associated with each option.[74] Thus, orthopaedic patients and surgeons should work together to identify the best management aligned with the goals of care. This shared decision-making (SDM) model involves surgeons and patients making use of CER to inform the treatment decision. Thus, SDM allows CER to return patient-centered practice, whereas CER provides the backbone of evidence to guide SDM discussions.[75,76]

SUMMARY

The recent emphasis on value-based health care has resulted in a shift to patient-centered care that prioritizes the patient experience over the surgeon evaluation. From utilization of the electronic medical record and establishment of multiple clinical registry databases in conjunction with the acquisition of patient-reported outcomes, the commitment to evaluating the success of orthopaedic procedures has dramatically increased in the past decade. Moreover, there has been a shift from statistically significant differences to identify various thresholds that establish true clinical benefit to the patient. Through the establishment of clinically meaningful endpoints following orthopaedic surgery, surgeons are now better equipped than before to lead conversations centered on SDM that will best educate and advise the patient to render true value-based health care.

REFERENCES

1. Sox HC: Comparative effectiveness research: A progress report. *Ann Intern Med* 2010;153(7):469-472.

2. Sox HC, Greenfield S: Comparative effectiveness research: A report from the institute of medicine. *Ann Intern Med* 2009;151(3):203-205.

3. Conway PH, Clancy C: Comparative-effectiveness research - Implications of the federal coordinating council's report. *N Engl J Med* 2009;361(4):328-330.

4. Iglehart JK: Prioritizing comparative-effectiveness research - IOM recommendations. *N Engl J Med* 2009;361(4):325-328.

5. Newhouse R, Barksdale DJ, Miller JA: The patient-centered outcomes research institute: Research done differently. *Nurs Res* 2015;64(1):72-77.

6. Hoerger M: Educating the psychology workforce in the age of the affordable care Act: A graduate course modeled after the priorities of the patient-centered outcomes research institute (PCORI). *Train Educ Prof Psychol* 2015;9(4):309-314.

7. United States Government Accountability Office: Comparative Effectiveness Research: Patient-Centered Outcomes Research Institute and HHS Continue Activities and Plan New Efforts [Internet]. GAO Highlights, 2020. Available at: https://www.gao.gov/assets/720/710713.pdf. Accessed October 4, 2023.

8. Armstrong K. Methods in comparative effectiveness research. *J Clin Oncol* 2012;30(34):4208-4214.

9. Anglemyer A, Horvath HT, Bero L: Healthcare outcomes assessed with observational study designs compared with those assessed in randomized trials. *Cochrane Database Syst Rev* 2014;2014(4):MR000034.

10. Schuemie MJ, Cepeda MS, Suchard MA, et al: How confident are we about observational findings in healthcare: A benchmark study. *Harv Data Sci Rev* 2020;2(1):10.1162/99608f92.

11. Danaei G, García Rodríguez LA, Cantero OF, Logan RW, Hernán MA: Electronic medical records can be used to emulate target trials of sustained treatment strategies. *J Clin Epidemiol* 2018;96:12-22.

12. Gensheimer SG, Wu AW, Snyder CF; PRO-EHR Users' Guide Steering Group, PRO-EHR Users' Guide Working GroupOh, the places we'll go: Patient-reported outcomes and electronic health records. *Patient* 2018;11(6):591-598.

13. Lake WB, Brooks NP, Resnick DK: Comparative effectiveness research in spine surgery. *J Comp Eff Res* 2013;2(1):45-51.

14. Lyman S, Lee YY, Franklin PD, Li W, Mayman DJ, Padgett DE: Validation of the HOOS, JR: A short-form hip replacement survey. *Clin Orthop Relat Res* 2016;474(6):1472-1482.

15. Mushlin AI, Ghomrawi HM: Comparative effectiveness research: A cornerstone of healthcare reform? *Trans Am Clin Climatol Assoc* 2010;121:141-154.

16. OME Cleveland Clinic Orthopaedics: Implementing a scientifically valid, cost-effective, and scalable data collection system at point of care: The Cleveland Clinic OME Cohort. *J Bone Joint Surg Am* 2019;101(5):458-464.

17. Gould D, Thuraisingam S, Shadbolt C, et al. Cohort profile: The St Vincent's Melbourne arthroplasty outcomes (SMART) registry, a pragmatic prospective database defining outcomes in total hip and knee replacement patients. *BMJ Open* 2021;11(1):e040408.

18. Concato J, Lawler EV, Lew RA, Gaziano JM, Aslan M, Huang GD: Observational methods in comparative effectiveness research. *Am J Med* 2010;123(12 suppl 1):e16-e23.

19. Ahmed S, Berzon RA, Revicki DA, et al: The use of patient-reported outcomes (PRO) within comparative effectiveness research: Implications for clinical practice and health care policy. *Med Care* 2012;50(12):1060-1070.

20. Nwachukwu BU, Patel BH, Lu Y, Allen AA, Williams RJ: Anterior cruciate ligament repair outcomes: An updated systematic review of recent literature. *Arthroscopy* 2019;35(7):2233-2247.

21. Makhni EC, Padaki AS, Petridis PD, et al: High variability in outcome reporting patterns in high-impact ACL literature. *J Bone Joint Surg Am* 2015;97(18):1529-1542.

22. Kemp JL, Collins NJ, Roos EM, Crossley KM: Psychometric properties of patient-reported outcome measures for hip arthroscopic surgery. *Am J Sports Med* 2013;41(9):2065-2073.

23. Al Mana L, Coughlin RP, Desai V, Simunovic N, Duong A, Ayeni OR: The hip labrum reconstruction: Indications and outcomes-an updated systematic review. *Curr Rev Musculoskelet Med* 2019;12(2):156-165.

24. Maldonado DR, Kyin C, Shapira J, et al: Defining the maximum outcome improvement of the modified Harris hip score, the nonarthritic hip score, the visual analog scale for pain, and the international hip outcome tool-12 in the arthroscopic management for femoroacetabular impingement syndrome and labral tear. *Arthroscopy* 2021;37(5):1477-1485.

25. Unger RZ, Burnham JM, Gammon L, Malempati CS, Jacobs CA, Makhni EC: The responsiveness of patient-reported outcome tools in shoulder surgery is dependent on the underlying pathological condition. *Am J Sports Med* 2019;47(1):241-247.

26. Nwachukwu BU, Schairer WW, Bernstein JL, Dodwell ER, Marx RG, Allen AA: Cost-effectiveness analyses in orthopaedic sports medicine: A systematic review. *Am J Sports Med* 2015;43(6):1530-1537.

27. Laucis NC, Hays RD, Bhattacharyya T: Scoring the SF-36 in orthopaedics: A brief guide. *J Bone Joint Surg Am* 2015;97(19):1628-1634.

28. Ramkumar PN, Karnuta JM, Haeberle HS, et al: Association between preoperative mental health and clinically meaningful outcomes after osteochondral allograft for cartilage defects of the knee: A machine learning analysis. *Am J Sports Med* 2021;49(4):948-957.

29. Kollmorgen RC, Hutyra CA, Green C, Lewis B, Olson SA, Mather RC: Relationship between PROMIS computer adaptive tests and legacy hip measures among patients presenting to a tertiary care hip preservation center. *Am J Sports Med* 2019;47(4):876-884.

30. Makhni EC, Meadows M, Hamamoto JT, Higgins JD, Romeo AA, Verma NN: Patient reported outcomes measurement information system (PROMIS) in the upper extremity: The future of outcomes reporting? *J Shoulder Elbow Surg* 2017;26(2):352-357.

31. Gire JD, Koltsov JCB, Segovia NA, Kenney DE, Yao J, Ladd AL: Single Assessment Numeric Evaluation (SANE) in hand surgery: Does a one-question outcome instrument compare favorably? *J Hand Surg Am* 2020;45(7):589-596.

32. Cella D, Riley W, Stone A, et al: The Patient-Reported Outcomes Measurement Information System (PROMIS) developed and tested its first wave of adult self-reported health outcome item banks: 2005-2008. *J Clin Epidemiol* 2010;63(11):1179-1194.

33. Cella D, Gershon R, Lai JS, Choi S: The future of outcomes measurement: Item banking, tailored short-forms, and computerized adaptive assessment. *Qual Life Res* 2007;16(suppl 1):133-141.

34. Roorda LD, Crins MH, Terwee CB: Clinimetrics: Patient-Reported Outcomes Measurement Information System (PROMIS®). *J Physiother* 2019;65(2):110.

35. Bykerk VP: Patient-reported outcomes measurement information system versus legacy instruments: Are they ready for prime time? *Rheum Dis Clin North Am* 2019;45(2):211-229.

36. Haws BE, Khechen B, Bawa MS, et al: The patient-reported outcomes measurement information system in spine surgery: A systematic review. *J Neurosurg Spine* 2019;30(3):405-413.

37. Tishelman JC, Vasquez-Montes D, Jevotovsky DS, et al: Patient-reported outcomes measurement information system instruments: Outperforming traditional quality of life measures in patients with back and neck pain. *J Neurosurg Spine* 2019;2019:1-6.

38. Kenney RJ, Houck J, Giordano BD, Baumhauer JF, Herbert M, Maloney MD: Do Patient Reported Outcome Measurement Information System (PROMIS) scales demonstrate responsiveness as well as disease-specific scales in patients undergoing knee arthroscopy? *Am J Sports Med* 2019;47(6):1396-1403.

39. Shamrock AG, Wolf BR, Ortiz SF, et al: Preoperative validation of the patient-reported outcomes measurement information system in patients with articular cartilage defects of the knee. *Arthroscopy* 2020;36(2):516-520.

40. Scott EJ, Westermann R, Glass NA, Hettrich C, Wolf BR, Bollier MJ: Performance of the PROMIS in patients after anterior cruciate ligament reconstruction. *Orthop J Sports Med* 2018;6(5):2325967118774509.

41. Trasolini NA, Korber S, Gipsman A, San AE, Weber AE, Hatch GFR: Performance of PROMIS computer adaptive testing as compared with established instruments for multiple-ligament knee injuries. *Orthop J Sports Med* 2019;7(9):2325967119867419.

42. Li DJ, Clohisy JC, Schwabe MT, Yanik EL, Pascual-Garrido C: PROMIS versus legacy patient-reported outcome measures in patients undergoing surgical treatment for symptomatic acetabular dysplasia. *Am J Sports Med* 2020;48(2):385-394.

43. Schwarz I, Smith JH, Houck DA, Frank RM, Bravman JT, McCarty EC: Use of the patient-reported outcomes measurement information system (PROMIS) for operative shoulder outcomes. *Orthop J Sports Med* 2020;8(6):2325967120924345.

44. Patterson BM, Orvets ND, Aleem AW, et al: Correlation of Patient-Reported Outcomes Measurement Information System (PROMIS) scores with legacy patient-reported outcome scores in patients undergoing rotator cuff repair. *J Shoulder Elbow Surg* 2018;27(6 suppl):S17-S23.

45. Nwachukwu BU, Rasio J, Beck EC, et al: Patient-reported outcomes measurement information system physical function has a lower effect size and is less responsive than legacy hip specific patient reported outcome measures following arthroscopic hip surgery. *Arthroscopy* 2020;36(12):2992-2997.

46. Matar RN, Shah NS, Grawe BM: Patient-reported outcomes measurement information system scores are inconsistently correlated with legacy patient-reported outcome measures in shoulder pathology: A systematic review. *Arthroscopy* 2021;37(4):1301-1309.e1.

47. Tenan MS, Galvin JW, Mauntel TC, et al: Generating the American Shoulder and Elbow Surgeons Score using multivariable predictive models and computer adaptive testing to reduce survey burden. *Am J Sports Med* 2021;49(3):764-772.

48. Banerjee S, Plummer O, Abboud JA, Deirmengian GK, Levicoff EA, Courtney PM: Accuracy and validity of computer adaptive testing for outcome assessment in patients undergoing total hip arthroplasty. *J Arthroplasty* 2020;35(3):756-761.

49. Banerjee S, Deirmengian GK, Levicoff E, Abboud JA, Plummer O, Courtney PM: Accuracy and validity of computer adaptive testing for outcome assessment in patients undergoing total knee arthroplasty. *J Arthroplasty* 2020;35(7):1819-1825.

50. Nwachukwu BU, Runyon RS, Kahlenberg CA, Gausden EB, Schairer WW, Allen AA: How are we measuring clinically important outcome for operative treatments in sports medicine? *Phys Sportsmed* 2017;45(2):159-164.

51. Katz NP, Paillard FC, Ekman E: Determining the clinical importance of treatment benefits for interventions for painful orthopedic conditions. *J Orthop Surg Res* 2015;10:24.

52. Sedaghat AR: Understanding the minimal clinically important difference (MCID) of patient-reported outcome measures. *Otolaryngol Head Neck Surg* 2019;161(4):551-560.

53. Nwachukwu BU, Chang B, Fields K, et al: Defining the "Substantial Clinical Benefit" after arthroscopic treatment of femoroacetabular impingement. *Am J Sports Med* 2017;45(6):1297-1303.

54. Rodríguez-Lozano C, Gantes MÁ, González B, et al: Patient-acceptable symptom state as an outcome measure in the daily care of patients with ankylosing spondylitis. *J Rheumatol* 2012;39(7):1424-1432.

55. Kivlan BR, Martin RL, Christoforetti JJ, et al: The patient acceptable symptomatic state of the 12-Item International Hip Outcome Tool at 1-year follow-up of hip-preservation surgery. *Arthroscopy* 2019;35(5):1457-1462.

56. Beck EC, Nwachukwu BU, Kunze KN, Chahla J, Nho SJ: How can we define clinically important improvement in pain scores after hip arthroscopy for femoroacetabular impingement syndrome? Minimum 2-year follow-up study. *Am J Sports Med* 2019;47(13):3133-3140.

57. Rosinsky PJ, Chen JW, Yelton MJ, et al: Does failure to meet threshold scores for mHHS and iHOT-12 correlate to secondary operations following hip arthroscopy? *J Hip Preserv Surg* 2020;7(2):272-280.

58. Kim DM, Kim TH, Kholinne E, et al: Minimal clinically important difference, substantial clinical benefit, and patient acceptable symptomatic state after arthroscopic rotator cuff repair. *Am J Sports Med* 2020;48(11):2650-2659.

59. Cleveland Clinic OME Sports Medicine; Bayomy AF, Schickendantz MS, et al: What are the predictors of poor patient-reported outcomes after shoulder instability surgery? *Orthop J Sports Med* 2020;8(12):2325967120966343.

60. Vega JF, Jacobs CA, Strnad GJ, et al: Prospective evaluation of the patient acceptable symptom state to identify clinically successful anterior cruciate ligament reconstruction. *Am J Sports Med* 2019;47(5):1159-1167.

61. Cristiani R, Mikkelsen C, Edman G, Forssblad M, Engström B, Stålman A: Age, gender, quadriceps strength and hop test performance are the most important factors affecting the achievement of a patient-acceptable symptom state after ACL reconstruction. *Knee Surg Sports Traumatol Arthrosc* 2020;28(2):369-380.

62. Okoroha KR, Beck EC, Nwachukwu BU, Kunze KN, Nho SJ: Defining minimal clinically important difference and patient acceptable symptom state after isolated endoscopic gluteus medius repair. *Am J Sports Med* 2019; 47(13):3141-3147.

63. Haunschild ED, Gilat R, Fu MC, et al: Establishing the minimal clinically important difference, patient acceptable symptomatic state, and substantial clinical benefit of the PROMIS Upper Extremity Questionnaire after rotator cuff repair. *Am J Sports Med* 2020;48(14):3439-3446.

64. Kuhns BD, Reuter J, Lawton D, Kenney RJ, Baumhauer JF, Giordano BD: Threshold values for success after hip arthroscopy using the patient-reported outcomes measurement information system assessment: Determining the minimum clinically important difference and patient acceptable symptomatic state. *Am J Sports Med* 2020;48(13):3280-3287.

65. Glassman SD, Copay AG, Berven SH, Polly DW, Subach BR, Carreon LY: Defining substantial clinical benefit following lumbar spine arthrodesis. *J Bone Joint Surg Am* 2008;90(9):1839-1847.

66. Wang D, Chang B, Coxe FR, et al: Clinically meaningful improvement after treatment of cartilage defects of the knee with osteochondral grafts. *Am J Sports Med* 2019;47(1):71-81.

67. Nwachukwu BU, Chang B, Adjei J, et al: Time required to achieve minimal clinically important difference and substantial clinical benefit after arthroscopic treatment of femoroacetabular impingement. *Am J Sports Med* 2018;46(11):2601-2606.

68. Martin RL, Kivlan BR, Christoforetti JJ, et al: Minimal clinically important difference and substantial clinical benefit values for a pain visual analog scale after hip arthroscopy. *Arthroscopy* 2019;35(7):2064-2069.

69. Nwachukwu BU, Chang B, Rotter BZ, Kelly BT, Ranawat AS, Nawabi DH: Minimal clinically important difference and substantial clinical benefit after revision hip arthroscopy. *Arthroscopy* 2018;34(6):1862-1868.

70. Nwachukwu BU, Chang B, Kahlenberg CA, et al: Arthroscopic treatment of femoroac-etabular impingement in adolescents provides clinically significant outcome improve-ment. *Arthroscopy* 2017;33(10):1812-1818.

71. Agarwalla A, Puzzitiello RN, Liu JN, et al: Timeline for maximal subjective out-come improvement after anterior cruciate ligament reconstruction. *Am J Sports Med* 2019;47(10):2501-2509.

72. Nwachukwu BU, Chang B, Voleti PB, et al: Preoperative short form health survey score is predictive of return to play and minimal clinically important difference at a minimum 2-year follow-up after anterior cruciate ligament reconstruction. *Am J Sports Med* 2017;45(12):2784-2790.

73. Jones IA, Togashi R, Heckmann N, Vangsness CT: Minimal clinically important difference (MCID) for patient-reported shoulder outcomes. *J Shoulder Elbow Surg* 2020;29(7):1484-1492.

74. Ward HH: A businessman's view of occupational health and human values. *Am J Ind Med* 1986;9(1):15-24.

75. Wilson CD, Probe RA: Shared decision-making in orthopaedic surgery. *J Am Acad Orthop Surg* 2020;28(23):e1032-e1041.

76. Elwyn G, Frosch D, Thomson R, et al: Shared decision making: A model for clinical practice. *J Gen Intern Med* 2012;27(10):1361-1367.

Telehealth in Orthopaedic Surgery

Melvin C. Makhni, MD, MBA
Harry M. Lightsey IV, MD
Caleb M. Yeung, MD

INTRODUCTION

The role of telehealth in value-based health care is evolving. Though the benefits and limitations of this form of care delivery are debated, the COVID-19 pandemic forced individuals and institutions to adopt telehealth, and state and federal governments to support its use. During this time, previous barriers to telehealth implementation were deconstructed to maintain a functioning health care system. Many of the projected benefits and limitations of telehealth were realized, and several unexpected developments also arose. Furthermore, many orthopaedic practices transformed their health care delivery pathways to offer virtual care to almost all patients; as the pandemic wore on, care gradually shifted back to the office setting. Continued shifts in the health care, legal, and technologic landscape will continue to affect the manner in which telehealth can be implemented in orthopaedic surgery. Optimal practices will continue to evolve to best care for patients in a safe, convenient, and cost-effective manner.

BACKGROUND

Despite the recent global focus on telehealth, no single definition exists to encapsulate its scope. This is largely because of the rapidly changing nature of technology. Various overlapping and sometimes interchangeable terms are used to refer to remote care delivery, including telemedicine, telehealth, e-health, and e-care. Other terms such as remote patient monitoring, mobile health, and digital health complicate matters further.

The National Academy of Medicine has defined telemedicine as the use of electronic information and communications technologies to provide and support health care when distance separates the participants.[1] Although many groups such as the Health and Human Services Department use the terms telemedicine and telehealth interchangeably, the American Telemedicine Association defines telehealth more broadly to encompass technology-enabled health and care management and delivery systems that extend capacity and access.[2]

None of the following authors nor any immediate family member has received anything of value from or has stock or stock options held in a commercial company or institution related directly or indirectly to the subject of this chapter: Dr. Makhni, Dr. Lightsey, and Dr. Yeung.

In this context, telemedicine refers to interactions between a patient and a clinician, or between two health care providers. This care can be delivered synchronously through real-time phone or video consultations, or asynchronously through means such as email or messaging. Telehealth refers to the entire spectrum of applications that contribute to remote care, including telemedicine as well as other facets such as artificial intelligence, virtual reality, and remote patient monitoring. Remote patient monitoring (RPM) uses various technologies to enable both real-time and longitudinal data collection to enhance health care monitoring.

HISTORY

Telehealth originated in the early 20th century. As early as 1906, Dr. Willem Einthoven practiced telecardiology by sending heart tracings from a local hospital to his laboratory more than 1 km away where a string galvanometer was located.[3] Throughout the 1920s to 1940s, telephone-mediated consultations became popular in the United States, Norway, Italy, and France.[4] The first radiographic images were transmitted in the 1950s. In the late 1960s, Massachusetts General Hospital paired with Logan International Airport to trial a telemedicine station designed to provide occupational health care to employees and to assist in the delivery of emergency medical attention.[5]

Advances in technology continued to drive telehealth development, broadening its capabilities. In the 1980s, digital transmission had progressed sufficiently to support videoconferencing, used primarily for peer-to-peer consultations. The 1990s and 2000s represented a watershed period for telehealth; during this timeframe, it became widely recognized as a viable health care platform deserving of federal investment.

In 2016, the Health Resources and Services Administration invested $16 million to expand telehealth in rural areas; more recently, the Health Resources and Services Administration reinforced this initiative, appropriating nearly $12 million to increase telehealth-based access to care in rural communities.[6] In March 2020, in response to the COVID-19 public health emergency, Congress passed the Coronavirus Aid, Relief, and Economic Security (CARES) Act. The CARES Act provided unprecedented levels of support for telehealth by expanding Medicare telehealth flexibilities as well as allocating billions of dollars to support increased telehealth capacities across the country.[7]

TELEHEALTH IN ORTHOPAEDICS: BEFORE COVID-19

Within orthopaedic surgery, telehealth was underutilized prior to the coronavirus pandemic despite multiple studies demonstrating its efficacy, cost-effectiveness, and patient satisfaction[8-20] (**Table 1**). This trend reflected the various challenges to widespread implementation, ranging from legislative barriers, practitioner hesitation, and technologic limitations.

Legislative Barriers

Prior to the coronavirus pandemic, federal and private payer endorsement of telehealth was curtailed by various restrictions on approved services and providers as well as permissible technology and prescribing capabilities (**Table 2**).

TABLE 1 Studies Supporting Telehealth in Orthopaedics Prior to COVID-19

Studies Demonstrating Efficacy and Accuracy

Bertani et al 2012	Prospective analysis of 48 teleconsultations for 39 patients for diagnostic and therapeutic problems. Teleconsultation modified surgical indications and technique in 77% of consultations. Clinical outcomes were "good" or "very good" in 81% of treated patients.
Good et al 2012	Prospective review of 36 patients with acromioclavicular joint hook plates comparing functional assessment using Skype versus outpatient visit. No significant differences were observed in Oxford and Constant shoulder score between modalities.
Zennaro et al 2014	Prospective study consisting of 42 children demonstrating a significant decrease in the number of consultations, faster activation of ancillary services (cast and plaster room), and a decrease in overall decision-making time when radiographs were available via an iPad.
Buvik et al 2016	Randomized trial consisting of 199 patients who underwent video-assisted remote consultation and 190 patients who underwent standard in-person consultation. Video consultations were noninferior; 98% of video visits were rated as "good" or "very good" by providers.

Studies Demonstrating Cost-Effectiveness

Harno et al 2001	Prospective study consisting of 419 patients demonstrating 45% savings in direct costs per patient for teleconsultation versus outpatient clinic visit.
Ohinmaa et al 2002	Randomized trial consisting of 145 patients demonstrating societal cost-savings with telemedicine at a threshold workload of more than 80 patients/year.
McGill and North 2012	Analysis of 27 videoconference fracture clinics and resultant cost savings; 21 transfers were avoided overall and in the final 5 months of the study, there was an overall savings of $11,334.
Buvik et al 2019	Randomized trial consisting of 389 patients demonstrating cost-effectiveness of video-assisted remote consultations versus in-person care as long as total consultations more than 151/year. Annual cost savings amounted to €18,616 ($20,869) for 300 consultations/year.
Sinha et al 2019	Nonrandomized study consisting of 116 patients comparing real-time video consultation (101 patients) with conventional outpatient clinic visits (66 patients) for pediatric fracture care. Telemedicine visits significantly decreased indirect and direct costs.

(Continued)

TABLE 1 Studies Supporting Telehealth in Orthopaedics Prior to COVID-19 (Continued)

Studies Demonstrating Patient Satisfaction

Good et al 2012	As mentioned previously, 93% of patients surveyed preferred Skype for follow-up due to convenience and cost savings.
Sharareh and Schwarzkopf 2014	Prospective study of 78 total joint arthroplasty patients, 34 of whom underwent telemedicine postoperative follow-up versus 44 patients undergoing standard follow-up. Telemedicine patients rated their postoperative care significantly higher than the nontelemedicine group and reported that Skype sessions increased their postoperative satisfaction.
Sathiyakumar et al 2015	Randomized pilot study consisting of 17 patients, 8 of whom had telemedicine follow-up and 9 of whom had in-person follow-up in an orthopaedic trauma setting. There was no significant difference in patient satisfaction. Furthermore, no patients in the telemedicine group took time off of work compared with 55.6% of patients in the control group.
Gilbert et al 2017	Systematic review of four qualitative studies. All studies demonstrated that the use of videoconferencing is "acceptable" to patients in an orthopaedic setting.
Sinha et al 2019	As noted previously. No significant difference was found in the overall quality of care provided and overall consult experience. Eight of 101 telemedicine patients preferred in-person follow-up as a next visit.
Buvik et al 2019	As noted previously. No difference was found in patient-reported satisfaction between video-assisted and standard consultations; 86% of videoconferencing patients preferred video-assisted consultation as their next visit.

Comprehensive legislative limitations on almost all aspects of care placed undue burden on health care facilities, providers, and patients and significantly contributed to overall underuse of telehealth.

Practitioner Reticence Prior to COVID-19

In 2016, a live poll during the American Orthopaedic Association Annual Meeting sought to investigate orthopaedic surgeons' use of and opinions on telehealth.[21] Although 96% of respondents believed in telehealth's clinical utility, only 42% and 38% reported using telephone or email correspondence to communicate with patients, respectively. Furthermore, although most providers chose video as their preferred mode of telecommunication, 27% of respondents expressed concerns over Health Insurance Portability and Accountability Act compliance and lack of training and 23% of respondents had questions regarding clinical appropriateness and reimbursement. A concern with successful backing and implementation was apparent; 42% of surgeons thought that their colleagues would be disinterested and 61% of surgeons thought that creating a coalition of providers willing to regularly use telehealth would take work.

Surgeon concern also stemmed from a fundamental limitation of the telehealth platform: inability to perform a physical examination. In a specialty wherein examination of musculoskeletal and spinal systems has traditionally been upheld as a key component of a complete patient assessment, the prospect of missing this information or performing limited virtual examinations was disconcerting. Such limitations also contributed to concern about increased medicolegal exposure. Additionally, with evidence to support the importance of the doctor-patient relationship in avoiding malpractice suits,[22,23] the idea of trying to develop this bond with virtual examinations discouraged surgeons.

Technologic Inefficiencies and Barriers to Implementation

Inefficiencies with telemedicine introduced through technology and its users served as additional deterrents to telehealth adoption. Difficulty connecting parties and unstable audiovisual streaming often result in frustrating and time-consuming delays. Furthermore, lack of familiarity with this technology by both practitioner and patient led to additional delays and avoidance. With the traditional system centered around face-to-face interactions and examinations, telehealth was deemed to be generally inefficient and unnecessary.

Tangible barriers to telehealth implementation have also complicated its appreciation. Prior to the pandemic, successful telehealth programs required substantial investment. Developing the infrastructure to support hardware while identifying and paying for software that satisfied security compliance, was integrated into existing electronic medical record systems, and had the capacity to archive encounter recordings was prohibitively expensive for most hospital groups and practices. These barriers, coupled with provider and patient apprehension, significantly contributed to telehealth's underutilization.

TELEHEALTH IN ORTHOPAEDICS: DURING COVID-19

The coronavirus pandemic necessitated rapid implementation of telehealth modalities in order to maintain a functioning health care system. Federal and state mandates comprehensively overturned legislative restrictions within their domains and private models largely mirrored these actions[24-26] (**Table 2**). In this unprecedented period, the US healthcare system adjusted to a new era of telehealth. Medicare increased covered services through various modalities and waived limitations on providers and patients. Medicaid established more state-level autonomy; for example, no federal approval was required for state programs to offer reimbursement parity.[27] Private insurers acted in kind; several payers began covering telehealth services at no cost to members.[28-30] Outside of the insurance realm, other government agencies adjusted policies to promote telehealth and continuity of care. The Drug Enforcement Administration permitted registered practitioners to issue prescriptions for controlled substances without in-person medical

TABLE 2 Legislative Changes Brought About by COVID-19

Subject	Pre-COVID-19 Legislation and Practice	COVID-19 Temporary Mandates[a]
Service restrictions	Centers for Medicare & Medicaid Services (CMS) maintained a list of approved telehealth services	135 new telehealth codes were added to this list
Provider restrictions	Limited to physicians, physician assistants, certified nurse anesthetists, certified nurse-midwives, clinical social workers, clinical psychologists, and registered dietitians	All providers eligible to bill Medicare to provide telehealth approved (added physical therapists, occupational therapists, speech language pathologists)
Geographic restrictions	Limited to rural health shortage areas	Waived
Originating site restrictions	Limited to specific healthcare facilities; home only approved for end-stage renal disease services	Waived
Payment parity	Distant site providers should be paid the amount equal to what they would have been paid in person	Providers use the place of service code for where they would have been in person; modifier 95 used to indicate telehealth
Licensing	Providers must be licensed in the state where the patient is located	Medicare requirements for out-of-state practitioner licensing waived; state and local licensing requirements unaffected
Audio-only services	Allowable telecommunication systems defined as synchronous audio-video interactions	Video requirement waived; 89 new codes added for allowable audio-only services
Provider applications	Formal enrollment process requiring written application and screening requirements; practitioners practicing primarily from home required to enroll their homes in Medicare as a practice location	Enrollment requirements waived; provider enrollment hotline established
Physician supervision	Residents involved in a service/procedure require the presence of a teaching physician during the key portions of the service	Direct supervision through interactive telecommunications technology permissible for both in-person and telehealth visits
	Non-physician clinicians require the presence and direct supervision of a physician when a service is provided	Direct supervision through interactive telecommunications technology permissible

	Pre-COVID-19 Legislation and	COVID-19 Temporary
TABLE 2 Legislative Changes Brought About by COVID-19 (Continued)		
Subject	**Practice**	**Mandates**[a]
Risk adjustment	Telehealth diagnoses did not qualify for Medicare risk adjustment programs	Overturned
Remote patient monitoring (RPM)	CMS allowed payment for RPM, inclusive of patient training time as well as time to analyze data and maintain treatment plans	RPM services deliverable to both new and established patients; days of data required to be collected per month shortened from 16 to 3; beneficiary consent obtainable by auxiliary staff
Controlled substance prescriptions	Drug Enforcement Administration (DEA) restricted telemedicine prescribing of controlled substances to DEA-registered hospitals and clinics	Waived as long as synchronous audio/video is used, the prescription is legitimate, and the prescriber is DEA-registered and practicing in accordance with state and federal law
Health Insurance Portability and Accountability Act (HIPAA) compliance	Technology platforms must meet select requirements to ensure patient privacy	Temporary enforcement discretion of HIPAA privacy rules allowing providers to use applications such as FaceTime, Zoom, or Skype

[a]Congress permitted the Centers for Medicare & Medicaid Service (CMS) to enable changes under 1135 authority and the Coronavirus Preparedness and Response Supplemental Appropriations Act.

Adapted from American Telehealth Association Permanent Policy Recommendations Chart. Telehealth Flexibilities During the COVID-19 Pandemic and the ATA's Recommendations for Permanent Policy. https://www.americantelemed.org/wp-content/uploads/2020/08/ATA-Permanent-Policy-Recommendations-Chart_Final-8.26.20-new.pdf

evaluations pending satisfaction of certain criteria.[31] The Office for Civil Rights redefined qualifications for Health Insurance Portability and Accountability Act violations to enable health care providers to use popular online communication technologies, including FaceTime or Skype.[32]

For all parties involved, the sudden shift to virtual care had drastic implications. Within orthopaedic surgery, most groups did not have existing telehealth programs; however, rapid adoption and adaption was necessary. In the early stages of the pandemic, Parisien et al[33] conducted a poll of 168 Electronic Residency Application Service participant orthopaedic programs aimed at assessing the prevalence of orthopaedic telehealth programs before and during the coronavirus pandemic. Prior to the pandemic, two programs in New York, one program in California, and no programs in Texas offered telehealth services. By March 26, 2020, 106 institutions offered telehealth services, 88 of which cited the pandemic as the impetus for implementation.

TELEHEALTH IN ORTHOPAEDICS: AFTER COVID-19

Telehealth's role in orthopaedics and in health care at large in the postpandemic period has yet to take shape. Many legislative leniencies were specifically designated as temporary mandates in response to the public health emergency.[34] As the pandemic wanes, federal and state-level actions will be critical to procuring the future of this platform. Accordingly, the American Telemedicine Association has led efforts to encourage permanent policy change with the ultimate goal of an integrated telehealth system.[35,36] Notable recommendations include continuation of the newly developed telehealth codes, permanent discontinuation of geographic and originating site restrictions, fair reimbursement of telehealth services, CMS reassessment and redetermination of acceptable telehealth practitioners, state-by-state determination of licensing requirements, and continuation of Drug Enforcement Administration prescribing flexibility maintaining the present protocol.

Although congressional and CMS legislative reformation will be critical in determining telehealth's utility and longevity, there remain significant challenges at hospital and individual levels. Although several studies have demonstrated telehealth's cost-effectiveness in various scenarios and settings,[12-16] a rigorous economic analysis of telehealth in its current form is missing from the literature. Complicating such an effort is the vast variability across the multitude of US health care groups and networks with regard to important cost considerations such as technology implementation and adaptability of existing systems.

At a more nuanced level, clinician and patient opinions of telehealth will determine its viability. For providers, telehealth offers promises of convenience, wider outreach, and possible financial gains depending on finalized reimbursement schemes; conversely, notable limitations such as inability to perform physical examinations, technologic inefficiencies, and medicolegal considerations weigh heavily against outright adoption. For patients, the potential cost savings, convenience, and increased accessibility to care must be balanced against a desire for many to be seen and evaluated in person.[37]

Greater implementation of telehealth in the postpandemic world is likely; however, the form that this will take will reflect the commitment to and investment in this platform at all levels. When it works well, telehealth is capable of promoting high-level, efficient, and cost-effective care to patients in need. Although there are various complexities surrounding telehealth, policymakers, administrators, and practitioners have a duty to explore its full potential. Similarly, patients also have a responsibility to adapt to a new system of care that carries with it the promises outlined previously and the potential to reshape the landscape of health care.

TELEHEALTH: FUTURE DIRECTIONS IN ORTHOPAEDICS

Telecommunications and Virtual Care

The value and utility of telehealth were demonstrated during the coronavirus pandemic. Although various specialties were more prepared than others for total telehealth conversion, surgical specialties encountered a novel predicament - diagnosing and treating patients without a physical examination. Within this arena, orthopaedic specialists found themselves uniquely challenged as the physical examination has long been upheld as a key component in the patient assessment. In response to this challenge, groups across various orthopaedic subspecialties began developing virtual examinations; to date, these examinations have yet to demonstrate diagnostic accuracy or validity.[38-42] However, this is an area of active research with prospective studies comparing virtual and in-person examinations showing promising results.[43]

Similarly, the full extent to which telemedicine and virtual visits can be used in the preoperative assessment of patients has yet to be determined. Without the ability to perform in-person examinations, some groups turned to a triage-based surgical approach. Within spine surgery, this consisted of using virtual visits to identify patients with pathology in need of urgent surgical intervention.[44,45] A different approach has explored the capability of virtual visits to develop accurate surgical plans without virtual examinations.[46] This finding could broaden the reach of surgeons and enhance their ability to provide meaningful consultations. Furthermore, patients would more easily be able to compare surgical plans across providers.

Technology and Remote Patient Monitoring

Technology is the foundation and driver of telehealth. Advances in telecommunications software and connectivity have drastically improved the interactive modalities of telehealth and enabled virtual visits to be an effective form of care during the coronavirus pandemic. Continued technologic developments in the telecommunications domain of telehealth will further solidify its role within the US healthcare system.

There have also been exciting developments within remote patient monitoring (RPM), which has increasingly merged with store-and-forward and mobile health modalities. Although RPM was initially described as a means to measure and track vital signs, blood glucose, and hearth rhythm data,[47] its role within orthopaedic surgery has been evolving with several promising innovations. Wearable technology and sensors permitting noninvasive monitoring and motion tracking have been shown to be effective in primary prevention of poor posture and strain-related spine injuries,[48-50] postoperative progress monitoring,[51-53] and in rehabilitation settings.[54-56] Advances in smartphone internal sensors and video capabilities have transformed self-care as well as engagement with clinicians. Furthermore, the field of smart implants capable of providing in vivo biomechanical feedback is promising. Although largely confined to laboratory settings at this stage, developments in

---

flexible sensors and microelectromechanical systems, in conjunction with efforts to decrease cost per implant, may soon make these devices clinically feasible.[57] In total, RPM promotes longitudinal as well as real-time data collection that is easily accessible to both patients and clinicians; in this way, RPM is redefining the physician-patient relationship and has direct applications within the telehealth framework.

SUMMARY

Telehealth is an evolving health care platform with origins dating back more than 100 years and rooted in innovations in radio and telephone technologies. Since that time, its value and utility within health care have expanded. Driven by technologic developments and bolstered at various stages by government investment, telehealth maintained its relevance as health care migrated toward the era of digital medicine and value-based care. Despite evidence supporting this system's clinical utility, telehealth within orthopaedic surgery was largely underutilized prior to the COVID-19 pandemic. This trend was multifactorial with barriers at federal, state, institutional, provider, and patient levels.

Many of these obstacles were abolished in order to maintain a functioning health care system during the COVID-19 pandemic; with these changes, the strengths and weaknesses of a largely untested telehealth system were experienced in full effect. Moving forward, much work remains in determining the role that telehealth will play in the postpandemic era. A coordinated effort at all levels will be necessary to truly understand and to critically evaluate key determinants such as clinical efficacy and diagnostic utility, cost-effectiveness, and accessibility and convenience for patients and clinicians. Ultimately, these considerations are fundamentally influenced by the underlying technology; advances in this arena will continue to maximize telehealth's promises while mitigating its drawbacks. In this way, though the COVID-19 pandemic incited a drastic change in the utilization of telehealth that revealed its potential, this system's technologic underpinnings will ensure its continued place in a health care system that increasingly upholds interconnected and value-based health care.

REFERENCES

1. Field MJ, ed: *Telemedicine: A Guide to Assessing Telecommunications in Health Care.* Institute of Medicine, National Academy Press, 1996.

2. Telehealth: Defining 21st Century Care. Available at: https://www.americantelemed.org/resource/why-telemedicine/. Accessed November 23, 2020.

3. Cooper JK: Electrocardiography 100 years ago. Origins, pioneers, and contributors. *N Engl J Med* 1986;315(7):461-464.

4. Ryu S, Peixoto PM, Won JH, Yule DI, Kinnally KW: Extracellular ATP and P2Y2 receptors mediate intercellular Ca(2+) waves induced by mechanical stimulation in submandibular gland cells: Role of mitochondrial regulation of store operated Ca(2+) entry. *Cell Calcium* 2010;47(1):65-76.

5. Murphy RL Jr, Bird KT: Telediagnosis: A new community health resource. Observations on the feasibility of telediagnosis based on 1000 patient transactions. *Am J Public Health* 1974;64(2):113-119.

6. HHS Awards over $35 million to Increase Access to High Quality Health Care in Rural Communities | .HHS.gov. Available at: https://www.hhs.gov/about/news/2020/08/20/hhs-awards-over-35-million-to-increase-access-to-high-quality-health-care-in-rural-communities.html. Accessed October 19, 2020.

7. COVID-19 | CARES Act Summary – Key Telehealth Provisions. Available at: https://info.americantelemed.org/covid-19-cares-act-summary. Accessed November 23, 2020.

8. Bertani A, Launay F, Candoni P, Mathieu L, Rongieras F, Chauvin F: Teleconsultation in paediatric orthopaedics in Djibouti: Evaluation of response performance. *Orthop Traumatol Surg Res* 2012;98(7):803-807.

9. Good DW, Lui DF, Leonard M, Morris S, McElwain JP: Skype: A tool for functional assessment in orthopaedic research. *J Telemed Telecare* 2012;18(2):94-98.

10. Zennaro F, Grosso D, Fascetta R, et al: Teleradiology for remote consultation using iPad improves the use of health system human resources for paediatric fractures: Prospective controlled study in a tertiary care hospital in Italy. *BMC Health Serv Res* 2014;14:327.

11. Buvik A, Bugge E, Knutsen G, Småbrekke A, Wilsgaard T: Quality of care for remote orthopaedic consultations using telemedicine: A randomised controlled trial. *BMC Health Serv Res* 2016;16(1):483.

12. Harno K, Arajärvi E, Paavola T, Carlson C, Viikinkoski P: Clinical effectiveness and cost analysis of patient referral by videoconferencing in orthopaedics. *J Telemed Telecare* 2001;7(4):219-225.

13. Ohinmaa A, Vuolio S, Haukipuro K, Winblad I: A cost-minimization analysis of orthopaedic consultations using videoconferencing in comparison with conventional consulting. *J Telemed Telecare* 2002;8(5):283-289.

14. McGill A, North J: An analysis of an ongoing trial of rural videoconference fracture clinics. *J Telemed Telecare* 2012;18(8):470-472.

15. Buvik A, Bergmo TS, Bugge E, Smaabrekke A, Wilsgaard T, Olsen JA: Cost-effectiveness of telemedicine in remote orthopedic consultations: Randomized controlled trial. *J Med Internet Res* 2019;21(2):e11330.

16. Sinha N, Cornell M, Wheatley B, Munley N, Seeley M: Looking through a different lens: Patient satisfaction with telemedicine in delivering pediatric fracture care. *J Am Acad Orthop Surg Glob Res Rev* 2019;3(9):e100.

17. Sharareh B, Schwarzkopf R: Effectiveness of telemedical applications in postoperative follow-up after total joint arthroplasty. *J Arthroplasty* 2014;29(5):918-922.e1.

18. Sathiyakumar V, Apfeld JC, Obremskey WT, Thakore RV, Sethi MK: Prospective randomized controlled trial using telemedicine for follow-ups in an orthopedic trauma population: A pilot study. *J Orthop Trauma* 2015;29(3):e139-e145.

19. Gilbert AW, Jaggi A, May CR: What is the patient acceptability of real time 1:1 videoconferencing in an orthopaedics setting? A systematic review. *Physiotherapy* 2018;104(2):178-186.

20. Buvik A, Bugge E, Knutsen G, Småbrekke A, Wilsgaard T: Patient reported outcomes with remote orthopaedic consultations by telemedicine: A randomised controlled trial. *J Telemed Telecare* 2019;25(8):451-459.

21. Wongworawat MD, Capistrant G, Stephenson JM: The opportunity awaits to lead orthopaedic telehealth innovation: AOA critical issues. *J Bone Joint Surg Am* 2017;99(17).e93,

22. Beckman HB, Markakis KM, Suchman AL, Frankel RM: The doctor-patient relationship and malpractice. Lessons from plaintiff depositions. *Arch Intern Med* 1994;154(12):1365-1370.

23. Huntington B, Kuhn N: Communication gaffes: A root cause of malpractice claims. *Proc (Bayl Univ Med Cent)* 2003;16(2):157-161.

24. COVID-19 telehealth coverage policies | CCHP Website. Available at: https://www.cchpca.org/resources/covid-19-telehealth-coverage-policies. Accessed October 6, 2020.

25. CMS. Physicians and Other Clinicians: CMS Flexibilities to Fight COVID-19. Available at: https://www.cms.gov/Medicare/Medicare-General-Information/Telehealth/Telehealth. Accessed October 6, 2020.

26. CMS Announces New COVID-19 Telehealth Flexibilities - ATA. Available at: https://www.americantelemed.org/policies/new-additional-rules-and-waivers-announced-by-cms/. Accessed October 6, 2020.

27. COVID-19 Frequently Asked Questions (FAQs) for State Medicaid and Children's Health Insurance Program (CHIP) Agencies. Available at: https://www.medicaid.gov/state-resource-center/disaster-response. Accessed October 6, 2020.

28. COVID-19 Telemedicine Coverage FAQs for Aetna Providers. Available at: https://www.aetna.com/health-care-professionals/covid-faq/telemedicine.html. Accessed October 14, 2020.

29. Blue Cross Blue Shield of Massachusetts expands coverage and access for members during the coronavirus pandemic. 2020. Available at: http://newsroom.bluecrossma.com/2020-03-18-Blue-Cross-Blue-Shield-of-Massachusetts-Expands-Coverage-and-Access-for-Members-During-the-Coronavirus-Pandemic. Accessed October 14, 2020.

30. Cigna Newsroom | Cigna Expands and Extends Its COVID-19 Relief Efforts for Medicare Advantage and Individual and Family Plans. Available at: https://www.cigna.com/newsroom/news-releases/2020/cigna-expands-and-extends-its-covid-19-relief-efforts-for-medicare-advantage-and-individual-and-family-plans. Accessed October 14, 2020.

31. Diversion Control Division D: How to Prescribe Controlled Substances to Patients During the COVID-19 Public Health Emergency. Available at: https://www.deadiversion.usdoj.gov/coronavirus.html. Accessed October 6, 2020.

32. Notification of Enforcement Discretion for Telehealth |.HHS.gov. Available at: https://www.hhs.gov/hipaa/for-professionals/special-topics/emergency-preparedness/notification-enforcement-discretion-telehealth/index.html. Accessed October 6, 2020.

33. Parisien RL, Shin M, Constant M, et al: Telehealth utilization in response to the novel coronavirus (COVID-19) pandemic in orthopaedic surgery. *J Am Acad Orthop Surg* 2020;28(11):e487-e492.

34. Telehealth Flexibilities During the COVID-19 Pandemic and the ATA's Recommendations for Permanent Policy. Available at: https://www.americantelemed.org/wp-content/uploads/2020/08/ATA-Permanent-Policy-Recommendations-Chart_Final-8.26.20-new.pdf. Accessed October 6, 2020.

35. American Telemedicine Association: Available at: https://www.americantelemed.org/wp-content/uploads/2020/09/PFS-CY2021_ATA-comments_9.24.20-FINAL-1.pdf. Accessed October 6, 2020.

36. American Telemedicine Association: Available at: https://www.americantelemed. org/wp-content/uploads/2020/04/COVID-4.0_ATA-letter-FINAL.pdf. Accessed October 6, 2020.

37. Makhni MC, Riew GJ, Sumathipala MG: Telemedicine in orthopaedic surgery: Challenges and opportunities. *J Bone Joint Surg Am* 2020;102(13), 1109-1115,

38. Tanaka MJ, Oh LS, Martin SD, Berkson EM: Telemedicine in the era of COVID-19: The virtual orthopaedic examination. *J Bone Joint Surg Am* 2020;102(12):e57.

39. Van Nest DS, Ilyas AM, Rivlin M: Telemedicine evaluation and techniques in hand surgery. *J Hand Surg Glob Online* 2020;2(4):240-245.

40. Yoon JW, Welch R, Alamin T, et al: Remote virtual spinal evaluation in the era of COVID-19. *Int J Spine Surg* 2020;14(3):433-440.

41. Iyer S, Shafi K, Lovecchio F, et al: The spine physical examination using telemedicine: Strategies and best practices. *Glob Spine J* 2022;12(1):8-14.

42. Satin AM, Lieberman IH: The virtual spine examination: Telemedicine in the era of COVID-19 and beyond. *Glob Spine J* 2021;11(6):966-974.

43. Donnally CJ 3rd, Vaccaro AR, Schroeder GD, Divi SN: Is evaluation with telemedicine sufficient before spine surgery? *Clin Spine Surg* 2021;34(10):359-362.

44. Rizkalla JM, Hotchkiss W, Clavenna A, Dossett A, Syed IY: Triaging spine surgery and treatment during the COVID-19 pandemic. *J Orthop* 2020;20:380-385.

45. Donnally CJ, Shenoy K, Vaccaro AR, Schroeder GD, Kepler CK: Triaging spine surgery in the COVID-19 era. *Clin Spine Surg* 2020;33(4):129-130.

46. Lightsey HM4th, Crawford AM, Xiong GX, Schoenfeld AJ, Simpson AK: Surgical plans generated from telemedicine visits are rarely changed after in person evaluation in spine patients. *Spine J* 2021;21(3):359-365.

47. Dias D, Paulo Silva Cunha J:Wearable health devices-vital sign monitoring, systems and technologies. *Sensors (Basel)* 2018;18(8):2414.

48. Wang Y, Zhou H, Yang Z, et al: An intelligent wearable device for human's cervical vertebra posture monitoring. *Annu Int Conf IEEE Eng Med Biol Soc* 2018;2018:3280-3283.

49. Voinea GD, Butnariu S, Mogan G: Measurement and geometric modelling of human spine posture for medical rehabilitation purposes using a wearable monitoring system based on inertial sensors. *Sensors (Basel)* 2016;17(1):3.

50. Yamamoto A, Nakamoto H, Yamaji T, et al: Method for measuring tri-axial lumbar motion angles using wearable sheet stretch sensors. *PLoS One* 2017;12(10):e0183651.

51. Mobbs RJ, Phan K, Maharaj M, Rao PJ: Physical activity measured with accelerometer and self-rated disability in lumbar spine surgery: A prospective study. *Glob Spine J* 2016;6(5):459-464.

52. Scheer JK, Bakhsheshian J, Keefe MK, et al: Initial experience with real-time continuous physical activity monitoring in patients undergoing spine surgery. *Clin Spine Surg* 2017;30(10):E1434-E1443.

53. Stienen MN, Rezaii PG, Ho AL, et al: Objective activity tracking in spine surgery: A prospective feasibility study with a low-cost consumer grade wearable accelerometer. *Sci Rep* 2020;10(1):4939.

54. Kairy D, Lehoux P, Vincent C, Visintin M: A systematic review of clinical outcomes, clinical process, healthcare utilization and costs associated with telerehabilitation. *Disabil Rehabil* 2009;31(6):427-447.

55. Wang Q, Chen W, Timmermans AAA, Karachristos C, Martens JB, Markopoulos P: Smart rehabilitation garment for posture monitoring. *Annu Int Conf IEEE Eng Med Biol Soc* 2015;2015:5736-5739.

56. Brogioli M, Schneider S, Popp WL, et al: Monitoring upper limb recovery after cervical spinal cord injury: Insights beyond assessment scores. *Front Neurol* 2016;7:142.

57. Ramakrishna VAS, Chamoli U, Rajan G, Mukhopadhyay SC, Prusty BG, Diwan AD: Smart orthopaedic implants: A targeted approach for continuous postoperative evaluation in the spine. *J Biomech* 2020;104:109690.

Index

Note: Page numbers followed by "*f*" indicate figures and "*t*" indicates tables.

A

AAOS. *See* American Academy of Orthopaedic Surgeons (AAOS)

ABC. *See* Activity-based costing (ABC)

ACA. *See* Affordable Care Act (ACA)

Accountable care organizations (ACOs), 6–7, 158, 218–219
  defining, 176, 178–179
  orthopaedic care and, 181–186
  orthopaedic surgeons in, 181
    bundled payment contracts, 182
    challenges and possible pitfalls, 183–186
    fee-for-service contracts, 182
    private practice/physician groups, 181–182
  overlap and integration of, 179–180
  precursors, 176–177
  rise of, 177–178

Activity-based costing (ABC), 4–5, 13

Acute Care Episode program, 7, 87

Administration champion, 267

Administrative claims-based outcomes, 17–18

Administrative service-only contract, 218

Advanced cost accounting platforms, 198–199

Advanced practice providers (APPs)
  clinic utilization, 283–286, 284*t*
  inpatient hospital utilization, 286–287
  nurse practitioners, 279*t*–280*t*, 281–282, 284*t*
  operating room utilization, 282–283
  physician assistants, 278–281, 279*t*–280*t*, 284*t*

Affordable Care Act (ACA), 91, 102, 109, 126, 158, 177

All-Inclusive Population-Based Payment (AIPBP), 159

Alternative payment models (APMs), 98, 99*f*, 101, 109–110, 125, 149, 157
  episodic bundled care, 110
  in musculoskeletal care, 126
  procedure-based, 126

Ambulatory surgery centers (ASCs)
  cost, 238–241
  history, 234–236
  legislation, 234–236
  origins of, 233
  policy, 234–236
  quality, 236–238

American Academy of Orthopaedic Surgeons (AAOS), 40–41, 58

American College of Surgeons, 20

American Joint Replacement Registry (AJRR), 32, 40–41

American Medical Association (AMA), 217

American Society of Actuaries, 220

American Society of Anesthesiologists
(ASA), 313
Argentine healthcare system,
317–319
Artificial intelligence, 199–202,
201*t*–202*t*, 289–290
ASCs. *See* Ambulatory surgical centers
(ASCs)
Australian Orthopaedic Association
National Joint Replacement
Registry, 34–35, 39

B

Balanced Budget Act (1997), 89
Balanced Budget Reduction Act
(1999), 90
Balance measures, 54
Better Health P4P program, 103–104
Blue Cross Blue Shield Physician
Group Incentive Program,
104
Bundled Payments for Care
Improvement (BPCI), 5, 7,
41, 101, 250, 255–257
for lower extremity joint
replacement, 111
reimbursement, models for, 110–111
Bundled Payments for Care
Improvement Advanced
(BPCI Advanced), 104,
113, 215

C

Capacity cost rates, 5
Capitated payment models, 155
Capitation, 225
CARES. *See* Coronavirus Aid, Relief,
and Economic Security
(CARES) Act
Cash pay, 90
CBEPs. *See* Condition-based bundled
episode payments (CBEPs)

Center for Medicare and Medicaid
Innovation (CMMI), 158
Centers for Medicare & Medicaid
Services (CMS), 85, 97, 189,
243*f*
accountable care organizations, 6,
158, 176, 178
alternative payment models, 109
Bundled Payments for Care
Improvement, 101, 110–111
Bundled Payments for Care
Improvement Advanced, 104
capitated payment models, 158
claims-based quality data, 18
Common Procedural Terminology
code, 87
Comprehensive Care for Joint
Replacement, 104, 111
conversion factor, 88
Health Care Payment Learning &
Action Network, 98
Inpatient Prospective Payment
System, 7, 17, 87
Medicare-Medicaid Financial
Alignment Initiative, 158
Medicare payments, 6
pay-for-performance, 102
proposed rule CMS-5529-P,
112, 114
Quality Payment Program, 102
Quality Rating System, 18
Relative Update Committee, 89
relative value unit, 12
total joint arthroplasty, 255
Change concepts, 54–55, 56*f*
Clinical outcomes measurement, 17
administrative claims-based
outcomes, 17–18
electronic clinical quality measures,
19–20
national ranking metrics, 18–19
National Surgical Quality
Improvement Program, 20
patient-centric outcomes, 20–25, 23*f*

MPP1123